THE NEW GENETICS OF MENTAL ILLNESS

THE MENTAL HEALTH FOUNDATION

The *Mental Health Foundation* (MHF) is Britain's leading grant-making charity concerned with promoting and encouraging pioneering research and community care projects in the field of mental health illness and mental handicap.

The Foundation aims to prevent mental disorders by funding and encouraging research into the causes of mental illness and mental handicap, and to improve the quality of life for mentally disordered people by funding and supporting pioneering and innovative community care schemes.

The Mental Health Foundation has several professional committees which meet at regular intervals to decide upon the allocation of funds to priority areas.

Apart from its interests in offering financial support, the Mental Health Foundation also runs regular seminars and conferences. These provide an arena for the exchange of information for a wide range of professionals.

THE NEW GENETICS OF MENTAL ILLNESS

Edited by

PETER McGUFFIN
MB, PhD, FRCP, MRCPsych

Professor, Department of Psychological Medicine, University of Wales College of Medicine, Heath Park, Cardiff

and

ROBIN MURRAY
MD, MPhil, FRCP, FRCPsych, DSc

Professor, Institute of Psychiatry, London

Butterworth–Heinemann

**The
Mental Health
Foundation**

Butterworth-Heinemann Ltd
Halley Court, Jordan Hill, Oxford OX2 8EJ

 PART OF REED INTERNATIONAL BOOKS

OXFORD   LONDON   GUILDFORD   BOSTON
MUNICH   NEW DELHI   SINGAPORE   SYDNEY
TOKYO   TORONTO   WELLINGTON

First published 1991

British Library Cataloguing in Publication Data
The new genetics of mental illness.
   1. Man. Mental disorders. Genetic aspects
   I. McGuffin, Peter   II. Murray, Robin
   616.89042

ISBN 0 7506 0029 2

Typeset by Latimer Trend & Company Ltd, Plymouth
Printed and bound in Great Britain by Redwood Press Ltd, Melksham,
Wilts.

Contents

Contributors

P. Bebbington
Reader and Honorary Consultant Psychiatrist, MRC Social Psychiatry Unit, Institute of Psychiatry, London

Aksel Bertelsen
Superintendent, Aarhus Psychiatric Hospital and Research Fellow, Institute of Psychiatry Demography, Statshospitalet, 8240 Risskov, Denmark

Françoise Clerget-Darpoux
Director of Research, INSERM U-155, Chateau de Longchamp, Bois de Boulogne, 75016, Paris

Lindon J. Eaves
Distinguished Professor, Department of Human Genetics and Department of Psychiatry, Medical College of Virginia, Virginia Commonwealth University, Richmond, Virginia, USA

J. H. Edwards
Professor of Genetics, University of Oxford, Honorary Consultant in Medical Genetics, Oxford Regional Health Authority, The Genetics Laboratory, Department of Biochemistry, University of Oxford

Anne E. Farmer
Senior Lecturer, Department of Postgraduate Education and Psychological Medicine, and Department of Psychological Medicine, University of Wales College of Medicine, Cardiff, Wales

Robert Goodman
Senior Lecturer, Institute of Psychiatry, Honorary Senior Lecturer, Institute of Child Health, Honorary Consultant, Maudsley Hospital and Great Ormond Street Hospital, London

I. I. Gottesman
Department of Psychology, University of Virginia, Charlottesville, USA

Hugh Gurling
Molecular Psychiatry Laboratory, Academic Department of Psychiatry, University College and Middlesex School of Medicine, London

J. Hardy
Senior Lecturer, Alzheimer's Disease Research Group, Departments of Biochemistry and Neurology, St. Mary's Hospital Medical School, London

Peter S. Harper
Professor of Medical Genetics, Institute of Medical Genetics, University of Wales College of Medicine, Cardiff

Ian Harvey
Research Psychiatrist, Institute of Psychiatry, De Crespigny Park, London

Andrew C. Heath
Associate Professor of Psychology and Genetics in Psychiatry, Department of Psychiatry, Washington University School of Medicine, St. Louis, Missouri, USA

Steve Hodgkinson
UFS Appointed Research Associate, Section of Psychiatric Genetics, Institute of Psychiatry and King's College Hospital Medical School, London

A. J. Holland
Senior Lecturer and Honorary Consultant Psychiatrist, Institute of Psychiatry, London

P. B. Jones
Research Psychiatrist and Honorary Senior Registrar, Genetics Section, Department of Psychological Medicine, King's College Hospital, Institute of Psychiatry, London

R. Katz
Assistant Professor, Department of Psychology, University of Toronto and Toronto General Hospital, Canada

Kenneth S. Kendler
Professor, Departments of Psychiatry and Human Genetics, Director, Psychiatric Genetics Program, Medical College of Virginia, Virginia Commonwealth University, Richmond, Virginia, USA

R. C. Kessler
Virginia Commonwealth University, Richmond, Virginia, USA

P. McGuffin
Department of Psychological Medicine, University of Wales College of Medicine, Cardiff

Michael J. Morris
Research Senior Registrar, Institute of Medical Genetics, University of Wales College of Medicine, Cardiff

Michael Mullan
Mental Health Foundation Research Fellow, Department of Biochemistry and Molecular Biology, St. Mary's Hospital Medical School, Norfolk Place, London

Robin Murray
Professor of Psychological Medicine, King's College Hospital and Department of Psychological Medicine, Institute of Psychiatry, London

Michael C. Neale
Research Assistant Professor, Department of Human Genetics, Medical College of Virginia, Virginia Commonwealth University, Richmond, Virginia, USA

M. J. Owen
Senior Lecturer in Neuropsychiatric Genetics, Institute of Medical Genetics and Department of Psychological Medicine, University of Wales College of Medicine, Cardiff

M. Potter
Senior Lecturer, Academic Department of Psychiatry, University College and Middlesex School of Medicine, London

T. Read
Academic Department of Psychiatry, University College and Middlesex School of Medicine, London

M. Rutter
Professor of Child Psychiatry and Director, MRC Child Psychiatry Unit, Institute of Psychiatry, London

Matthew P. Sargeant
Formerly Research Worker and Senior Registrar, University of Wales College of Medicine, Cardiff; presently Consultant Psychiatrist, St. Tydfils Hospital, Merthyr Tydfil, Mid Glamorgan, Wales

J. L. Treasure
Senior Lecturer, Institute of Psychiatry, London

S. A. Whatley
Senior Lecturer in Molecular Neurobiology, Department of Neuroscience, Institute of Psychiatry, London

Maureen Williams
Principal Psychologist, King's College Hospital, London

Alan F. Wright
Senior Clinical Scientist, MRC Human Genetics Unit, Western General Hospital, Edinburgh

Preface

Human genetics is still a young science. The term 'genetics' was first coined by Bateson in 1905 and even though essential pioneering work was carried out by Galton , Mendel and others in the 19th century, almost the entire development of the subject has taken place in the 20th. Growth in knowledge has occurred at a remarkable rate with a pronounced acceleration over the past 20 years following the advent of the so-called 'new genetics' of recombinant DNA technology. One of the welcome side effects of the recent advances has been an increased public awareness of the importance of genetics and a new optimism about what the subject has to offer. Such optimism has affected the attitudes of both psychiatrists and behavioural scientists; where it was once thought that searching for a genetic aetiology for psychiatric disorders was hopelessly pessimistic, there is now widespread enthusiasm for using molecular biological approaches to resolve many aetiological issues which in the past seemed intractable. Indeed if anything, we appear to have reached a stage where, in some quarters, the willingness to invoke genetic explanations overcomes the more common-sense view that psychiatric disorders probably result from a complex interplay between genotype and environment.

We are aware of the dangers of intemperate optimism, and in calling this book *The New Genetics of Mental Illness* we are not aiming to mislead the reader into thinking that it is only about the application of molecular biology to psychiatry. Instead we are endeavouring to point out that the renaissance in psychiatric genetics depends for its continued success on the application of a wide range of techniques which do justice to the complicated nature of the subject. Molecular genetics certainly figures large but in addition some of what is new in this book includes the application of 'classic' methods of study to hitherto under-explored areas. We also introduce the reader to new quantitative methods which are presented in a non-technical, and we hope, accessible way. Other novel aspects include attempts to integrate purely genetic approaches with quite different research strategies ranging from life event studies to the investigation of brain development.

Because we are attempting to present an integrated picture of modern psychiatric genetics, we deliberately have not divided the book into sections. However, the chapters are arranged thematically starting with basics in biology and quantitative models before moving on to theoretical and practical aspects of linkage analysis. In turn, selected clinical syndromes are considered beginning with schizophrenia and affective disorders, and followed by alcoholism, eating disorders and important aspects of childhood and developmental disorders. Finally, we turn to dementia, and conclude with Huntington's disease which is so far the only disorder of psychiatric relevance where recombinant DNA technology has had a major impact on strategies for predictive testing and prevention. Huntington's disease is, of course, rarer than most of the other conditions discussed and differs from them in having a simple mendelian mode of transmission. Nevertheless it occupies an important place because the lessons learned so far and the difficulties encountered in prediction and prevention can potentially inform future work in other neuropsychiatric disorders.

Like other volumes in this series, this book was planned in parallel with a Mental Health Foundation Conference. However, as with these previous volumes the aim has been to produce not merely a record of the conference proceedings but a book which has a life of its own. To this end we commissioned additional chapters on topics of importance which could not be covered at the conference. Our work both as editors and conference organizers has been greatly aided by the efficient administrative skills of Deirdre Laing of the Mental Health Foundation.

Peter McGuffin and Robin M. Murray,
September, 1990.

1 *The cell, molecular biology and the new genetics*

S. A. WHATLEY AND M. J. OWEN

THE STRUCTURE AND FUNCTION OF CHROMOSOMES

Our knowledge of the hereditable make-up of the cell is derived classically from studies of its chromosomes. These had long been observed as thread-like structures which stained with various dyes within the dividing nucleus. It had been known since the nineteenth century that the nuclei of cells from higher organisms contain a fixed number of chromosomes. It was careful observations of their behaviour during the processes of cell division and gametogenesis that allowed the physical basis of Mendel's laws to be understood.

Cell division and the preservation of chromosomal number—mitosis

Before cell division, each nuclear chromosome duplicates to form two identical chromatids. These subsequently separate to become chromosomes in their own right, thus doubling the normal chromosome complement of the cell. When the cell divides, one of each pair of chromatids segregates into each daughter cell. The result is that the original chromosome number, and composition, of the parent is exactly duplicated in the progeny. This process is termed mitosis and is shown diagrammatically in Fig. 1.1. During the early stages of mitosis (prophase), the lengthwise division of each chromosome into two pairs of chromatids is apparent, sister chromatids being joined together at the centromere. Although duplication of each chromosome occurs early in mitosis, it is only during the later stages that the sister chromatids are actually able to separate. Before this they tend to be twisted together as well as being attached to each other at the centromere, which appears to control the movement of the chromosomes during mitosis. Most of our information is derived from the observation of chromosomes in early metaphase, when sister chromatids are most clearly visible. The position of the centromere on the chromosome is fixed and characteristic of each chromosome. Depending on whether it is sited centrally, off-centre or terminally, the chromosome is said to be metacentric, acrocentric or telocentric. This, together with

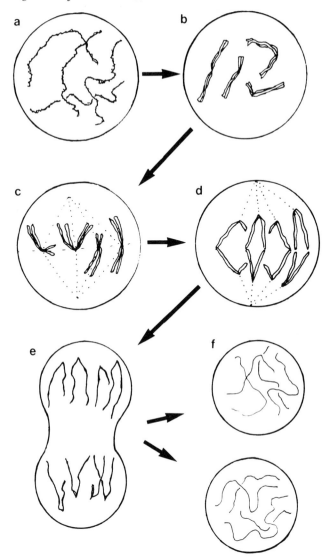

Fig. 1.1   *Mitosis—the appearance of the nucleus: a, prophase; b, early metaphase; c, late metaphase; d, anaphase; e, start of telophase; f, telophase completed*

differences in size, allows us to discriminate between chromosomes. Chromosomes are conventionally ordered by decreasing size from 1 to 22 in man. In higher animals and plants, each specific chromosome is present in two copies, termed a 'homologous pair', and the cell is classified as diploid.

Gametogenesis and the reduction of chromosomal number—meiosis

An important exception to the behaviour of chromosomes during normal cell division was discovered when gametogenesis was studied in higher organisms. In this case, two cell divisions occur in the parent cell. However, because the chromosomes only duplicate once, the number of chromosomes in the final progeny is reduced to half that in the parent. This process is termed meiosis, and is shown diagrammatically in Fig. 1.2. Meiosis is more complex than mitosis, the main difference being that not only are sister chromatids paired during the first division but homologous chromosomes also come together, giving rise to a quadruple structure during diakinesis. During the ensuing two divisions, both sister chromatids and homologous pairs are separated and pass to different daughters. Gametes therefore have only one chromosome of each kind and are said to be haploid.

Chromosomes and the laws of heredity

These observations have important implications for understanding the physical basis of inheritance. Union of sperm and egg during fertilization restores the diploid state and results in a fertilized egg in which each homologous pair of chromosomes comprises one chromosome derived from the male sperm and one derived from the female egg.

Hereditary transmission through sperm and egg was known by 1860, and, as sperm consist mainly of nucleus, it was postulated that this structure was responsible for the transmission of characteristics to the offspring. Some time passed before the chromosomes were identified as its active principle, however, and this involved linking the laws of chromosome segregation to the laws of heredity discovered by Mendel.

Mendel's experiments with plant breeding drew him to a major interpretation, which was that traits are controlled by pairs of factors (which we now call genes)—one derived from the male and one from the female. However, the significance of these laws was not appreciated until it was observed that the diploid cell contains two morphologically similar sets of chromosomes, and that during gametogenesis each gamete receives only one chromosome of each homologous pair. The geneticist Sutton explained Mendel's laws by suggesting that the hereditary factors are part of the chromosomes themselves. He proposed that genes governing alternative characteristics are carried on a specific pair of chromosomes and that entirely different characteristics were carried on different chromosomes. Although specific proof was not yet available, Sutton's hypothesis was of fundamental importance in the field of genetics.

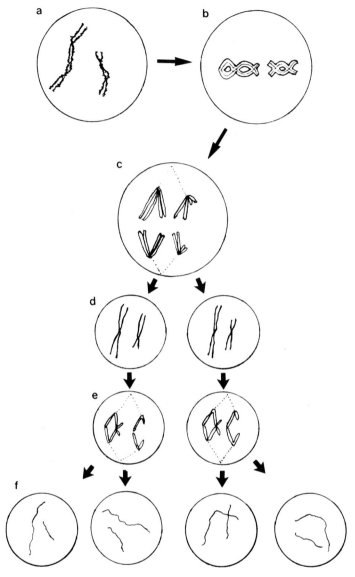

Fig. 1.2 *Meiosis—nuclear events: a, prophase 1 (pachytene); b, metaphase 1 (diakinesis); c, anaphase 1; d, metaphase 2 (after first telophase); e, anaphase 2; f, telophase 2*

Chromosomal determination of sex

There is one important exception to the rule that the chromosomes of higher animals and plants are paired within the diploid nucleus: one chromosome does not always have a homologous copy. This was therefore termed the accessory chromosome (we now call it the X chromosome). The significance of this phenomenon was appreciated when it was realized that the distribution of this chromosome is sex-specific. Cells of the female contain two X chromosomes, whereas those of the male contain only one. Furthermore, in some species including humans, male cells contain a unique chromosome, termed the Y chromosome. During egg production in the female the two X chromosomes are divided between the gametes such that each egg contains only one. In the male, X and Y chromosomes segregate during gametogenesis so that half the sperm contain a single X chromosome and half contain a Y chromosome. This provides a simple method of sex determination: fertilization of an egg by an X chromosome-containing sperm results in an XX zygote, which will be female; fertilization by a sperm containing a Y chromosome will result in an XY zygote, which will be male. These observations provided the first association of a specific chromosome with an hereditary trait and account for the fact that male and female offspring are created in roughly equal numbers.

Chromosomal analysis—the search for the basis of genetic disorders

The understanding of Mendel's laws of heredity with reference to chromosomal behaviour during meiosis greatly encouraged speculation as to the chemical basis of genes and their actions. It was some years before this came to fruition. However, in the meantime, a great deal was learned by studying the gross structure of chromosomes and by correlating chromosomal abnormalities with genetic abnormalities. Early identification of paired chromosomes during mitosis gave way to more sophisticated methods of studying their structure by using banding techniques. These rely on dyes that differentially stain parts of the chromosome, resulting in a characteristic pattern of bands across the width of each chromosome. Chromosomes that have been stained in this way are easily distinguished from their non-homologous neighbours, thus allowing gross analysis of chromosomal composition. The chromosomal complement of an individual is called the *karyotpe* and its morphological analysis is known as 'karyotyping'. Each species has a characteristic karyotype consisting of a set of paired chromosomes, termed the autosomes, together with the sex chromosomes, X and Y.

The normal human complement is a total of 46 chromosomes comprising 22 pairs of autosomes together with two sex chromosomes, XX or XY, depending on sex. Abnormal karyotypes containing extra copies of a chromosome (termed trisomy when involving the autosomes) can be easily detected. Indeed the genetic basis of Down's syndrome (trisomy 21) was elucidated by karyotyping before the chemical structure of deoxyribonucleic acid (DNA) was known. In addition, chromosomal abnormalities, such as deletions or duplications of part of a chromosome, can be detected using high-resolution banding methods, as can translocations of parts of one chromosome to a non-homologous neighbour. This has greatly enhanced our understanding of many disorders, especially certain types of cancer. As we shall see, cytogenetics may yet play an important role in elucidating the genetic basis of some psychiatric disorders.

GENETICS AND THE MOLECULAR BASIS OF HEREDITY

The structure of DNA

Genetic traits are not always independently inherited. Sometimes they tend to be coinherited because the genes that control their expression are close together on the same chromosome, a phenomenon known as *linkage*. As more traits became known it was possible to construct linkage maps of groups of genes that are related in this way. As may be expected, the number of separate linkage groups corresponds to the number of chromosomes in the cell. This further enhanced the concept of chromosomal inheritance, and in the process geneticists were able to designate the order of the genes on each chromosome. The linearity of genetic information has proved its single most important property in aiding our understanding of both its molecular and organizational character.

Watson and Crick (1953) were able to use the available evidence from genetics and chemistry to propose a model for the structure of the hereditary material of chromosomes, the DNA, which is both simple and elegant. This was able to accommodate the linear nature of genetic information, to elucidate the basis for the self-replicating nature of chromosomes and, as it soon became apparent, to allow an understanding of how genetic information is read. This model is briefly described below.

DNA is made up of two chains of nucleotide bases wrapped around each other in the form of a double helix, which is held together by hydrogen bonding between the bases (Fig. 1.3). There are four bases in DNA: adenine (A), guanine (G), cytosine (C) and thymine (T), which can lie in any order along the sugar–phosphate backbone. Because of their particular steric properties (i.e. the molecular shape and structure), A always pairs with T and C with G. This means that one strand contains a sequence of bases complementary to the other and that each strand can always be copied using the complementary strand as a template. This allows the reduplication of the double helix before cell division. Genetic information is encoded by the sequence of bases along the DNA, but to be useful it has first to be read (transcription) and then to be decoded (translation).

Genetic information is transported from the cell nucleus to the cytoplasm by a type of ribonucleic acid (RNA) known as *messenger RNA* (mRNA). This is copied directly from one strand of the DNA (Fig. 1.4). Each molecule of mRNA therefore contains bases in a sequence complementary to that found on the portion of the DNA molecule (gene) from which it was copied. The transfer of genetic information from the gene to mRNA is known as *transcription*. Once in the cytoplasm, mRNA then acts

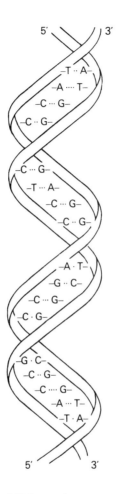

Fig. 1.3 *The structure of DNA: DNA comprises two antiparallel strands in the form of a double helix. The four bases in DNA are adenine (A), guanine (G), cytosine (C) and thymine (T)*

as a template from which protein molecules are assembled. This is done with the protein synthesizing machinery of the cell, its basic unit being the ribosome. Assembly is based simply upon the sequential reading of groups of three bases: each triplet sequence codes for a particular amino acid with some acting as start and stop signals. The amino acids, which are the building blocks of the proteins, are themselves polymerized sequentially until the protein product is finished. The end result is the conversion of linear genetic information encoded in the DNA into either an enzyme or a structural protein.

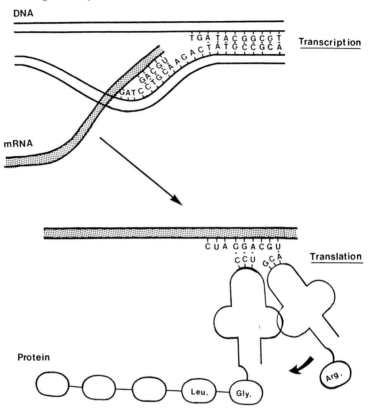

Fig. 1.4 *The flow of genetic information in the cell. The linear information contained in the base sequence of DNA (see Fig. 1.3) is converted to structural information by the process of transcription of DNA to mRNA followed by translation of mRNA into protein (in which Leu is leucine, Gly, glycine and Arg, arginine, for example) (reproduced from Whatley et al., 1989)*

This simple view was accepted as a complete picture until quite recently. However, it has become clear that, although basically correct, these processes are much more complex than was originally thought, particularly when one considers eukaryotic, or higher, organisms. Thus much of the DNA of higher organisms does not appear to encode structural information but, for example, exists to regulate the expression of coding regions (so-called enhancer or promoter regions). In addition, much is considered to be 'junk' DNA serving no purpose as far as we know at present. Even within genes that code for a single protein it is clear that there are stretches of intervening non-coding regions (introns), which separate coding regions (exons). On transcription of the gene, the initial transcript of RNA is processed in a complex manner, which involves 'splicing' out non-coding regions as well as making other post-transcriptional modifications (e.g. addition of poly(A), and end 'capping'), before the mature mRNA is released into the cytoplasm. This processing is itself regulated by sequence information, such as specific base sequences at the so-called splice 'junctions' (Fig. 1.5).

Organization of the DNA sequence in eukaryotes

Although the genetic code is based upon a simple reading of triplet codons, this provides potentially for a huge diversity of genetic information. As proteins are themselves polymers comprising a linear sequence of amino acids, their structure and function depend both upon size and amino acid sequence. For a protein of 100 amino acids there are therefore potentially 23^{100} combinations using 23 different amino acids as building blocks. If we consider the base sequence of the DNA that could code for this hypothetical protein (300 bases long), there are potentially 4^{300} combinations of the four bases (although we would have to exclude combinations containing start and stop signals). The potential diversity contained within a large polymer made of only four bases is thus staggering in size. Indeed, if we consider DNA as a random mixture of polymerized nucleotides, in a genome the size of the human (3×10^9 base pairs per haploid genome) we would expect any specific, 17 base-pair sequence to be represented only once in the genome by chance.

In fact the genome of an organism is not a random collection of bases, as the base sequence is subject to powerful selective pressure. However, where sequences do occur more than once in the genome, this will be the result of positive molecular mechanisms within the cell. The organization of sequences in higher organisms can be classified into three kinds: unique, repetitive and highly repetitive (Table 1.1). It is beyond the scope of this

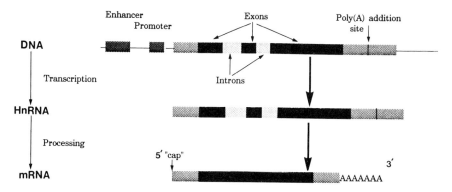

Fig. 1.5 *The structure of a typical eukaryotic gene. Genes are characterized by a promoter close to the start of transcription as well as enhancer sequences which may be at various sites including within the gene itself or 'downstream' of it. After transcription, specific signal sequences control processing of the mRNA precursor HnRNA. These include 'splicing' out of non-coding introns between coding exons and addition of the poly(A) tail. The 5 'cap' is essential for efficient translation of the mature mRNA*

Table 1.1 DNA sequence organization in eukaryotes

Sequence type	Number of copies	Approximate proportion of total genome (%)
Highly repetitive	10^6	10
Middle repetitive	10^5–10^3	20
Unique	5	70

chapter to discuss the significance of this classification fully, but it is worth pointing out here that protein-coding regions of DNA are generally contained in the unique class of DNA.

DNA mutations, genetic disease and variation of the human genome

It is obvious that changes in the sequence of bases in coding regions of DNA can have deleterious effects on cellular structure and metabolism. Point mutation, which is the substitution of one base for another, is common and can cause an amino acid substitution in the protein that may change its chemical properties. Similarly, the production of a novel stop signal will cause premature termination of protein synthesis. In addition, changes outside coding regions can also have a profound effect on gene expression. For example, a mutation at a promoter sequence may abolish transcription of a gene and one at a splice junction may result in abberant processing of the mRNA.

Point mutations are themselves just one of a number of ways of disrupting gene activity: others include deletions (loss of a base sequence), insertions (the gaining of a piece of DNA), frameshift mutations (the loss of one base, causing the triplet code to be read out of frame) and translocations (the breaking of a chromosome and its rejoining at a different site on a different chromosome). These deleterious changes will tend to be selected against in the ensuing population through a reduction in the fitness of the organism.

Not all changes in DNA are deleterious, however. Some changes may be advantageous to the organism, for example, if they improve the properties of an enzyme. These will confer a selective advantage upon the progeny of the organism, and hence will tend to spread within the population. There is also another class of mutations that have little or no effect. Some base substitutions will not change the amino acid composition of a particular protein because of the redundancy of the genetic code (the use of more than one triplet for a particular amino acid). Similarly, some amino acid changes may not change protein function, particularly if one amino acid is replaced by another with similar chemical and physical properties. It is also evident that changes in non-coding regions of DNA may also have no net effect. Such 'neutral' changes in DNA (Kimura, 1979) may be carried passively in the population, their frequency changing through random processes. The result is that comparison of any one individual's DNA with another reveals a difference in base sequence at approximately every 10^3 base pairs.

Once again, neutral changes in DNA structure are not restricted to base substitutions. Variation of a different type also occurs frequently at genetic loci which contain a short sequence of bases that is repeated along the DNA. These are termed *tandem repeats* to distinguish them from sequences which are duplicated at different genetic loci. Once a tandem repeat has been established in the genome there is a tendency for unequal crossing over to occur during genetic recombination. This results in variation between individuals in the lengths of the tandem repeats at that site, coined 'variable number tandem repeats' or VNTRs (Nakamura *et al.*, 1987). This variation in both the base sequence and repetitive length of DNA between individuals has proved extremely useful in the study of genetic disease and will be discussed more fully later.

THE NEW GENETICS

Whereas classical genetics makes inferences from an examination of the phenotype, recent advances in molecular biology have provided techniques that enable the progressive characterization of genetic disorders more directly in terms of both genotypic and endophenotypic abnormality. Genotypic, of course, refers to studies of DNA itself, whereas endophenotypic consists in the definition of alterations in its expression.

The study of DNA

All the cells of an individual person have essentially the same genotype. DNA can be obtained and prepared most conveniently from peripheral blood leucocytes. However, one of the daunting aspects of the study of this genetic material is its sheer size in molecular terms (about 10^8 base pairs of DNA per chromosome). Two characteristics of DNA, however, have proved particularly useful in its study. The first, as explained above, is the linear nature of genetic information, which enables us to place an order both on the base sequence of DNA and on the sequence of genes in the chromosome. The second is the concept of complementarity between two DNA strands, which was also discussed above. DNA has the property that above a certain temperature it 'melts' or 'denatures', i.e. the two strands of the helix will separate. This is a reversible process, and under the correct conditions the strands will 'hybridize' or 'renature' back together again. However, because of the constraints of base pairing (A to T and G to C), a certain sequence of DNA will only recognize, and hence hybridize to, its corresponding complementary partner (although a certain amount of mismatch is possible). Thus, in general, a purified, single-stranded sequence of DNA will recognize only its complementary sequence of DNA, even in a complex mixture. Similarly, a purified RNA sequence will recognize only the DNA sequence from which it was transcribed, and vice versa. Thus purified sequences can be used as detectors or 'probes' for the corresponding sequences in a mixture of nucleic acids. These properties of DNA had been known for a long time, but several developments have allowed us to exploit them, as outlined next.

Restriction enzymes

A key development in modern molecular genetics has been the discovery of restriction enzymes (or restriction endonucleases), which cut DNA not at random but where specific base sequences occur in the molecule. Each restriction enzyme recognizes a different sequence of bases. This results in fragments of easily manageable size (usually 10^3–10^4 base pairs). It is relevant to point out that this size is of the order of what is expected for some genes and therefore digestion by restriction enzymes enables genes to be handled more or less in isolation rather than as part of a single, very long molecule.

Molecular cloning

The second major development has been in the ability to purify specific pieces of DNA in order to use them as gene 'probes'. There are two main types of gene probe. First, they may be made from genomic DNA extracted and digested with restriction enzymes. Secondly, they can be made from complementary DNA (cDNA), which is synthesized from mRNA by the action of an enzyme called reverse transcriptase. cDNA probes therefore represent copies of the coding sequences of genes. These DNA pieces can be inserted into the genome of vectors, such as bacterial plasmids (again using restriction enzymes), which have the ability to replicate freely within bacteria such as *Escherichia coli* and from which they can be recovered. The preparation is treated in such a way that only one DNA fragment is inserted into each bacterium. If the collection of bacteria is then diluted and plated out, individual bacteria will give rise to colonies, each containing many copies of the DNA fragment that was inserted into the founder. This process is known as 'molecular cloning' and can be considered as a process of biological purification and amplification of specific DNA fragments (see Fig. 1.6). The collection of bacterial colonies from a particular source is termed a 'library', in which there is a certain probability that any given sequence from the starting DNA mixture will be represented.

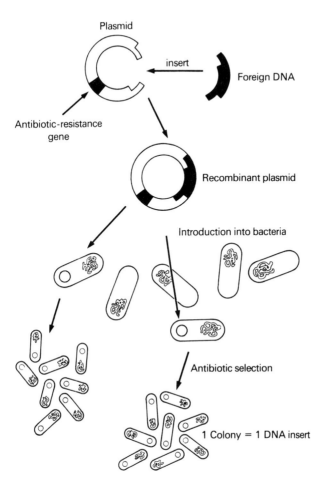

Fig. 1.6 *Bacterial cloning. Foreign DNA is inserted into a bacterial plasmid which contains an antibiotic-resistance gene. On transfection, bacteria that contain plasmid are able to grow in the presence of antibiotics whereas those without plasmids cannot. Plating bacteria on antibiotic selective medium therefore produces colonies, each of which is derived from a single bacterium and which contains a pure population of recombinant plasmid (reproduced from Whatley et al., 1989)*

Southern blotting

These technological advances are combined in one of the most fundamental techniques of molecular genetics which is called Southern blotting after its inventor E. M. Southern. First, genomic DNA is cut with a restriction enzyme. This produces a large number of different-sized DNA fragments, which can be separated according to their size by electrophoresis on an agarose gel. Because of the specificity of the enzyme, only a few particular sizes of fragment will contain the DNA region of interest. In order to detect these fragments, the DNA has to be treated with alkali to denature it to single-stranded DNA. It is then transferred to a membrane sheet of either nitrocellulose or modified nylon by a blotting procedure. This results in a copy of the gel that retains the electrophoretically produced arrangement of DNA fragments. The blot is then exposed to a DNA 'probe' that has been radioactively labelled for easy detection. The DNA probe will bind to that part of the filter containing its complementary sequence but surplus DNA probe will not bind elsewhere and can be washed away. The position on the membrane of the fragments containing the region of DNA to be analysed, whose sequence corresponds to that of the probe, can then be determined by autoradiography (see Fig. 1.7).

Southern blotting can therefore detect a sequence of interest in a starting sample of DNA and can also provide information about the surrounding region in terms of the size of DNA contained between the flanking, enzyme recognition sites.

The complete characterization of a piece of DNA requires knowledge of its exact base sequence. Once again, until recently this was a daunting prospect, but techniques are now available to determine the base sequence

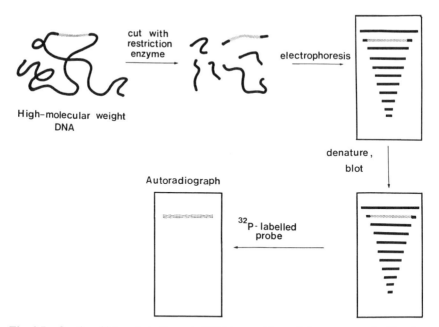

Fig. 1.7   *Southern blot analysis. Genomic DNA is cut with restriction enzyme and subjected to agarose gel electrophoresis. The gel is then blotted on to nitrocellulose, producing a replica that can be hybridized to a suitable radiolabelled probe. If the probe is complementary to the shaded piece of DNA, the position of this particular fragment will show up on subsequent autoradiography (reproduced from Whatley* et al., *1989)*

of any purified piece of DNA by either chemical or enzymatic means. The only factor limiting the analysis of base sequence is that it is labour intensive and time consuming, which sets an upper limit (ca. 10^5 base pairs) on the size of DNA conveniently studied. This has not deterred the proposal that the whole of the human genome should be sequenced in the near future, and with this in prospect, attempts are being made to speed up the process of DNA sequencing by several orders of magnitude, using automated techniques.

THE APPLICATION OF MOLECULAR GENETICS TO THE STUDY OF DISEASE

As described above, there is considerable genetic variation between individuals at the level of the base sequence of DNA, most of which is undetectable phenotypically. A powerful aspect of the new genetic techniques is their ability to detect and exploit these variations. We are able therefore to study either the mutations that give rise to a particular defect or simply to use genetic variation to mark the location of mutations without detailed analysis of the molecular pathology.

The characterization of causal mutations

In the case of diseases for which a genetic locus has already been identified, it is now a relatively simple task to characterize the abnormality at the molecular level. Gross deletions may be identified, by Southern blotting techniques, from alterations in the size of the band detected by a probe for the disease gene. Point mutations may be detected by DNA sequencing. Alternatively, where a specific mutation is known to exist in the population, short oligonucleotide probes can be synthesized, which can distinguish between the normal and mutated DNA sequence by their hybridization characteristics. This is based on the observation that mismatches between probe and a particular sequence tend to lower the melting temperature of the hybrid duplex, and this effect is more marked the shorter the probe length. Appropriate washing conditions can be selected that will 'melt off' mismatched hybrids but leave perfect matches intact. This technique has been used in the prenatal diagnosis of phenylketonuria (DiLella *et al.*, 1987).

Genetic markers and disease

Genetic variation can also be exploited to give rise to a number of types of markers that can be used to distinguish specific alleles of a particular DNA sequence. These markers may not be directly related to the mutation that causes a particular disorder, but are useful in several ways. First, they enable the detection of carriers and prenatal diagnosis where the marker is close to a known mutation site, even if the detailed molecular pathology is not known. Secondly, they enable the location of a disease gene to be determined without any prior knowledge as to its whereabouts (see below).

Restriction fragment length polymorphisms

We have seen that restriction enzymes cleave DNA at specific base sequences. However, as discussed above, there is considerable variation in base sequence between individuals (except in identical twins), which can be due either to base substitutions or to variability in the length of repetitive DNA sequences. The result of this is that fragments produced by digestion of one individual's DNA by a restriction enzyme will not be the same as those produced by digestion of DNA from someone else. This is due to two mechanisms: (a) the gain and loss of restriction enzyme recognition sites through base changes; or (b), variations between individuals in the number of bases between the same recognition sites, resulting often from variable lengths of tandemly repeated DNA. This is illustrated in Fig. 1.8. Variations in the size of specific restriction fragments labelled by a given probe after Southern blotting are termed restriction fragment length polymorphisms (RFLPs). In such instances, the polymorphic site is either within or, more usually, close to the sequence recognized by the probe. As they are generally inherited in a simple Mendelian fashion, RFLPs can be used as genetic markers; the different alleles of the markers can be distinguished and their inheritance followed through families.

Linkage analysis using RFLPs and 'reverse genetics'

In the case of many inherited diseases, including most of those of relevance to psychiatry, the biochemical abnormality responsible is not known and cannot therefore be used as a starting-point from which to identify the exact molecular defect. However, it is in such seemingly hopeless circumstances that the power of molecular genetics is greatest. Starting only with the knowledge that a disease is genetic and of its mode of transmission, it is now possible to locate the genetic abnormality responsible. The key to this so-called reverse genetics lies in the use of RFLPs as genetic markers in linkage studies.

In such studies, DNA is extracted from the members of families containing several individuals with the disease in question. The aim is to find an RFLP in which alleles tend to segregate with the illness. In other words, one variant of the polymorphism will be present in affected but not unaffected members of a particular family more often than would be expected by chance. If this happens, it suggests that the marker allele and the pathological gene are close enough on the same chromosome to render separation during meiosis (recombination) unlikely. The frequency of recombination is therefore a measure of the physical distance separating the two loci.

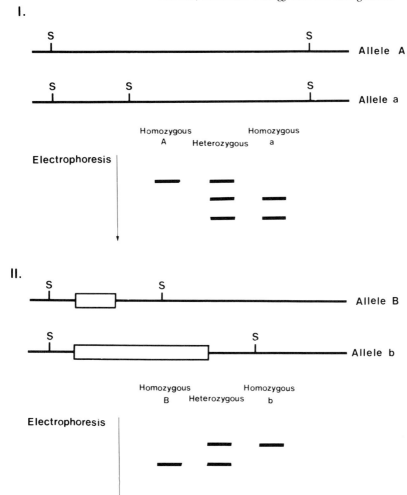

Fig. 1.8 *Restriction fragment length polymorphisms (RFLPs). RFLPs are of two main types: (I) random alteration in the base sequence on this piece of DNA have resulted in the formation of two alleles—allele A contains two recognition sites (S) for a particular restriction enzyme; allele a has an additional recognition site. Restriction enzyme digestion therefore produces one fragment from allele A, but two smaller fragments from allele a. (II) Unequal crossing over has produced a variable length in this tandemly repeated DNA sequence (indicated by box). Illustrated are two alleles (B, b) with identical restriction-enzyme recognition sites in the unique sequence but which have varying lengths of DNA between them. The electrophoresis profiles show the pattern of fragments produced after digestion by restriction enzyme of DNA from individuals representing the different possible combinations of genotype. This fragment pattern can therefore be used to analyse the genotype of a particular individual at this locus using a DNA probe for the region between the end-restriction sites*

Broadly, there are three strategies that can be employed in attempts to find linkage using RFLPs. In the first, which we may call *the random search method*, unknown pieces of DNA, selected at random, are used as probes to detect and follow polymorphisms in families that are multiply affected by the disease in question. The identities and positions in the genome of these 'anonymous markers' are then determined only if linkage is established. It was this method that Gusella *et al.* (1983, 1984) used to locate the gene for Huntington's disease on chromosome 4. Recently this has been superseded by the *systematic search method*. This has been made possible by the availability of systematically constructed linkage maps of the human genome. These consist of collections of largely anonymous markers whose chromosomal positions have been mapped, which are polymorphic and which have been assembled so that they are approximately evenly spaced throughout the genome. These probes are separated by a distance that allows detection of linkage between them and any intervening marker. This enables a systematic search to be made for linkage, a strategy recently successful in the case of Freidreich's ataxia (Chamberlain *et al.*, 1988).

In the second strategy, a candidate gene whose involvement in the disease is suspected *a priori* may be used as a probe. For example, genes coding for various enzymes involved in the biosynthesis and metabolism of monoamine neurotransmitters might be relevant to psychiatric disorders. Obviously this approach is something of a shot in the dark but it can allow a definitive answer to be obtained to the question: is a mutation in this gene responsible for this disease?

In the third strategy, attention may be concentrated upon probes that label a particular part of the genome such as a particular chromosome or chromosomal region. The association between Down's syndrome and Alzheimer's disease led to the successful search for linkage in familial Alzheimer's disease on chromosome 21 (St. George-Hyslop *et al.*, 1987; Goate *et al.*, 1989).

Another way in which interest may be focused upon a particular chromosomal region is when cases of a disease are identified in association with a gross, cytogenetically identifiable, chromosomal abnormality such as a translocation or a deletion. The study of cases with deletions greatly facilitated the identification of the gene for Duchenne muscular dystrophy (Monaco *et al.*, 1985, 1986). It was the discovery of two related individuals with schizophrenia associated with an unbalanced translocation of chromosome 5 that prompted investigators to look for linkage to markers from this region (Basset *et al.*, 1988). This approach offers a potentially powerful method of locating disease genes without the necessity for a lengthy, labour-intensive, systematic search. However, there is always the danger that researchers will be misled by either a chance association or in cases where there is a more complex causal relationship between the chromosomal abnormality and the disease in question.

Linkage analysis relies upon the ability to detect cosegregation of marker alleles with those of the disease gene. In order for a marker to be 'informative' for a particular meiosis, the individual concerned must be heterozygous at the marker locus. Consequently, the usefulness of a given genetic marker for linkage analysis, known as 'informativeness', depends upon the frequency with which it is heterozygous in the population. The majority of DNA markers that arise from single base substitutions are biallelic, which limits their informativeness. However, markers that rely on length polymorphisms of tandemly repeated sequences (VNTRs) are often extensively polymorphic (Jeffreys *et al.*, 1985; Nakamura *et al.*, 1987). The use of probes for detecting VNTRs typically generates multiallelic systems that are highly informative. More recently, it has been discovered that 'microsatellite' repeats, such as (AC)n, are highly polymorphic (Litt and Luty, 1989; Weber and May, 1989). These can readily be detected by sequencing methodology after amplification of the region concerned by the polymerase chain reaction (PCR).

Another approach is to use methods that detect DNA sequence polymorphisms but which do not rely on the alteration in size of restriction fragments. For example, techniques have been developed that allow the identification of mismatches between a single strand of DNA and a reference strand (Myers *et al.*, 1988). In addition, methods relying on the direct sequencing of PCR-amplified DNA are also being developed.

In psychiatric disease, suitable families are difficult to identify and time consuming to trace and assess. Methods that will allow the maximum information to be obtained from each family will therefore be particularly important.

Diseases with apparently complex patterns of inheritance

It is apparent from the above discussion that linkage analysis requires the disease under study to show Mendelian transmission. At first sight this might seem to preclude its application to the majority of psychiatric disorders. However, for a number of disorders, such as schizophrenia, affective disorder and Alzheimer's disease, pedigrees have been reported in which various family members are affected and in which Mendelian transmission appears to be taking place. These pedigrees are certainly atypical and raise questions of aetiological heterogeneity. However, they do suggest that single genes of major effect might be operating, at least in these families, and that the application of linkage analysis may therefore be appropriate. This assumption is central to much current work in psychiatric molecular genetics. We should therefore remember that its validity can only be established by the unequivocal demonstration of linkage, as there are explanations other than single gene effects for the clustering of cases in such highly selected families.

If linkage can be established, then this should ultimately lead to the precise definition of the molecular defect in these cases (see below). Once this has occurred it should be possible to determine the immediate biochemical consequences. From here we may hope to follow the sequence of changes that finally results in the phenotype. This will represent a major advance in our understanding of the biology of mental illness. Even if the majority of cases do not turn out to have such a simple genetic cause, the insights gained from the study of these atypical cases should serve as a second starting point from which to study the pathophysiology of cases with more complex causes.

From linkage to the genetic defect

The discovery of DNA polymorphisms that are tightly linked to a disease may, as we have seen, permit prenatal and presymptomatic diagnosis. However, for a number of reasons, which include the probable existence of heterogeneity as well as ethical considerations, it seems unlikely that these will prove to be the major benefits resulting from the discovery of linkage in most of the common psychiatric disorders (for a fuller discussion, see Owen and Whatley, 1988). Rather, the importance of demonstrating linkage lies in the fact that this is the first step towards identifying the defective gene itself. As we have seen, once this has been achieved it is relatively straightforward to characterize the defect at a molecular level. We shall now outline some of the methods that may be used to move from linked marker to the gene.

The first step consists in further genetic mapping using linkage analysis of multiply affected families. The aim now is to identify probes that recognize loci that are closer to the disease gene than existing linked markers. New markers can be generated from the chromosome, or chromosomal region, in question, for example from libraries constructed from somatic cell hybrids or flow-sorted chromosomes. In time, markers flanking the disease locus can be identified and subsequent genetic mapping will result in the progressive reduction of the region known to contain it. Human genetic mapping, however, is limited in its resolution. RFLPs are not 'informative' in every family, although here, as we have seen, the situation is improving all the time as the known number of highly informative markers increases. Another limitation arises from the simple fact that humans breed slowly compared with, say, drosophila. Human pedigrees therefore contain relatively few meioses and many must be studied in order to gain detailed genetic maps. Thus, in most human genetic illnesses, one is fortunate to define the disease locus with a resolution of 1 cm. First-generation, molecular genetic techniques of cloning, sequencing and Southern blotting on conventional agarose gel electrophoresis can only readily analyse distances of up to a hundred kilobase pairs (kbp). In man, 1000 kbp, or 1 megabase (mbp), correspond to approximately 1 cm. Thus there is a gap in resolution between first-generation molecular techniques and genetic mapping. This gap might well turn out to be even larger for the majority of psychiatric illness, where factors such as the rarity of suitable pedigrees, age-dependent penetrance, variability in phenotypic expression and diagnostic uncertainty will all tend to reduce the accuracy of genetic mapping. It therefore seems likely that, even if linkage can be definitely established, for many psychiatric disorders it will only be possible to estimate the location of the disease gene to within several million base pairs.

Fortunately, the gap in resolution is continually being narrowed by the rapid development of new techniques. From the side of DNA cloning, it is being narrowed through the development of techniques for chromosome jumping (Poustka *et al.*, 1986), which allow distances of several hundred kilobases to be covered in a single step; and through the construction of yeast artificial chromosomes (YACs), which allow fragments of up to 500 kbp or more to be cloned (Anand *et al.*, 1989). It is also being reduced from the side of physical mapping by the use of pulsed-field gel electrophoresis (PFGE), which allows very large, as well as small, DNA fragments to be separated (Smith *et al.*, 1988). In contrast to standard gel electrophoresis, where a unidirectional electric field is applied, in the pulse-field gel DNA is subjected to two alternating, pulsed fields applied at 90° or more to each other. Quite how this allows the resolution of very large molecules whereas conventional electrophoresis does not is unclear, but it probably results from the fact that molecules differ in their ability to reorientate to changed direction as a function of their length. Resolution of DNA molecules of between 500 kbp and 9 mbp has been achieved using such techniques, whereas conventional agarose gel electrophoresis has an upper limit of about 20 kbp. PFGE therefore extends very considerably the usefulness of Southern blotting for mapping the genome. For such analysis, restriction enzymes that recognize very rare sites in the human genome—the so-called 'rare cutters'—are used to generate very large fragments of DNA. These large fragments can then be resolved by PFGE before Southern blotting.

The development of these and other techniques is rapidly enabling molecular analysis to cover the same order of genomic distances as classical genetic techniques. It is now relatively easy to detect the propinquity of two markers and estimate directly the physical distance between them. The region of interest can be further analysed and various strategies used to detect the genes amongst the non-coding sequences that make up the greater part of DNA. Sites of rare-cutter restriction enzymes cluser in 'CpG islands' that mark the location of at least a subset of genes (Bird, 1986). Genes can also be detected using 'shorter range' techniques, such as the demonstration of conservation in non-human species and finding homologous sequences in cDNA libraries. However, these techniques are extremely laborious and it would take several years of work by a large team to identify all the genes within 1 megabase of DNA using current methods. For psychiatric diseases, as we have seen, it may not even be possible to define the region containing the disease gene this precisely by genetic means. The problem is not so much that the newer techniques of molecular genetics (such as PFGE) cannot cope with such distances but that they will prove a lure to characterize the region completely, an exercise which is likely to throw up an enormous amount of information. Much is thus likely to be learned about the structure and function of the region concerned. However, the search for the disease gene within the linked region may well be considerably more complex than the original search for linkage. The hope at this point is that there will be affected individuals who have easily identifiable genetic lesions, such as deletions, duplications or chromosomal translocations, which will further define the location of the disease gene, as occurred in the case of Duchenne muscular dystrophy (Monaco *et al.*, 1985, 1986)—and, indeed, such individuals have been identified for schizophrenia. Moreover, we should not lose sight of the fact that molecular techniques are advancing at prodigious speed. In particular, the development of techniques that allow the rapid identification of genes within large regions of the genome will be crucial to the successful application of reverse genetics to psychiatric disorders.

The pure reverse genetic approach aims to identify a genetic defect without reference to prior knowledge of the disease process. It is at this stage that a certain amount of prior knowledge may be of help. Although up until now, candidate genes have not provided us with loci that are consistent with a primary causal role in psychiatric disease, this does not mean that a functional approach should be abandoned. Studies of the biological basis of psychiatric disorder should continue in parallel with genetic studies, and at some stage the two will presumably converge. Apart from functional systems, such as neurotransmitter-related enzymes and receptors, which have been investigated in psychiatric illness and which have been studied by biochemical and pharmacological means, molecular biology also enables us to identify new candidates by the analysis of the expression of the genome in disorders with a genetic component.

THE STUDY OF GENE EXPRESSION

The identification of endophenotypes is important because this is likely to throw light upon pathological processes within the cell that, in turn, may have therapeutic implications. Indeed, in disorders with a complex genetic component, or those where the environmental determinants are more distinctive than the genetic, the characterization of endophenotypes is arguably more likely to be of therapeutic relevance than an understanding of the genotype. Moreover, in psychiatry, where precise definitions of categories of exophenotype are difficult and consequently there are interminable arguments about diagnostic concepts, the need for endophe-notypic characterization is especially pressing. In a disorder in which there is a genetic component the analysis of genes expressed in the condition may help to give such endophenotypic characterization. This has the advantage that functional aspects of the genome are being studied rather than purely structural aspects, as outlined above. The strategy used in this case is to identify genes whose expression is altered in the disease state by comparison of their relative abundance between control and affected individuals. In many cases it is found that a mutation causing a condition can completely block the read-out of the affected gene, which results in the absence of that mRNA in the cell. The converse of this is that genes under- or overexpressed in the relevant tissue in a condition may lead us to the genetic defect. As it is not always apparent how structural changes in DNA give rise to functional changes, it is likely that studies of gene expression will be very valuable as a complement to purely genetic ones, and may serve to identify the causal gene in a particular chromosomal region that has been implicated by purely genetic analysis.

We can use either a random search method or test the expression of candidate genes for the illness (such as the dopamine D_2 receptor for schizophrenia). In the cell, mRNA exists as a mixture of many different sequences, each destined to be translated into separate proteins. It can be extracted easily from brain tissue, either post-mortem or from neuro-surgical specimens. As in the case of DNA, the complexity of this mixture used to be a severe handicap to its analysis, but the ability to purify individual species by molecular cloning has made the task much easier. In addition, the development of the techniques of cloning and gel electro-phoresis has enabled us to study the relative abundance of many mRNA species simultaneously. Therefore, as with DNA-analysis, we can search for genes whose expressions change without *a priori* assumptions about what those genes are.

The random search method relies on the analysis of the relative abundance of the various mRNAs in the brain. Thus mRNAs can be used as templates to construct cDNA libraries specific to different regions of the brain, and to compare libraries from control and diseased individuals. Any clones that appear to be expressed at different levels in the illness can then be used as candidate gene probes in DNA studies. mRNA mixtures may also be analysed by first using them to direct protein synthesis in a cell-free system. The protein products are then analysed themselves by two-dimensional gel electrophoresis. It may thus be possible to characterize a specific protein or proteins involved in the pathogenesis of a disease.

The use of candidate genes relies on hybridization of a probe for the gene with the mRNA mixture to assess the abundance of its complemen-tary mRNA. This is again rather a shot in the dark, but it gives a very quick answer as to whether the relative expression of a certain gene is altered in a particular state. Such quantitative hybridization experiments can be done either in solution or with the mRNA bound to a filter after size separation in a gel (a 'Northern' blot). In addition, the technique of in situ hybridization allows the abundance of a particular mRNA to be assessed in a fixed preparation such as a tissue slice. Here the hybridization of a gene probe occurs to immobilized mRNA molecules in the preparation in the same way as to RNA bound to a nylon membrane. For in situ hybridiza-tion, gene probes are radiolabelled with short-range radioactive isotopes such as ^{3}H or ^{35}S, to enable fine resolution of label detection after autoradiography. Thus gene probes can be used as cytochemical markers in a similar fashion to immunological probes in immunohistochemistry. This obviously increases greatly the range of information obtainable about gene expression and offers the ability to identify changes in gene expression in small anatomical regions or groups of cells. For example, the expression of the gene for the precursor protein of brain amyloid has been studied in various brain regions in Alzheimer's disease (Cohen *et al.*, 1988; Higgins *et al.*, 1988).

There are several disadvantages to the study of gene expression, the most obvious of which is that mRNA populations reflect the pattern of gene expression only at the time the RNA was extracted. It is certainly possible that some mental illnesses result from abnormalities of gene expression that only occur at certain stages in development. Moreover, gene expression may also be influenced by factors such as medication and agonal state, for which controls are needed. The study of mRNA also has advantages, however. It is theoretically possible for a disease to have a fairly complex genetic basis, for example involving several regulator genes at widely separate loci, but for the disorder in expression to be fairly simple. Moreover, the study of an endophenotype allows the identification of state as well as trait markers, which might well afford insight into the biological basis of a relapsing and remitting condition. Perhaps more importantly we may be able to identify by these means groups of genes which are coordinately controlled, or which have effects on specific cellular functions in nerves. Thus we may be able to link functionally genes from different chromosomal loci.

CONCLUSIONS

We have briefly introduced some of the techniques of molecular genetics and indicated their application and relevance to psychiatric disorders. As we have seen, it is now possible to analyse the structure of human genes directly, and to determine the underlying molecular pathology of single gene disorders. Molecular genetics has also provided us with a series of DNA markers scattered throughout the human genome to which we can link genes for disorders of completely unknown aetiology. Furthermore, it is now possible to proceed from the demonstration of linkage to the identification of the causal mutation. There are problems associated with the application of these techniques to the common mental disorders whose solution is now the major challenge facing psychiatric genetics. However, in view of the prodigious rate of current technological advance, we can regard the future with optimism.

REFERENCES

Anand R., Villosante A., Tyler-Smith C. (1989). Construction of yeast artificial chromosome libraries with large inserts using fractionation of pulsed field gel electrophoresis. *Nucleic Acids Research*; 17: 3425–31.

Bassett A. S., McGillivray B. C., Jones B. D., Pantzar K. T. (1988). Partial trisomy chromosome 5 cosegregating with schizophrenia. *Lancet*; i: 799–801.

Bird A. P. (1986). CpG-rich islands and the function of DNA methylation. *Nature*; 12: 209–13.

Chamberlain S., Shaw J., Rowland A. *et al.* (1988). Mapping of mutation causing Friedreich's ataxia to human chromosome 9. *Nature*; 334: 248–50.

Cohen M. L., Golde T. E., Usiak M. F. *et al.* (1988). *In situ* hybridisation of nucleus basalis neurons shows increased B amyloid mRNA in Alzheimer's disease. *Proceedings of the National Academy of Sciences (USA)*; 85: 1227–31.

DiLella A. G., Morvit J., Brayton K., Woo S. L. C. (1987). An amino acid substitution involved in phenylketonuria is in linkage disequilibrium with DNA haplotype 2. *Nature*; 327: 333–6.

Goate A. M., Owen M. J., James L. A. *et al.* (1989). Predisposing locus for Alzheimer's disease on chromosome 21. *Lancet*; i: 352–5.

Gusela J. F., Tanzi R. E., Anderson M. A. *et al.* (1984). DNA markers for nervous system disease. *Science*; 225: 1320–6.

Gusela J. F., Wexler N. S., Conneally P. M. *et al.* (1983). A polymorphic DNA marker genetically linked to Huntington's disease. *Nature*; 306: 234–8.

Higgins G. A., Lewis D. A., Bahmanyar S. *et al.* (1988). Differential regulation of amyloid B protein mRNA expression within hippocampal neuronal subpopulation in Alzheimer's disease. *Proceedings of the National Academy of Sciences (USA)*; 85: 1292–301.

Jeffreg A. J., Wilson V., Thien S. L. (1985). Hypervariable 'minisatellite' regions in human DNA. *Nature*; 314: 397–401.

Kimura M. (1979). The neutral theory of molecular evolution. *Scientific American*; 241: 98–100.

Litt M., Luty J. A. (1989). A hypervariable microsatellite revealed by *in vitro* amplification of a dinucleaotide repeat within the cardiac muscle actin gene. *American Journal of Human Genetics*; 44: 397–401.

Monaco A. P., Bertelson C. J., Middlesworth W. *et al.* (1985). Detection of deletions spanning the Duchenne muscular dystrophy locus using a tightly linked DNA segment. *Nature*; 316: 842–5.

Monaco A. P., Neve R. L., Colletti-Feeno C. *et al.* (1986). Isolation of candidate cDNAs for portions of the Duchenne muscular dystrophy gene. *Nature*; 323: 646–50.

Myers R. M., Sheffield V. C., Cox D. R. (1988). Detection of single base changes in DNA: ribonuclease cleavage and denaturing gradient gel electrophoresis. In: *Genome Analysis: A Practical Approach* (Davies K. E., ed.), pp. 95–139. Oxford: IRL Press.

Nakamura A., Leppart M., O'Connell P. *et al.* (1987). Variable number of tandem repeats (VNTR) markers for human gene mapping. *Science*; 235: 1616–22.

Owen M. J., Whatley S. A. (1988). Polymorphic DNA markers and mental disease. *Psychological Medicine*; 18: 529–33.

Poustka A., Pohl T., Barlow D. P. *et al.* (1986). Molecular approaches to mammalian genetics. In: *Cold Spring Harbor Symposia of Quantitative Biology*, 51 (part 1), pp. 131–9.

St. George-Hyslop P. H., Tanzi R. E., Polinsky R. J. *et al.* (1987). The genetic defect causing familial Alzheimer's disease maps on chromosome 21. *Science*; **235**: 885–90.

Smith C. L., Klco G. R., Cantor C. R. (1988). Pulsed-field gel electrophoresis and the technology of large DNA molecules. In: *Genome Analysis: A Practical Approach* (Davies K. E., ed.), pp. 41–72. Oxford: IRL Press.

Watson J. D., Crick F. H. E. (1953). A structure for deoxyribose nucleic acid. *Nature*; **171**: 737–8.

Weber J., May P. E. (1989). Abundant class of human DNA polymorphisms which can be typed using the polymerase chain reaction. *American Journal of Human Genetics*; **14**: 388–96.

Whatley S. A., Owen M. J., Murray R. M. (1989). The new genetics and neuropsychiatric disorders. In: *The Bridge between Neurology and Psychiatry* (Reynolds E. H., Trimble M. R., eds.), pp. 353–79. Edinburgh: Churchill Livingstone.

2 Genetic models of madness

PETER McGUFFIN

The term 'model' is used quite frequently in psychiatry, often in a broad and fairly inexact way to describe general concepts of mental illness. Thus it is not uncommon to hear clinicians speaking of the 'medical model' and contrasting this with the 'psychoanalytical model' or the 'behavioural model'. More strictly, in scientific discourse, a model is a theoretical representation of something that we cannot view directly but whose workings can be better understood by postulating that it has a certain form. A well-known example from physics would be Bohr's model of the atom. This is now known to be an over-simple representation, but the concept of a central nucleus about which electrons orbit in a planet-like fashion provides us with an easy to grasp, mental picture of something that is unobservable by direct means. Similarly, in genetics, although methods now exist for directly investigating genotypes at a molecular level, we still need to construct models to represent the ways in which genes and the environment may combine together to produce complex phenotypes. This is so because examining the genotype does not usually, in itself, offer a complete explanation of observed phenotypes; genetic endowment is much more like the recipe for a cake than the blueprint for a machine (Dawkins, 1986).

The most precise models used in genetics, and the ones that have the greatest predictive potential, are usually described in mathematical terms. Unfortunately, mathematical language is often off-putting for the clinician and is therefore seen by some as a source of obfuscation rather than clarification. However, most currently useful models can be described without resorting to complicated mathematical notation and so an attempt will be made in this chapter to describe genetic models of mental illness, their uses and their benefits with (almost) no algebra.

At the simplest level, our picture of how a phenotype, the thing we observe, is produced, is illustrated in Fig. 2.1. There are separate contributions from the genotype and the environment; the environment can be thought of as having two major components, *common* environment, which is shared within families, and environment that is *special* to the individual and not shared by relatives. Clearly, genes and the common environment can both contribute to familiality. Thus clustering in families is necessary to the inference that a trait is genetic but it is not enough.

It has long been established that some forms of mental illness tend to

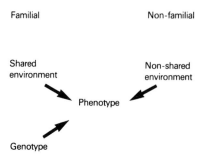

Fig. 2.1   *Contributions to the phenotype*

run in families and much effort has been expended in determining whether this is mainly caused by genetic influences, common environment, or a combination of the two. This has been an essential endeavour and, it could be argued, one that has produced the hardest evidence that we have concerning the aetiology of disorders such as schizophrenia and manic-depressive illness. The fact that most familial mental illness, with rare exceptions such as Huntington's chorea, does not show regular Mendelian patterns of segregation has resulted in much controversy and confusion; indeed, it is precisely for this reason that more complicated models are necessary. However, it should also be pointed out that it is not difficult to find traits that have the superficial appearance of a regular Mendelian pattern of transmission but that are almost certainly not due to simple monogenic inheritance. The ability to roll the tongue was at one stage frequently cited in elementary texts as an example of autosomal-dominant inheritance. However, this is almost certainly an over-simplification (Fogle, 1987). More blatant examples of the simulation of Mendelism have been discussed by Edwards (1960), and elsewhere by Lilienfeld (1959), who demonstrated that attending medical school runs in families in a fashion compatible with autosomal-recessive transmission. We have recently been able partially to replicate this finding using more modern and more complex methods of segregation analysis (McGuffin and Huckle, 1990). Most medically qualified readers will probably personally know other families in which attending medical school follows a more 'dominant-like' pattern of inheritance!

We can, of course, help ourselves to avoid spurious inferences about genetic markers in complex traits by resorting to twin and adoption studies, the classical methods of distinguishing genetic and environmental sources of familiality. It has long been theoretically possible to use a third method, a search for linkage or association with genetic markers, to demonstrate the genetic basis for a familial trait, but it is only comparatively recently—with the discovery of many genetic polymorphisms, including those resulting from recombinant DNA technology (Chapter 1)—that this approach has become practicable. The use of genetic markers in psychiatric research is a focus of much attention (see Chapters 7, 11) and provides a further reason for producing adequate theoretical models. While it is possible, without much knowledge of formal genetics, to interpret the results of twin and adoption studies at a fairly rudimentary level (i.e. suggesting presence or absence of a genetic effect), it would not be wise to attempt a linkage study without having a reasonable grasp of the plausible models of transmission for the disorder under investigation (see Chapter 13).

SIMPLE GENETIC MODELS AND IRREGULAR TRAITS

It is logical to start with simple models where genes are considered as the sole source of resemblance among relatives. It is also convenient to adopt the terminology of Morton (1982), who distinguishes *regular* phenotypes, which conform to a simple, Mendelian pattern of transmission, from *irregular* phenotypes, which do not. However, it is important in doing so to remember that an observed pattern of transmission depends on how the phenotype is defined, detected or measured. One phenomenon that may lead to the appearance of irregularity in a monogenic disorder is variable *expressivity*. For example, the peripheral form of neurofibromatosis can manifest as just a few *café-au-lait* spots rather than the full-blown picture with multiple tumours of the skin and systemic involvement. Similarly, Huntington's disease in its early stages can show considerable variability in expression, some cases presenting with movement disorder, others with cognitive deterioration, and yet others with alteration of personality and disturbance of mood. It has been suggested that the transmission of schizophrenia could be explained by a simple dominant gene with a very broad range of expressivity. Heston (1970) suggested that 'schizoid disease' might be manifest in the relatives of schizophrenics not just as schizophrenia or schizoid traits but as a wide range of psychological attitudes including some relatives who are particularly gifted and creative. This appealing hypothesis would, however, require that all monozygotic co-twins of schizophrenics would show schizoid disease and this appears not to be the case (Gottesman and Shields, 1982).

A rather different phenomenon, which also leads to irregular patterns of transmission, is that of incomplete *penetrance*. Penetrance is the probability of manifesting a particular phenotype, given a certain genotype. Therefore, for regular traits, penetrance is always either zero or one. However, it is perhaps helpful in attempting to understand the concept of penetrance if we remember that dominance and recessivity are properties of the phenotype which we observe rather than intrinsic properties of the underlying genotype. For example, it is possible to detect a heterozygous 'carrier' status for various recessive disorders. Suppose in such conditions we were arbitrarily to reclassify all carriers as well as all homozygotes showing the full-blown disorder as 'affected'. Hence by redefining the phenotype we would convert from a recessive to a dominant condition. Both autosomal-dominant and recessive inheritance can be considered as subsets of a *general single locus* (GSL) model (Table 2.1). Here we consider a single locus where A_1 is the normal allele, and A_2 is the mutant or 'disease' allele. The three genotypes, A_1A_1, A_1A_2 and A_2A_2, have penetrances of f_1, f_2 and f_3, respectively. It follows that if $f_1 = 0$ and $f_2 = f_3 = 1$, the disease is a regular dominant with no non-genetic/sporadic cases. If $f_1 = f_2 = 0$, and $f_3 = 1$, then the disease is regular recessive with no sporadics. However, under the GSL model, the penetrances may take any value between 0 and 1. An earlier example of a model of this type being applied in psychiatry (although using a slightly different notation), was Slater's (1958) monogenic hypothesis concerning the transmission of schizophrenia. Here it was proposed that all A_2A_2 homozygotes were affected (i.e. $f_3 = 1$), there were no sporadics ($f_1 = 0$), and there was a low penetrance in heterozygotes (f_2) of around 20%. Although on superficial examination the results are plausible, Slater did not attempt a formal goodness-of-fit test. Had he done so he would have unfortunately found that the fit is very poor (McGuffin, 1990).

It has been pointed out (James, 1971) that using incidence data (i.e. morbidity risks) in pairs of relatives can be misleading when the aim is to attempt a goodness-of-fit of the GSL model. It can be shown that having estimated the population frequency of the disease (K_p), observations on pairs of relatives can yield estimates of two further parameters, the variance due to additive gene effects (V_A) and the variance due to dominance (V_d). It is possible to derive expressions relating each of these three known values to the parameters of the GSL model. There are actually four parameters to be considered, q, the frequency in the population of A_2 and the penetrances f_1, f_2 and f_3, which we have already defined. However, we are then left with

Table 2.1 Penetrances (probabilities of being affected) in simple Mendelian and general single major locus (GSL) models of disease

	Genotypes		
Model	A_1A_1	A_1A_2	A_2A_2
Recessive	0	0	1
Dominant	0	1	1
General	$0 \leqslant f_1 \leqslant 1$	$0 \leqslant f_2 \leqslant 1$	$0 \leqslant f_3 \leqslant 1$

Note: A penetrance of 1 means that all individuals of this phenotype are affected while zero penetrance means that none are affected. However, in the general model the penetrances (f_1, f_2 or f_3) can theoretically take any value between 0 and 1.

three known values and four unknowns so that it is impossible to arrive at a unique solution. One way around the problem was proposed by Suarez *et al.* (1976), who showed that if the parameters of the GSL model are all constrained within the biologically meaningful limits of 0 and 1, then the area of fit to the model can be graphically delineated so that it may then be possible mathematically to exclude GSL inheritance. This test was applied to all the available published data on schizophrenia concerning twins and other pairs of relatives, producing results that appeared incompatible with the GSL model (O'Rourke *et al.*, 1982). No formal statistical test was made in this attempted refutation but subsequently McGue *et al.* (1985) tested the goodness-of-fit of the GSL model using a similar, combined data set. Again, parameters were constrained to within biologically meaningful limits, and it was possible convincingly to exclude this mode of transmission for schizophrenia.

It should again be noted that the GSL model as defined here is classified as 'simple' because of the hypothesis that a genetic factor provides the sole source of resemblance between relatives. Hence penetrances are regarded as parameters that are characteristic of the whole population and are therefore uncorrelated within families. (It would therefore make no real sense to talk about 'high penetrance' and 'low penetrance' families.) An alternative, simple hypothesis is to consider that liability to develop the disease is continuously distributed in the population and is contributed to by the predominantly additive effects of multiple genes at different loci. Liability would then tend to be normally distributed (or could be readily transformed to a normal distribution), but only those individuals whose liability at some point exceeded a certain threshold would manifest the disorder (Fig. 2.2). It is then assumed that the relatives of affected individuals have an increased mean liability compared with the population as a whole, with the result that more relatives lie beyond the threshold and manifest the disorder. By knowing the frequency of the disorder in the population and in relatives, it is possible to calculate the *correlation in liability* (Falconer, 1965; Reich *et al.*, 1972), which provides a useful measure of the strength of familial association. Moreover, as we are here assuming that the only source of familial resemblance is polygenic, it is quite simple to obtain an estimate of *heritability*. Heritability is the proportion of total phenotypic variance that can be accounted for by additive genetic effects and, under a pure polygenic model, is simply the correlation in liability divided by the *coefficient of relationship*. This is the average proportion of genes held in common and is thus one for monozygotic twins, a half for dizygotic twins and full siblings and a quarter for half-siblings, and so on. Again, it was in an attempt to explain the transmission of schizophrenia that a polygenic threshold model was first used in psychiatry (Gottesman and Shields, 1967). As with Slater's early application of a single gene model, no goodness-of-fit test was applied. However, it has since been shown that a pure polygenic model, unlike the pure GSL model, does fit the observed risks in a combined European data

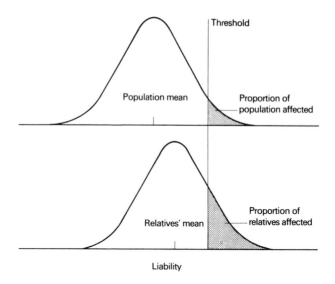

Fig. 2.2   *The liability/threshold model*

set of various classes of relatives of schizophrenic patients (McGue *et al.*, 1985).

In addition, some consider that the polygenic model has greater appeal than the GSL model because it allows a disorder like schizophrenia to be considered as a 'semi-continuous' trait rather than a simply dichotomous one. Thus, if severity of illness can be equated with severity on a liability scale, this might explain why concordance in twins or first-degree relatives increases with the severity of the illness of the proband. Similarly, the liability/threshold concept could explain why the risk of schizophrenia for an individual increases with the number of affected relatives. The persistence of schizophrenia in the population, despite the selective disadvantages conferred by the condition (i.e. the reduced probability of producing offspring), is also more easily explicable in terms of a polygenic than a GSL model. However, one major drawback of a pure polygenic model is that it allows only genes as a source of resemblance between relatives and does not take into account the effects discussed earlier of shared family environment (Fig. 2.1) or transmission of environmental influences from parent to child (cultural transmission). In order for such effects to be incorporated we need to consider more complex models that are truly multifactorial.

MULTIFACTORIAL MODELS

Multifactorial models have been introduced, not as has sometimes been suggested as a cloak for ignorance, but as a means of trying to do full justice

to the possible effects of the interplay between genes, the family environment and the cultural transmission of complex traits. As already pointed
out, it is well known that certain traits and some diseases may cluster in
families for reasons that are not mainly genetic. We might expect,
returning to our earlier example, that attending medical school shows
strong familiality because of the effects of cultural transmission and shared
environment. This would include such factors as style of upbringing,
parental expectation and the offspring's emulation of parents or elder
siblings. However, genes may contribute indirectly, for example, via an
influence on intellectual abilities. Tuberculosis provides a different example of a trait that in the past was found to be aggregated in families,
presumably mainly because of contagion. Here again, genes may still
contribute by conferring susceptibility to the tubercle bacillus. For a
dichotomous trait, such as the presence or absence of mental illness, the
most useful approach is to extend the concept of the liability/threshold
model such that liability can be contributed by multiple genetic and
family–environmental effects (which again are assumed to combine in a
predominantly additive fashion). It then becomes a matter of interest to ask
how much liability is contributed by genes, how much is contributed by
environment and what sort of environment? The 'how much' is usually
expressed in terms of proportion of variance accounted for. I have already
mentioned and defined heritability but another quantity of interest is the
proportion of variance accounted for by common family environment.

A frequently used way of partitioning phenotypic variance involves path
analysis. A straightforward path model accounting for the sources of
resemblance between siblings is shown in Fig. 2.3. The calculus of path
analysis dictates that the expected correlation between variables is the sum
of the permissible paths connecting them. Suppose that siblings 1 and 2
were actually dizygotic twins, then the phenotypic correlation (r_{dz}) is given
by the path via father's genotype, $h \times \frac{1}{2} \times \frac{1}{2} \times h$, the path via the
mother's genotype, $h \times \frac{1}{2} \times \frac{1}{2} \times h$, plus the path via common environ-

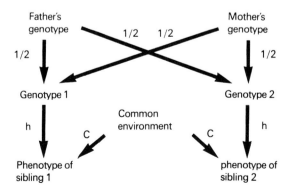

Fig. 2.3 *A path model of sources of resemblance in siblings or twins*

ment, $c \times c$. Thus the sum is $\frac{1}{4} h^2 + \frac{1}{4} h^2 + c^2 = \frac{1}{2} h^2 + c^2$. If siblings 1 and 2 are monozygotic twins, then genotypes 1 and 2 are identical so that the phenotypic correlation (r_{mz}) is given by:

$$r_{mz} = h^2 + c^2$$

Some examples of the results of applying this type of multifactorial model are summarized in Table 2.2. We can examine the contributors to the variance of continuously distributed traits such as intelligence quotient (IQ) and personality. Similarly, if they are considered as threshold traits, the same sort of treatment can be applied to affective disorders, schizophrenia and tuberculosis. In Table 2.2 I have taken the correlations computed by Loehlin and Nichols (1976) for IQ in their well-known twin study as an example. The data here suggest that IQ is very strongly familial, with only 16% of the variance accounted for by non-shared environment. Just under half of the total variance is genetic and this is in good agreement with recent estimates produced by more complicated analyses (Rice *et al.*, 1980). For personality I have taken correlations for female twins computed by Eaves and Young (1981), using the extraversion (E) scale of Eysenck and Eysenck (1975). The greater part of the variance is genetic, but a substantial proportion, over a third, is environmental. It should be noted, however, that the environmental variance is entirely of a non-familial type so that the contribution of common environment to the variance is approximately 0. At first sight this is a rather surprising result but it accords well with the findings from reared-apart twins and is consistent with the results of nearly all recent genetic studies of personality traits (Henderson, 1982; Plomin, 1990). The provocative issues concerning the effects of family environment on personality and temperament are discussed further in Chapter 14.

For affective disorders, the results are probably more in keeping with

Table 2.2 Genetic and environmental contribution to the variance

Trait	Additive genetic (h^2)	Common environment (c^2)	Non-shared environment
IQ	0.48	0.36	0.16
Personality (E)	0.66	0	0.34
Manic-depressive psycho-sis	0.86	0.07	0.07
Major depression	0.52	0.30	0.18
Neurotic depression	0.08	0.54	0.38
Schizophrenia	0.63	0.29	0.08
Tuberculosis	0.06	0.62	0.32

See text for explanation of calculations and sources of data.

most readers' intuitive expectations. The data are based on calculations carried out by McGuffin and Katz (1989), who used their own preliminary data for twins, together with those of Bertelsen *et al.* (1977) and Torgersen (1986). It appears that all forms of affective disorder are substantially familial in that the combined effects of genes and common environment far outweigh non-familial environment. However, for manic-depressive psychosis, it is genes that make the major contribution, with a heritability in excess of 80%, while for neurotic depression, heritability is small and family environment is the largest contributor to variation in liability. Major affective disorder occupies an intermediate position and appears to be substantially influenced both by genetic factors and common family environment.

The estimates for schizophrenia and tuberculosis are taken directly from a paper by McGue *et al.* (1985) in which a more complex but, in principle, fairly similar path model was adopted to analyse twin and family data from a variety of published sources. The data for tuberculosis were analysed alongside those for schizophrenia because, as we have noted, tuberculosis is often identified as being a familial disorder, moreover one which has a high monozygotic concordance in some twin studies. As mentioned earlier, tuberculosis is one of those traits where one might spuriously infer a substantial genetic component. It is therefore reassuring that the analysis of McGue *et al.* showed that the major contribution to the variance, as one would expect with an infection, comes from shared family environment rather than from genes. In the case of schizophrenia, by contrast, the largest contribution to the variance comes from genes, with the suggestion of a more modest role for common environment.

Straightforward path models of this type have been applied elsewhere in this book, (for example, Chapter 13), and it is not too difficult to extend the approach to examine the effects of associated traits (for example, Chapter 10). More complex and arguably more realistic models can be produced using essentially the same principles but taking into account such factors as positive correlations between spouses reflecting assortative mating and the transmission of environmental effects from parents to offspring ('cultural' transmission). Ideally, direct measures of environmental effects, 'environmental indices', can also be incorporated (Rice *et al.*, 1978; Rao *et al.*, 1979).

One drawback of presenting data in the style of Table 2.2 is that it does not tell us how confident we can be about our estimates of the influence of genetic and environmental factors or indeed whether we could explain the data just as well by dropping out one or other of the factors. The traditional way of dealing with this problem is, of course, to calculate the standard errors and hence produce confidence limits for the estimates of the parameters. However, with the advent of high-speed computers, it has become relatively easy and practicable to apply a more satisfactory approach, hence iterative model fitting (involving a repetitive search for the best fit) has become generally adopted as the standard way to test the applicability of quantitative genetic hypotheses. It is therefore worthwhile digressing slightly to consider the broad principles.

ITERATIVE MODEL FITTING

A schematic representation of iterative model fitting is given in Fig. 2.4. Essentially, the process involves a repetitive search for the values of the model parameters that give the optimum fit. In carrying this out the researcher provides the main computer program with the relevant data and supplies starting values for the parameters that are effectively his or her best guess at what the 'correct' values should be. This information determines the initial value of a mathematical function supplied by the investigator, the form of which depends upon the model being tested. Usually the mathematical function is either a chi square or a log likelihood. The optimization routine then calculates 'improved' estimates of the values that will bring about either an increase in the likelihood or a decrease in the chi square. (It should be noted that likelihood and chi square are inversely related. The size of chi square depends on the magnitude of the difference between observed and expected values and is therefore at a minimum when these are closely similar. 'Likelihood' refers to the likelihood of a certain hypothesis given the observed data, and it is therefore maximized when observed and expected values are in close agreement.) Iteration ceases when either the *maximum likelihood* or the *minimum chi square* is obtained, so providing the 'best fit' estimates of the model parameters.

Table 2.3 summarizes the results of a worked example of iterative fitting of the type of simple path model described earlier. I have taken the

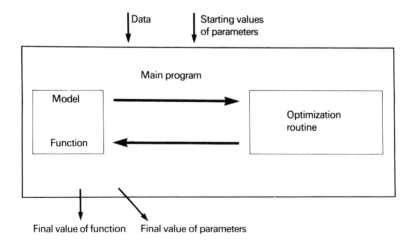

Fig. 2.4   *Iterative model fitting*

Table 2.3 Fitting a path model to twin data on major affective disorder

Model	Parameter estimates			
	h^2	c^2	χ^2	p
No transmission	[0]	[0]	399.50	0.000
Additive genetic effects only				
(G)	0.84	[0]	3.98	<0.05
Family environment only (C)	[0]	0.70	8.28	<0.005
G and C	0.51	0.31	0.0	

h^2 = heritability; c^2 = variance contributed by family environment; parameters in square brackets are fixed.

preliminary twin data on concordance for major affective disorder reported by McGuffin and Katz (1989). Here the proband-wise concordance for monozygotic twins was 32 out of 62 (53%) while that for dizygotic twins was 22 out of 79 (28%). The sample was obtained by screening all probands on the Maudsley Hospital Twin Register with a primary diagnosis of depression. It was found that 53% fulfilled the American Psychiatric Association (1980) *Diagnostic and Statistical Manual of Mental Disorders* (DSM-III) criteria for major depression. As the register provides a representative sample of patients (selected only for the fact of being born a twin), we can use this figure as an approximate estimate of the proportion of Maudsley patients with a diagnosis of depression who have had DSM-III major affective disorder. Then, taking the risk of being treated for depression up to age 65 as being 8.9% (Sturt *et al.*, 1984), we obtain an approximate population risk of major affective disorder of 8.9% × 53% = 4.7%. From this and the monozygotic and dizygotic concordances we can calculate correlations in liability and use these in the model-fitting exercise. The results shown in Table 2.3 enable a comparison between a full model, in which both additive genetic effects (G) and family environmental effects (C) are brought into play, and reduced models where only C has an influence (and the heritability is fixed at 0) or when only G has an effect (and common environment is fixed at 0). Comparison is made by taking the difference in the chi square values between the full model and the sub-models, where degrees of freedom (d.f.) are equal to the difference in the number of parameters. As we can see from the table, the full model is superior to both the additive genetic model (χ^2 = 3.98; d.f. = 1; $p<0.05$) and the family environment model (χ^2 = 8.28; d.f. = 1; $p<0.005$). A 'no transmission' model, in which both heritability and common environment are fixed at 0, provides a very poor fit indeed (χ^2 = 399.5; p = 0.000). We can therefore conclude that there is familial transmission of major affective disorder and that both genetic effects and family environment are significant contributors to this familiality.

It should be noted that in this exercise, the computer program minimized a chi square function. In the alternative procedure, where a likelihood is maximized, comparison of models is carried out using a *likelihood ratio test*. This depends on the fact that if L_1 is the log likelihood for a certain model and L_2 is the log likelihood of a second model, which is a subset of the first, then $-2(L_1 - L_2)$ is approximately distributed as a chi square. Again degrees of freedom equal the difference in the number of parameters.

SEGREGATION ANALYSIS

So far the discussion of applying genetic models in psychiatric disorders has focused on methods that use incidence data on pairs of relatives. However, if the aim is primarily to discover the most likely mode of transmission and to resolve major gene effects rather than to partition sources of variation, a more powerful approach is to carry out complex segregation analysis in which information from entire pedigrees is used. Probably the most commonly applied procedures are based on the mixed model of Morton and MacLean (1974), where it is postulated that liability to develop the disorder is given by a combination of a major gene effect, a multifactorial effect and a residual environmental component. It can be readily appreciated that this is effectively a combination of the multifactorial threshold model described earlier and the GSL model. The mixed model is illustrated in Fig. 2.5. The main parameters are a gene frequency (q), a displacement between the mean liability values of two homozygotes (*t*) and a dominance deviation that gives the heterozygote mean value relative to the means of the two homozygotes (*d*). The multifactorial effect is parameterized as the proportion of liability variance contributed by non-major gene familial factors, the 'multifactorial heritability' (H). Applying

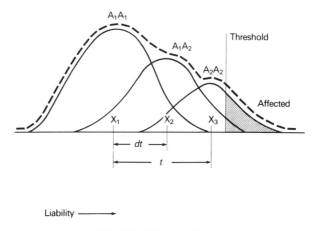

Fig. 2.5   *The mixed model*

the mixed model provides a more comprehensive and satisfactory strategy than piecemeal attempts to fit single-gene, multifactorial or 'oligogenic' models involving two or more loci. Full use is made of the potential of iterative model-fitting strategies, as described earlier. The standard procedure is then to test the full, mixed model against the reduced models, which are its subsets.

An example is the study of Rice *et al.* (1987), which carried out a mixed-model analysis of the transmission of affective disorder in families ascertained through probands with bipolar illness. These investigators controlled for the effects of birth cohort and age of onset and were able to show that the mixed model was superior to the multifactorial but did not offer any appreciable advantage over a major locus model. Thus, on grounds of parsimony, the major locus explanation would be favoured. Similar results, analysing the family data of bipolar probands, were obtained by O'Rourke *et al.* (1983). However, it is possible to incorporate a further check on the plausibility of major gene transmission by carrying out tests of transmission probabilities (Elston and Stewart, 1971). If we use the same notation as we did earlier in describing the GSL model, we could consider a locus with two alleles, A_1 and A_2. The probabilities of parents transmitting the allele A_1 to their offspring are 1, $\frac{1}{2}$, and 0, for parents of the types A_1A_1, A_1A_2 and A_2A_2. Lalouel *et al.* (1983) have incorporated the notion of transmission probabilities together with mixed-model concepts to produce a 'unified' model. Therefore, if there is evidence of a major locus effect resulting from mixed-model analysis, it is then possible to test for deviation from Mendelian expectations by iterating on the transmission probabilities. When Rice *et al.* (1987) analysed their data, removing constraints on the probabilities of transmission of the major gene, the log likelihood increased, giving a result for the likelihood ratio test that was highly significant when compared with the Mendelian, major gene model. This therefore casts some doubt on the prospect that all familial bipolar disorders can be explained on the basis of a single, major gene.

The application of a similar analytic approach to the transmission of schizophrenia has, if anything, been more disappointing. Carter and Chung (1980) studied the relatives of schizophrenic probands identified through hospital records. It was impossible to resolve multifactorial and single-gene inheritance statistically but the results could be interpreted as at least suggesting multifactorial inheritance. Risch and Baron (1984) obtained more extensive diagnostic data on 79 nuclear families where the probands were a consecutive series of admissions for schizophrenia. With a straightforward, affected/unaffected dichotomy, it was not possible to distinguish between models but when a multiple threshold approach was adopted, with three categories of graded severity, it was possible to reject pure, single-gene models but not a mixed model or pure polygenic inheritance. Risch and Baron concluded that a recessive single locus with a high gene frequency, low penetrance and a multifactorial background might account for the transmission of schizophrenia. This study underlines the fact that it is often difficult to resolve genetic models by segregation analysis when dealing with a complex disorder and relying purely on 'affection status' (i.e. when the only information is whether an individual is ill or not ill). Grading the level of severity or, better still, developing some reliable, continuous measure that might be correlated with liability, can potentially increase the power to resolve models. It would therefore be of great benefit, if we return to schizophrenia as an example, to be able to devise a measure that quantifies schizotypal traits consistently and reliably and is able to produce high average scores in both affected and non-schizophrenic relatives of schizophrenics. So far this has proved remarkably difficult (Gottesman, 1987).

THE BENEFITS AND LIMITATIONS OF QUANTITATIVE MODELS

The main thesis in this chapter is that in dealing with complex phenotypes such as mental disorders, it is necessary to start from the premise that the phenotypes we observe are products both of genotypes and the environment to which the genotypes are exposed. Quantitative analyses then proceed in one of two main directions, either first to evaluate the relative importance of the genetic and environmental components or, second, to attempt to explore the genetic component further and, in particular, to resolve major locus effects. However, the whole idea of applying quantitative models to psychiatric disorders is sometimes viewed with suspicion, either because of their apparent complexity or because they can be misused.

Studies focusing on heritability in particular have frequently provoked controversy (see, for example, Wahlsten, 1990). However, much of this derives from mistaken ideas about the very concept of heritability (McGuffin and Katz, 1990). As discussed earlier, heritability is the proportion of variance accounted for in the *population*. It does not have a simple meaning at an individual level, so that it would be ludicrous to estimate that the heritability of schizophrenia was around 70% and then suggest that 70% of the cause of an individual patient's illness is genetic! Similarly, heritability is specific to the population in which it is estimated. Other populations may differ with respect to genetic or environmental variance, or both, and hence the ratio of genetic to total phenotypic variance may differ too. A further, rather more technical shortcoming, is that commonly applied models require the prior assumption that non-additive genetic factors are negligible and therefore ignore dominance and epistatis (i.e. gene–gene interactions) as well as non-additive, gene–environment interactions (Wahlsten, 1990). Despite these shortcomings, estimating heritability and other major components of variance can have practical benefits. In Chapter 15 it is shown how heritability or associated measures of the strength of genetic factors can be used as a tool in the refinement of phenotypes. Similarly, analyses which reveal that most of the variance in liability to bipolar disorder can be accounted for by genes, while neurotic depression probably receives a large input from common family environment, provide us with clear leads for further studies. Bipolar disorder becomes an obvious focus for more purely genetic strategies including those using genetic linkage markers (Chapter 11), while in less severe forms of affective illness, it will be profitable to attempt to study the coaction of family–environmental factors and social stressors (Chapter 9). Thus estimation of variance components can give valuable insights, providing the estimates themselves are not awarded undue respect. Thus it is of no interest whatsoever to know that the heritability of major affective disorder is 'really' 0.6 rather than 0.4, but it is potentially of considerable value to know that both genes and family environment make a significant and substantial contribution. Discovering this is a necessary first step in unravelling the complicated relationship between nature and nurture.

Studies that attempt to elucidate mode of transmission are in most respects less controversial. However, in some senses, attempts to resolve major gene effects by purely statistical methods have been disappointing. Such studies have, however, informed us about the plausible models that can be invoked in the transmission of schizophrenia or major affective disorder. Knowing this is essential and again must be seen as a necessary first step before proceeding with more ambitious work which seeks to establish the molecular biological basis of inheritance. Thus, even though it is possible to carry out non-parametric methods of analysis in studies of genetic linkage markers (Chapter 3), it will be misleading to suggest that any form of linkage analysis can be completely 'model free', as the very aim of detecting linkage presumes that major gene effects exist. In conclusion, the construction of a quantitative model, no matter how cleverly built, is not an end in itself. Rather such models are a necessary part of the equipment of a modern geneticist setting out to study psychiatric disorders or other common diseases of complex aetiology.

REFERENCES

American Psychiatric Association (1980). *DSM III: Diagnostic and Statistical Manual of Mental Disorders*. Washington DC: APA.

Bertelsen A., Harvald B., Hauge M. (1977). A Danish twin study of manic depressive disorders. *British Journal of Psychiatry*; **130**: 330–51.

Carter C. L., Chung C. S. (1980). Segregation analysis of schizophrenia under a mixed model. *Human Heredity*; **30**: 350–6.

Dawkins R. (1986). *The Blind Watchmaker*. London: Penguin.

Edwards J. H. (1960). The simulation of Mendelism. *Acta Genetica*; **10**: 63–70.

Elston R. L., Stewart J. (1971). A general model for genetic analysis of pedigree data. *Human Heredity*; **21**: 523–42.

Eysenck H. J., Eysenck S. B. G. (1975). *Manual of the Eysenck Personality Questionnaire*. London: Hodder and Stoughton.

Falconer D. S. (1965). The inheritance of liability to certain diseases, estimated from the incidence among relatives. *Annals of Human Genetics*; **29**: 51–76.

Fogle T. A. (1987). The phenotypic deception: influences of classical genetics on genetic paradigms. *Perspectives in Biology and Medicine*; **31**: 65–81.

Gottesman I. I. (1987). The borderlands of psychosis or the fringes of lunacy. *British Medical Bulletin*; **43**: 557–69.

Gottesman I. I., Shields J. (1967). A polygenic theory of schizophrenia. *Proceedings of the National Academy of Sciences (USA)*; **58**: 199–205.

Gottesman I. I., Shields J. (1982). *Schizophrenia, the Epigenetic Puzzle*. Cambridge: Cambridge University Press.

Henderson N. D. (1982). Human behaviour genetics. *Annual Review of Psychology*; **33**: 403–40.

Heston L. L. (1970). The genetics of schizophrenia and schizoid disease. *Science*; **167**: 249–56.

James J. (1971). Frequency in relatives for an all-or-none trait. *Annals of Human Genetics*; **35**: 47–9.

Lalouel J. M., Rao D. L., Morton N. E., Elston R. L. (1983). A unified model for complex segregation analysis. *American Journal of Human Genetics*; **26**: 484–503.

Lilienfield A. M. (1959). A methodological problem in testing a recessive genetic hypothesis in human disease. *American Journal of Public Health*; **49**: 199–204.

Loehlin J. C., Nichols R. C. (1976). *Heredity, Environment and Personality: a Study of 850 Sets of Twins*. Austin and London: University of Texas Press.

McGue M., Gottesman I. I., Rao D. C. (1985). Resolving genetic models for the transmission of schizophrenia. *Genetic Epidemiology*; **2**: 99–110.

McGuffin P. (1990). Models of heritability and genetic transmission. In: *Search for the Causes of Schizophrenia 2* (Hafner H., Gattaz W., eds.). Heidelberg: Springer-Verlag.

McGuffin P., Huckle P. (1990). Simulation of Mendelism revisited. The recessive gene for attending medical school. *American Journal of Human Genetics* **46**: 994–9.

McGuffin P., Katz R. (1989). The genetics of depression: current approaches. *British Journal of Psychiatry*; **155** (suppl. 6): 18–20.

McGuffin P., Katz R. (1990). Who believes in estimating heritability as an end in itself? (Commentary on Wahlsten). *Behavioural and Brain Sciences* **13**: 141–2.

Morton N. E. (1982). *Outline of Genetic Epidemiology*. Basel: Karger.

Morton N. E., MacLean C. J. (1974). Analysis of family resemblance. III. Complex segregation analysis of quantitative traits. *American Journal of Human Genetics*; **26**: 489–503.

O'Rourke D. H., Gottesman I. I., Suarez B. K. *et al.* (1982). Refutation of the single locus model in the aetiology of schizophrenia. *American Journal of Human Genetics*; **33**: 630–49.

O'Rourke D. H., McGuffin P., Reich T. (1983). Genetic analysis of manic depressive illness. *American Journal of Physical Anthropology*; **62**: 51–9.

Plomin R. (1990). The role of inheritance in behavior. *Science*, **248**: 183–8.

Rao D. C., Morton N. E., Cloninger C. R. (1979). Path analysis under generalised assortative mating—I. Theory. *Genetic Research (Cambridge)*; **33**: 175–88.

Reich T., James J. W., Morris C. A. (1972). The use of multiple thresholds in determining the mode of transmission and semi-continuous traits. *Annals of Human Genetics*; **36**: 163–84.

Rice J., Cloninger C. R., Reich T. (1978). Multifactorial inheritance with cultural transmission and assortative mating. I. Description and basis properties of the unitary models. *American Journal of Human Genetics*; **30**: 618–43.

Rice J., Cloninger C. R., Reich T. (1980). Analysis of behaviour traits in the presence of cultural transmission and assortative mating: applications to I.Q. and S.E.S. *Behaviour Genetics*; **10**: 73–92.

Rice J. P., Reich T., Andreasen N. C. *et al.* (1987). The familial transmission of bipolar illness. *Archives of General Psychiatry*; **44**: 441–7.

Risch N., Baron M. (1984). Segregation analysis of schizophrenia and related disorders. *American Journal of Human Genetics*; **36**: 1039–59.

Slater E. (1958). The monogenic theory of schizophrenia. *Acta Genetica*; **8**: 50–6.

Sturt E., Kumakara N., Der G. (1984). How depressing life is—lifelong morbidity risk for depressive disorder in the general population. *Journal of Affective Disorders*; **7**: 109–22.

Suarez B. K., Reich T., Trost J. (1976). Limits of the genetic two allele single major locus model with incomplete penetrance. *Annals of Human Genetics*; **12**: 309–26.

Torgersen S. (1986). Genetic factors in moderately severe and mild affective disorders. *Archives of General Psychiatry*; **43**: 222–6.

Wahlsten D. (1990). Insensitivity of the analysis of variance to heredity-environment interaction. *Behavioural and Brain Sciences* **13**: 109–20.

3 The uses and abuses of linkage analysis in neuropsychiatric disorder

FRANÇOISE CLERGET-DARPOUX

INTRODUCTION

Many psychiatric diseases, and in particular affective disorders and schizophrenia, are known to cluster in families. Moreover, twin studies, adoption studies and path analyses have shown that this family clustering is due—at least partially—to genetic factors (Gottesman *et al.*, 1982; McGuffin and Katz, 1989).

Having established the existence of such factors, genetic epidemiology can propose inheritance models for genetic susceptibility, and then discriminate the most adequate one among them. Segregation analysis is the most common way of testing a mode of inheritance. It relies on a sample of families segregating the disease, and aims at determining whether or not there is a factor that plays a 'major role' and whether it is transmitted in a Mendelian manner.

In many diseases for which the existence of a genetic component has been established, segregation analysis is not able to demonstrate the role of a major gene. This is the case for affective disorders and schizophrenia (O'Rourke *et al.*, 1982; Goldin *et al.*, 1983). These diseases, with complex aetiological backgrounds, involve the participation of several interacting factors and are often also likely to be heterogeneous.

Thus, to study these complex diseases, new strategies have been developed, which take advantage of the information provided by so-called genetic markers in families of affected individuals. A genetic marker is a polymorphic gene, i.e. one with multiple allelic forms of expression. One knows the frequencies and dominance relationships of the alleles, as well as the location of the gene on the genome. For example, the ABO blood group system or the HLA system may be considered genetic markers. Thanks to molecular technology, the number of genetic markers is increasing very rapidly and there will soon be markers for any part of the genome.

Information from genetic markers can be used at a population level through association studies and at the family level through linkage studies. Only linkage studies will be presented and discussed in this chapter.

LINKAGE STUDIES

At family level a genetic marker can be informative if the disease and the marker do not segregate independently. An illustration of non-independent segregation of a complex disease and a genetic marker is shown in the pedigree published by Mendlewicz *et al.* in 1980 (Fig. 3.1).

In this pedigree we can observe the segregation of a psychiatric illness— affective disorder with bipolar and unipolar types—and the segregation of another disease, the glucose-6-phosphate dehydrogenase (G6PD) deficiency. The enzyme G6PD may be considered the genetic marker. This gene is located on the X chromosome and the deficiency is due to a rare recessive allele. Males carrying the deficient allele are affected and carrier females are mothers of affected males. In this pedigree nearly all of the individuals over 20 years of age having the deficient allele for G6PD also have the affective disorder and vice versa.

Several methods may be used to test non-independent segregation, including parametric methods requiring disease models, such as the lod score (Morton, 1955), and non-parametric methods such as the sib pair (Penrose, 1935) or the affected pedigree member (Weeks and Lange, 1988).

Parametric method

The most widely used parametric method for testing non-independence or 'linkage' is the lod score. It is not a new approach, as it was first proposed in 1955 by N. Morton. It is important to stress that it was initially

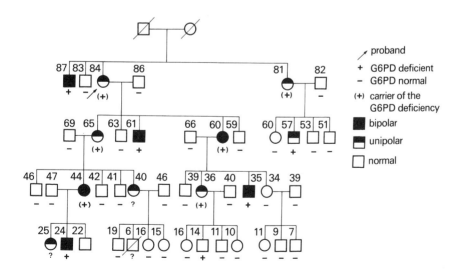

Fig. 3.1 *Cosegregation of affective disorder and glucose-6-phosphate dehydrogenase (G6PD) deficiency (from Mendlewicz et al., 1980)*

developed to locate genes with a known mode of inheritance and not for testing linkage between a complex disease and a genetic marker.

In the usual conditions, i.e. when the disease is monogenic with well-specified genetic parameters (disease allele frequency, dominance relationship between normal and disease alleles, penetrance value), the lod score method can be applied to a sample of families where the segregation of the disease and of a genetic marker is observed. It is then possible to test if the disease and the marker are transmitted independently, i.e. to test the recombination fraction between the disease locus and the marker locus equal to $\frac{1}{2}$, against the linkage at $\theta_1 < \frac{1}{2}$, by comparing the likelihoods $L(\theta = \frac{1}{2})$ and $L(\theta = \theta_1)$. This is equivalent to comparing the probability of observing the data under $\theta = \frac{1}{2}$ or $\theta = \theta_1$. For a given family sample, the lod score is defined as the decimal logarithm of the ratio of the two likelihoods,

$$Z(\theta_1) = \log_{10} [L(\theta_1)/L(\theta = \tfrac{1}{2})]$$

If the lod score $Z(\theta_1)$ is greater than or equal to 3, linkage is concluded. Given the sequential nature of the lod score test, the stopping criterion of 3 was shown by Morton to correspond to a reliability of the test of greater than 95% for autosomal loci. The advantage of a sequential procedure is that the number of observations required to detect linkage at a given value θ_1 is minimal. The lod score computation, however, is not restricted to a unique value θ_1 but to a set of θ values ranging between 0 and $\frac{1}{2}$. To conclude linkage, the critical value of 3 is then applied to the maximum $Z_{max}(\theta)$ of the lod function over the interval $[0, \frac{1}{2}]$. In addition, the test is not carried out in a sequential way and is more similar to a classical test procedure based on a fixed sample size (Chotai, 1984). However, the value of 3 has been chosen in order to make the test very conservative.

When a conclusion of linkage is reached, the estimate of the recombination fraction is the value that maximizes the lod score function or, equivalently, the value for which the probability of observing the given data is maximum. For more details, interested readers may refer to the book edited by J. Ott (1985). Several computer programs are available for computing the likelihood of recombination fractions or lod scores: LIPED (Ott, 1976); PAP (Hasstedt and Cartwright, 1981); FAP (Neugebauer *et al.*, 1984); LINKAGE (Lathrop and Lalouel, 1984).

It is important to note that the computations of $L(\theta_1)$ and $L(\theta = \frac{1}{2})$ and thus of $Z(\theta_1)$ are made under certain assumptions, in particular concerning the mode of inheritance of the disease. These assumptions are necessary to infer the probabilities of genotypes from the observed phenotypes. What happens if these assumptions are incorrect?

We have studied the effect of different kinds of error in modelling the genetic component of a disease when using the lod score method (Clerget-Darpoux and Bonaiti-Pellié, 1980; Clerget-Darpoux, 1982; Clerget-Darpoux *et al.*, 1986). More specifically, we studied the effect of:

1. using wrong genetic parameters for the disease locus (allele frequencies, penetrance values);
2. ignoring an interaction between the disease locus and the marker locus;
3. ignoring an association between alleles for the disease and the marker loci.

We showed that the estimated recombination fraction is very sensitive to the specification of the genetic parameters at the disease locus and may be highly biased when the genetic model is badly specified. The results of two lod-score analyses done on 52 HLA-typed families with insulin-dependent diabetes, shown in Table 3.1, illustrate this effect. In both analyses, the disease is assumed to result from a recessive disease allele but in the first one the disease allele frequency (q) is taken to be equal to 0.065 and the penetrance value (f), i.e. the probability for an individual having the disease allele twice to be affected, is taken to be 0.50, whereas in the second analysis, $q = 0.35$ and $f = 0.20$.

The location of the disease locus is very different according to the values used. While in the first case the disease locus is far from the HLA marker ($\theta = 0.11$), in the second, when the disease allele is assumed to be very common ($q = 0.35$), the disease locus is within the HLA system ($\theta = 0$).

Let us consider an interaction between the alleles at the marker locus and those at an unlinked disease locus, which is equivalent to assuming a two-locus disease model in which one locus is unlinked and the other is strictly linked to the marker. If the lod-score analysis is performed under a one-locus disease model, ignoring this interaction we would wrongly conclude that there was a loose linkage or, in other words, the existence of a disease locus linked to the marker but located at a large recombination fraction.

Estimating a recombination fraction seems meaningless when doing a lod-score analysis between a disease with an unknown mode of inheritance and a genetic marker. The robustness of lod-score estimator can be improved, however, by using the information from several genetic markers simultaneously.

Table 3.1 Effect of the specification of the genetic parameters on the estimate of the recombination fraction $\hat{\theta}$

Disease	Number of families	Parameters		Z_{MAX}	$\hat{\theta}$
Insulin-dependent diabetes	52	Recessive	$q = 0.065$ $f = 0.50$	6.83	0.11
		Recessive	$q = 0.35$ $f = 0.20$	7.45	0.00

Multipoint mapping

If we consider three loci A, B, C in this order on the same chromosome pair and if θ_{AB}, θ_{BC}, θ_{AC} are respectively the recombination fractions between A and B, B and C, and A and C, one generally has: $\theta_{AC} \neq \theta_{AB} + \theta_{AC}$.

Thus, it is useful to define a mapping function that is an additive function of the recombination fraction and depends on assumptions about the occurrence of crossovers (Sturt and Smith, 1976). If we assume that crossovers occur independently from each other (no interference), then:

$$\theta_{AC} = \theta_{AB} + \theta_{BC} - 2\theta_{AB}\theta_{BC} \qquad (1)$$

The function $x(\theta) = -\frac{1}{2} Ln (1 - 2\theta)$, called the Haldane mapping function, is additive:

$$x(\theta_{AC}) = x(\theta_{AB}) + x(\theta_{BC})$$

and x measures the genetic distance expressed in morgan (M) units. When there is no independence of crossover events (interference), the relation (1) does not hold, and:

$$\theta_{AC} = \theta_{AB} + \theta_{BC} - 2C\theta_{AB}\theta_{BC}$$

where C is called the coincidence coefficient. If $C > 1$, there is a negative interference and if $C < 1$, there is a positive interference. Crossovers in the segment AB respectively decrease and increase the probability of crossovers in segment BC. A test of interference may be made by a likelihood ratio. In practice, because the power to detect interference is low, the mapping function is chosen before the analysis.

For a given mapping function, the likelihood of different possible orders for the loci studied can be computed, and one may compare the relative likelihoods or location scores and test the different orders (Lathrop et al., 1984a,b). A goodness-of-fit test for each order can also be made, as proposed by Ott and Lathrop (1987), retaining as possible orders only those which fit the data. The number of orders to consider increases quickly with the number of loci studied. Several algorithms have now been proposed for ordering loci (Lander and Green, 1987; Thompson, 1987; Lathrop and Lalouel, 1988; Hazout et al., 1989). Besides, mapping exclusion is also important when establishing a genetic map, and a computer program may be used to display exclusion areas (Edwards, 1987).

Using two genetic markers A and B at a known genetic distance will not only increase the power of detecting linkage if the putative disease locus D lies between the two markers (Lander and Botstein, 1986), but also because, given the constraint $x(\theta_{AB}) = x(\theta_{AD}) + x(\theta_{DB})$, the recombination fraction estimates θ_{AD} and θ_{DB} will be less sensitive to an incorrect parametrization of the disease locus. It should be noted, however, that the significance level of a linkage test corresponding to a lod score value of 3 is not the same if the lod score is computed between a disease locus and one genetic marker or between a disease locus and two genetic markers.

Another important effect of erroneous modelling is that it decreases the maximum lod score (or at least the expected one). This effect is particularly important when a gametic disequilibrium between alleles at the disease and marker loci is ignored. Two consequences can result from this observation. Using the wrong genetic model for the disease may lead to an erroneous rejection of linkage for a given recombination fraction θ, but it does not artifically increase evidence for linkage. This is, however, true only in expectation.

It is also important to note the sensitivity of the lod score to misclassification (Skolnick *et al.*, 1984). This sensitivity is very dependent on the genetic parameters specified in the linkage analysis. For example, one individual misclassified into affected/unaffected will influence the lod score differently under high and low penetrance. This observation is important with respect to the use of different criteria for classification in lod score analyses. As explained below, doing so modifies the significance of a maximum lod score and this effect is more important under high rather than low penetrance.

Non-parametric methods

Other approaches, such as the sib pair method, first proposed by Penrose (1935) and repeat statistics (Green and Woodrow, 1977; Weeks and Lange, 1988), may be used for testing linkage. Such approaches may be particularly interesting when testing linkage between a marker locus and a disease with an unknown mode of inheritance. They are indeed independent of the genetic model underlying the disease.

An extension of the sib pair method (Day and Simons, 1976; Thomson and Bodmer, 1977; Suarez, 1978) has been widely used for testing linkage between the HLA marker and many diseases. The distribution of the number of shared haplotypes in a sample of affected sib pairs is compared to the one expected under independent transmission of the disease and of the marker. In the case of the HLA marker, which is highly polymorphic, each parent of a sib pair can be assumed to be HLA heterozygous (ab) and different from his (her) spouse (cd). In the case of independent transmission of the marker and the disease, if one of the affected sibs is ac, the probability for the second sib of sharing two HLA haplotypes (i.e. to be ac) is $\frac{1}{4}$, that of sharing one haplotype (ad or bc) is $\frac{1}{2}$, and that of sharing no haplotype is $\frac{1}{4}$. An HLA haplotype shared by two sibs corresponds necessarily to a unique haplotype found in one parent. Two sibs with the same HLA genotype can be considered as identical by descent.

On the other hand, if we consider a less polymorphic marker with two alleles A_1 and A_2, two sibs having A_1A_2 have not necessarily inherited the same alleles A_1 and A_2. For example, if both parents are A_1A_2, one of the sibs may have inherited the maternal A_1 and the paternal A_2 but the reverse may be true for the second sib. For a less polymorphic marker, the information used is not the identity by descent but the identity by state.

Weeks and Lange (1988) have proposed the use of a variable Z measuring the degree of identity by state observed between all affected members of the same pedigree. Note that the probability of identity by state for one allele is a function of both the probability of identity by descent and the probability of random identity. For a sample of pedigrees with affected individuals, the observed value of Z may be compared to its value expected under independent segregation.

These parametric and non-parametric approaches each have their advantages and inconveniences. As mentioned above, erroneous specification of the genetic model in the lod score method decreases the power for detecting linkage. Similarly, the information provided by non-affected individuals is lost in non-parametric methods. In particular, let us consider two individuals from the same pedigree having the same allele. The probability of this allele being identical by descent or randomly will be computed without considering if intermediate-linked individuals in the pedigree have or do not have this allele. Comparisons of the loss of power with different approaches are only possible in specific situations.

ILLUSTRATION AND INTERPRETATION

Table 3.2 shows several examples of reported linkage between genetic markers and complex neuropsychiatric diseases using a lod score method.

A non-independent segregation of a disease and a genetic marker shows that at least one gene is involved in the aetiology of the disease. This gene is necessarily located on the same chromosome pair as the genetic marker at a recombination fraction smaller than 0.50, and eventually is confounded with the marker. However, interpretation has to be very cautious, especially with regard to three aspects: the significance levels, the population to which one is entitled to apply the conclusions, and the possible inferences on the aetiology of the disease in question.

Table 3.2 Reported linkage between markers and complex neuropsychiatric diseases

Affective disorders	Chromosome X
	G6PD, Xg, colour blindness; Mendlewicz and Fleiss (1974), Mendlewicz *et al.* (1980, 1987), Baron (1977), Baron *et al.* (1987)
	Chromosome 11
	INS, H*ras*; Egeland *et al.*, (1987)
Schizophrenia	Chromosome 5
	D5SM76, D5S39; Sherrington *et al.* (1988)
Alzheimer's disease	Chromosome 21
	D21S16; St. George-Hyslop *et al.* (1987), Goate *et al.* (1989)

It is important to note that when the mode of inheritance of a disease is not perfectly known, it is very tempting to perform lod score analysis using different genetic models or parameter values, different diagnostic criteria for classifying into affected/unaffected individuals, and different genetic markers. We must then deal with the problem of multiple testing, as the statistical significance of a maximum lod score greater than 3 is not the same when we do one or several tests.

Let us assume that we are testing H_0 with a type 1 error $\alpha = 5\%$. This means that when H_0 is correct, five results in every hundred (1 in 20) are expected to fall outside the confidence limits. Thus, when making one comparison on 20 random samples, or 20 independent comparisons on one sample, one difference is expected to be observed. If we make several tests simultaneously and if these tests are independent, it is possible to give the type-one error or conversely, for a given type-one error, to know the lod score criteria to be used. Thompson (1984) provided such criteria when testing linkage between a disease locus and several independent genetic markers. Determining the significance of multiple tests, however, is far more complicated and general rules cannot be given if the tests are dependent, as is the case when using different diagnostic criteria or several, linked, genetic markers (Clerget-Darpoux *et al.*, 1990).

Replication studies are often necessary to obtain good significance levels and to be confident of the existence of a positive linkage between a complex disease and a genetic marker. Replication must be done on an independent family sample using the same genetic model, the same diagnostic classification, and the same genetic marker for which a positive linkage was concluded in the first study.

At present, replications of positive findings in psychiatric diseases have not been very encouraging. For affective disorders, Gershon *et al.* (1979), Leckman *et al.* (1979) and Kidd *et al.* (1984) reject linkage with markers of the X chromosome; Hodgkinson *et al.* (1987) and Detera-Wadleigh *et al.* (1987) with markers of chromosome 11. For schizophrenia, Kennedy *et al.* (1988) and St. Clair *et al.* (1989) reject close linkage with markers of chromosome 5: D5S76, D5S39. Schellenberg *et al.* (1988) and Pericak-Vance *et al.* (1988) fail to replicate linkage between Alzheimer's disease and markers of chromosome 21.

Heterogeneity in the aetiology of the disease might explain these discrepancies. They show the importance both of comparing the selection criteria of the families studied and of describing the population of patients concerned by the conclusions of a linkage analysis. It would be erroneous to extend the role of a genetic factor demonstrated in a given pedigree or family sample to a larger population.

Two different tests have been proposed to search for linkage heterogeneity in a family sample. The first one was developed by Morton (1956) and the other by Smith (1963). They have been called, respectively, the 'predivided sample test' and the 'admixture test'. In the predivided sample test, the family sample is subdivided into m subsamples according to a specific criterion. Let $Z_i(\theta)$ be the lod score of the ith subsample, r_i the value of θ that maximizes this lod score function, and r the value of θ that maximizes the lod score of the total sample. To test the homogeneity of the recombination fractions between all the subsamples, we may use the quantity $2L_n(10)[\Sigma_i Z_i(r_i) - Z(r)]$, which approximately follows a chi-square distribution, with $m-1$ degrees of freedom. In the admixture test, it is assumed that the sample contains two kinds of families: those where the disease is determined at a locus linked to the marker with a recombination fraction θ, in a proportion α, and the other $1-\alpha$ families where the disease segregates independently of the marker. Let $L(\alpha,\theta)$ be the likelihood of α,θ. Under the null hypothesis of homogeneity ($\alpha=1$), the quantity: -2 [max $Ln(\alpha=1,\theta) -$ max $Ln(\alpha,\theta)$] follows asymptotically a chi-square distribution with one degree of freedom. In other words, if this quantity is larger than 3.84, we will conclude to the existence of heterogeneity with a type-one error of 5%.

Strategies for both replicating a positive finding of linkage and for determining the proportion of patients concerned by this linkage are necessary. We have considered this question in two studies. In the first one (Clerget-Darpoux et al., 1987), we studied the power to detect hetero-geneity in the presence of linkage and the robustness of the 'admixture test' when disease modelling is erroneous. We found the test highly sensitive to the disease modelling when a constraint is fixed on the recombination fraction between the genetic marker and the putative disease locus. However, the use of such constraints may be not only logical if we use a 'candidate' gene (potential involvement of this gene in the disease) as a marker, but also necessary if we want to have sufficient power. Using two genetic markers at a known genetic distance will also increase the power of detecting heterogeneity (Lander and Botstein, 1986; Martinez and Goldin, 1989).

In the second study (Leboyer et al., 1990), we proposed strategies for the replication of linkage between affective disorders and markers of chromosome X and 11. These strategies are proposed for nuclear families assuming different degrees of heterogeneity. The test gives the average number of families required to replicate linkage, given the size of the sibship, the number of affected individuals in the sibship and the parental status for the disease.

Both studies show not only the value of using genetic markers in a candidate-gene region, but also the precautions necessary in interpreting the results.

If a positive linkage is shown, further studies are needed before drawing conclusions on the nature and the importance of the genetic factor shown by the linkage study. In particular, it is misleading to use the terminology 'major gene for the disease' before demonstrating that this gene is involved in a majority of the affected individuals. Even if this is the case, other factors may play very important parts and may even be necessary to the development of the disease. Let us consider the example of leprosy, for which linkage with the HLA marker has already been established in a sample of affected families (De Vries *et al.*, 1980). Such linkage may be due to a differential immune response to the leprosy bacillus but the bacillus is obviously necessary for the development of the disease. Similarly, linkage is observed between the HLA marker and narcolepsy: affected sibs always share an HLA haplotype. In addition, except in very rare cases, narcolepsy develops only in individuals bearing the DR_2 antigen, demonstrating the role of this antigen or of a very strictly linked factor. However, as the risk of getting the disease for a DR_2-positive sib of a patient is less than 2%, this also indicates that other factors have important roles in the aetiology of the disease.

To avoid erroneous interpretations, and considering the current state of our knowledge, it seems particularly important, when studying complex diseases, better to define what is meant by a major gene.

The usefulness as well as the limitations of genetic marker information in the study of complex disorders is well illustrated by the contribution of the HLA marker to the understanding of type 1 diabetes. Indeed, until recently, it was unclear if the different types of diabetes mellitus had different causes. It is now well established that insulin-dependent diabetes (type 1 diabetes) is associated with HLA antigens and does not segregate independently of this marker in families, but that this is not the case for the other types of diabetes. In Caucasian populations, type 1 diabetes is associated with the DR_3 and DR_4 antigens (Svejgaard *et al.*, 1980). For example, in a sample of 266 French patients, 95% had either the DR_3 antigen or the DR_4 antigen versus 32% in a control sample. Moreover, 27% of these patients had the genotype DR_3DR_4 versus 3% in the control sample.

Apart from these associations, a non-independent segregation of the HLA marker and type 1 diabetes has also been found. In a large sample of 185 affected sib pairs, 56% are HLA identical, 38% semi-identical and 6% different, which is statistically very different from the 25%, 50,% 25% proportions expected in the case of independent transmission.

These well-established observations have been very useful in demonstrating the role of genetic factors located in the HLA region in the aetiology of type 1 diabetes. But the exact manner in which these and other interacting factors participate in the aetiology is still puzzling.

CONCLUSION

The strategies of genetic epidemiology are not the same for diseases with simple modes of inheritance and for diseases with complex modes of inheritance. With simple modes, the information provided by the segregation of the disease in families is sufficient to establish the role of a disease gene. The marker information will enable us to locate the disease locus. It may then be possible to determine the defective DNA sequence and even to determine its activity. For diseases with complex aetiology, the trait segregation is not enough to infer the way susceptibility to the disease is inherited. The additional information provided by genetic markers may be useful in showing the role of one factor and in subdividing a heterogeneous group of patients into subgroups that are homogeneous for at least one factor. In this way it becomes more realistic to study the role of other potential factors.

REFERENCES

Baron M. (1977). Linkage between an X-chromosome marker (deutan color blindness) and bipolar affective illness. *Archives of General Psychiatry*; **24**: 721–7.

Baron M., Rish N., Hamburger R. *et al.* (1987). Genetic linkage between X chromosome markers and bipolar affective illness. *Nature*; **326**: 289–92.

Chotai J. (1984). On the lod score method in linkage analysis. *Annals of Human Genetics*; **48**: 359–78.

Clerget-Darpoux F. (1982). Bias of the estimated recombination fraction and lod score due to an association between a disease gene and a marker gene. *Annals of Human Genetics*; **46**: 363–72.

Clerget-Darpoux F., Bonaiti-Pellié C. (1980). Epistasis effect: an alternative to the hypothesis of linkage disequilibrium in HLA-associated diseases. *Annals of Human Genetics*; **44**: 195–204.

Clerget-Darpoux F., Babron M-C., Bonaiti C. (1987). Power and robustness of the linkage homogenity test in genetic analysis of common disorders. *Journal of Psychiatric Research*; **21**: 625–30.

Clerget-Darpoux F., Bonaiti-Pellié C., Hochez J. (1986). Effects of misspecifying genetic parameters in lod score analysis. *Biometrics*; **42**: 393–9.

Clerget-Darpoux F., Babron M. C., Bonaiti-Pellié (1990). Assessing the effect of multiple linkage tests in complex diseases. *Genetic Epidemiology*; **7**: 245–53.

Day N. E., Simons M. J. (1976). Disease susceptibility genes—their identification by multiple case family studies. *Tissue Antigens*; **8**: 109–19.

Detera-Wadleigh S. D., Berrettini W. H., Goldin L. *et al.* (1987). Close linkage of C-Harvey-ras and the insulin gene to affective disorders is ruled out in three North American pedigrees. *Nature*; **325**: 806–8.

De Vries R. P. P., Mehra N. K., Vaidya M. C. *et al.* (1980). HLA linked control susceptibility to tuberculoid leprosy. *Tissue Antigens*; **16**: 294–304.

Edwards J. H. (1987). Exclusion mapping. *Journal of Medical Genetics*; **24**: 539–43.

Egeland J. A., Gerhard D. S., Pauls D. L. *et al.* (1987). Bipolar affective disorders linked to DNA markers on chromosome 11. *Nature*; **325**: 783–7.

Gershon E. S., Targum S. D., Matthysse S., Bunney W. E. (1979). Color blindness not closely linked to bipolar illness. *Archives of General Psychiatry*; **36**: 1423–30.

Goate A. M., Owen M. J., James L. A. *et al.* (1989). Predisposing locus for Alzheimer's disease on chromosome 21. *Lancet*; **i**: 352–5.

Goldin L. R., Gershon E. S., Targum S. D. *et al.* (1983). Segregation and linkage analyses in families of patients with bipolar, unipolar, and schizoaffective mood disorders. *American Journal of Human Genetics*; **35**: 274–87.

Gottesman I. I., Shields J., Hanson D. R., eds. (1982). *Schizophrenia. The Epigenetic Puzzle*. Cambridge: Cambridge University Press.

Green J. R., Woodrow J. C. (1977). Sibling method for detecting HLA-linked genes in disease. *Tissue Antigens*; **9**: 31–5.

Hasstedt S., Cartwright P. (1981). University of Utah (Salt Lake City), Department of Medical Biophysics and Computing, Technical Report 13: PAP—Pedigree Analysis Package.

Hazout S., Babron M-C., Clerget-Darpoux F. (1989). 'Pairwise Permutation' algorithm for ordering loci. In: *Multipoint Mapping and Linkage Based upon Affected Pedigree Members* (Elston R. C., Spence M. A., Hodge S. E., MacCluer J. W., eds.). New York: Alan R. Liss (in press).

Hodgkinson S., Sherrington R., Gurling H. *et al.* (1987). Molecular genetic evidence of heterogeneity in manic depression. *Nature*; **325**: 805–6.

Kennedy J. L., Giuffra L. A., Moises H. W. *et al.* (1988). Evidence against linkage of schizophrenia to markers on chromosome 5 in a northern Swedish pedigree. *Nature*; **336**: 167–70.

Kidd K. K., Egeland J., Molthan L. *et al.* (1984). Amish study. IV: Genetic linkage study of pedigrees of bipolar probands. *American Journal of Psychiatry*; **141**: 1042–8.

Lander E. S., Botstein D. (1986). Strategies for studying heterogeneous genetic traits in humans by using a linkage map of restriction fragment length polymorphisms. *Proceedings of the National Academy of Sciences (USA)*; **83**: 7353–7.

Lander E. S., Green P. (1987). Construction of multilocus genetic linkage maps in humans. *Proceedings of the National Academy of Sciences (USA)*; **84**: 2363–7.

Lathrop G. M., Lalouel J. M. (1984). Easy calculations of lod scores and genetic risks on small computers. *American Journal of Human Genetics*; **36**: 460–5.

Lathrop G. M., Lalouel J. M. (1988). Efficient computations in multilocus linkage analysis. *American Journal of Human Genetics*; **42**: 498–505.

Lathrop G. M., Chotai J., Ott J., Lalouel J. M. (1984a). Tests of gene order from three-locus linkage data. *Annals of Human Genetics*; **51**: 235–49.

Lathrop G. M., Lalouel J. M., Julier C., Ott J. (1984b). Strategies for multilocus linkage analysis in humans. *Proceedings of the National Academy of Sciences (USA)*; **81**: 3443–6.

Leboyer M., Babron M. C., Clerget-Darpoux F. (1990). Sampling strategy in linkage studies of affective disorders. *Psychological Medicine*; **20**: 573–9.

Leckman J., Gershon E. S., McGinniss M. H. *et al.* (1979). New data do not suggest linkage between the Xg blood group and bipolar illness. *Archives of General Psychiatry*; **36**: 1436–41.

McGuffin P., Katz R. (1989). The genetics of depression and manic-depressive disorder. *British Journal of Psychiatry*; **155**: 294–304.

Martinez M., Goldin L. R. (1989). The detection of linkage and heterogeneity in nuclear families for complex disorders: one versus two linked marker loci, *American Journal of Human Genetics*; **44**: 552–9.

Mendlewicz J., Fleiss J. L. (1974). Linkage studies with X-chromosome markers in bipolar (manic-depressive) and unipolar depressive illness. *Journal of Biological Psychiatry*; **9**: 261–94.

Mendlewicz J., Linkowski P., Wilmotte J. (1980). Linkage between glucose-6-phosphate dehydrogenase deficiency and manic-depressive illness: new evidence. *British Journal of Psychiatry*; **137**: 337–42.

Mendlewicz J., Simon P., Sevy S. *et al.* (1987). Polymorphic DNA marker on X chromosome and manic depression. *Lancet*: 1230–2.

Morton N. E. (1955). Sequential tests for the detection of linkage. *American Journal of Human Genetics*; 7: 277–318.

Morton N. E. (1956). The detection and estimation of linkage between the genes for elliptocytosis and the Rh blood type. *American Journal of Human Genetics*; 8: 80–96.

Neugebauer M., Willems J., Baur M. P. (1984). Analysis of multilocus pedigree data by computer. In: *Histocompatibility Testing 1984* (Albert E. D., Baur M. P., Mayr W. R., eds.), pp. 333–41. Berlin, Heidelberg: Springer-Verlag.

O'Rourke D. H., Gottesman I. I., Suarez B. K. *et al.* (1982). Refutation of the general single locus model in the aetiology of schizophrenia. *American Journal of Human Genetics*; 34: 630–49.

Ott J. (1976). A computer program for linkage analysis of general human pedigrees. *American Journal of Human Genetics*; 28: 528–9.

Ott J., ed. (1985). *Analysis of Human Genetic Linkage*. Baltimore and London: Johns Hopkins University Press.

Ott J., Lathrop G. M. (1987). Goodness-of-fit tests for locus order in three-point mapping. *Genetic Epidemiology*; 4: 51–7.

Penrose L. S. (1935). The detection of autosomal linkage in data which consist of pairs of brothers and sisters of unspecified parentage. *Annals of Eugenics*; 6: 133–8.

Pericak-Vance M. A., Yamaoka L. H., Haynes C. S. *et al.* (1988). Genetic linkage studies in late-onset Alzheimer's disease families. In: *Genetics and Alzheimer's Disease* (Sinet P. M., Lamour Y., Christen Y., eds.), pp. 116–23. Berlin, Heidelberg: Springer-Verlag.

St. Clair D., Blackwood D., Muir W. *et al.* (1989). Absence of linkage of chromosome 5q11–q13 markers to schizophrenia in Scottish families. *Nature* 339: 305–9.

St. George-Hyslop P. H., Tanzi R., Polinsky R. J. *et al.* (1987). The genetic defect causing familial Alzheimer's disease maps on chromosome 21. *Science*; 235: 885–90.

Schellenberg G. D., Bird T. D., Wijsman W. M. *et al.* (1988). Absence of linkage of chromosome 21q21 markers to familial Alzheimer's disease. *Science*; 241: 1507–10.

Sherrington R., Brynjolfsson J., Petursson H. *et al.* (1988). Localization of a susceptibility locus for schizophrenia on chromosome 5. *Nature*; 336: 164–7.

Skolnick M. H., Thomson E. A., Bishop D. T., Cannon L. A. (1984). Possible linkage of a breast cancer-susceptibility locus to the ABO locus: sensitivity of lod scores to a single new recombinant observation. *Genetic Epidemiology*; 1: 363–73.

Smith C. A. B. (1963). Testing for heterogeneity of recombination fraction values in human genetics. *Annals of Human Genetics*; 27: 175–82.

Sturt E., Smith C. A. B. (1976). The relationship between chromatid interference and the mapping function. *Cytogenetics and Cellular Genetics*; 17: 212–20.

Suarez B. K. (1978). The affected sib pair IBD distribution for HLA-linked disease susceptibility genes. *Tissue Antigens*; 12: 87–93.

Svejgaard A., Platz P., Ryder L. P. (1980). Insulin-dependent Diabetes Mellitus. Joint Report in: Histocampatibility Testing (Terasaki P. I. ed). pp. 1638–56. Berlin: Springer-Verlag.

Thompson E. A. (1984). Interpretation of lod scores with a set of marker loci. *Genetic Epidemiology*; 1: 357–63.

Thompson E. A. (1987). Crossover counts and likelihood in multipoint linkage analysis. *IMA Journal of Mathematics and Applied Medicine and Biology*; 4: 93–108.

Thomson G., Bodmer W. (1977). The genetics of HLA and disease associations. In: *Measuring Selection in Natural Populations* (Christiansen F. B., Fenchel T., eds.), pp. 545–64. Berlin: Springer-Verlag.

Weeks D. E., Lange K. (1988). The affected-pedigree-member method of linkage analysis. *American Journal of Human Genetics*; 42: 315–26.

4 *The formal problems of linkage*

J. H. EDWARDS

The traditional approach to medical problems is aptly summarized by Socrates' contribution to Plato's *Phaedrus*:

To look at natural phenomena we must first consider both true logic and the approach of Hippocrates. First are the phenomena simple or complex in their origin and in their actions? And, if simple, study their basis and also on what they act, and by what means. And if complex, to enumerate the elements one by one, and to know what each does, and how it causes suffering.

The essential features are the use of reason disciplined and constrained by reality. In the case of medicine, there must also be the appreciation that treatment is the primary aim. However, as was clear to Hippocrates, some disorders are resistant to treatment but amenable to prevention.

Over two thousand years later, Comings (1980) produced an editorial in the *American Journal of Human Genetics* on the paper of Botstein *et al.* (1980), which had proposed the use of random DNA linkage markers in all genetic diseases where the biochemical defect is unknown. Comings stated:

But we now have the ironic situation of being able to jump right to the bottom line without reading the rest of the page, that is, without needing to identify the primary gene product or the basic biochemical mechanism of the disease. The technical capability of doing this is now available. Since the degree of departure from previous approaches and the potential of this procedure are so great, one will not be guilty of hyperbole in calling it the 'New Genetics'.

This break with tradition offered death before birth by indirect and necessarily inexact methods. The main burden of the article of Botstein *et al.* was to elaborate the use of numerous arbitrary markers to define a linkage map from which loci relating to Mendelian disorders could be defined. The various logical errors, which lead to a gross overestimate of both the reliability and the precision of linkage analysis, were dwarfed by the clarity of the exposition and the grandeur of the claims. However, no claim was made for non-Mendelian disorders, which lead to most of our morbidity in body and mind, and include the commoner psychoses and malformations.

The attraction of a standardized technique, Southern blot analysis (see Chapter 1), offered an approach to those disorders in which the tissue at fault was inaccessible or absent. These could be investigated by using blood, whose study previously had not revealed any consistent abnormality on analysis of protein and smaller molecules.

THE APPLICATION OF NEW METHODS

The approach outlined above led to several books of great clarity, including those of Weatherall (1982, 1985) and Emery (1984), and the general adoption of the term 'New Genetics' to cover any technique relating to DNA variants. This profoundly influenced the deployment of major resources, improving the precision of some prenatal and carrier diagnoses and providing the framework within which a number of Mendelian disorders were localized to within a few megabases. In addition, a number of disorders with a somewhat diffuse manifestation were shown to be determined, in most families with several cases, by mutations at a single locus. Examples include early-onset Alzheimer's disease (see Chapter 17), atopy, Battens's disease and Friedreich's ataxia.

Even more recently we have the crowning and solitary achievement of the definition of a gene, that related to cystic fibrosis, by linkage methods alone (Kerem *et al.*, 1989). This will allow indirect methods of prenatal diagnosis by defining nearby loci to be replaced with direct methods. It will also allow the screening of parents. This is important because currently 80% of children with cystic fibrosis are the first to be affected in a sibship.

These successes have led to an increasing use of the approach and its extension to non-Mendelian orders (notwithstanding the lack of precision of linkage analysis, even in Mendelian disorders). The problems of resolving power were exemplified by Sturtevant (1916), who introduced the concept of deducing gene order by an efficient numerical analysis of six loci in over 16 000 fruit flies. Haldane (1919) clarified the relationship of recombination and distance, introducing the much misunderstood term centimorgan, while Fisher (1922) (discussed by Smith [1989] and Edwards [1989]) showed both how to define position within order and estimate its precision.

The eventual success in cystic fibrosis involved work with thousands of families in one of the commonest Mendelian disorders with fairly distinctive signs and symptoms. In spite of these advantages, the high technical and moral standards of those participating, and the advantages, when living parents are needed, of working with disorders of children, the numbers required were large. In retrospect, it seems likely that if adequate funding had been diverted to the search for concomitant translocations, or to characterizing the elusive serum proteins associated with the disease and its carriers, the gene would have been found earlier.

The attractions of a direct attack on the nucleus, which could be applied to any Mendelian disorder and handled by laboratories without advanced expertise in biochemistry, have had a wide appeal. However, there are newer techniques, which include site-directed mutagenesis, the direct infection of the mouse germ-line with segments of human DNA, the amplification of genes provided by a single sperm, and the synthesis of the active parts of genes from the leakage of inappropriate transcripts from all cells. These should allow RNA, whose production is mainly confined to the brain, to be analysed from cells in the blood, or from cell lines established from blood during life or from skin after death, including fetal death.

THE PROBLEMS OF STUDYING THE PSYCHOSES

The psychoses are peculiarly difficult to study directly. Their well-established familial tendency has been documented but provides little evidence of mechanism (Gottesman and Shields, 1982). Even the apparently simple problem of whether the predisposition is usually acquired from one parent or both is unresolved. The term multifactorial has been used, but this means little except non-Mendelian, and adjectives that cover substantial majorities are of little value in science, which must divide to conquer. A study of tissues outside the brain has been unrewarding; the brain after death has left few consistent traces of abnormality and during life is protected from biopsy both by its own softness and by the hardness of the skull, not to mention the ethical objections. There are no wholly satisfactory animal models, although animals will respond to drugs known to induce or control psychotic behaviour in man. Even when biopsy material can be obtained, the entanglement of the neural and other processes would make the separation of different cells difficult. The study of other tissues, including blood, has been unrewarding. Given these difficulties, and the failure of understanding of even so simple a functional change as sleep, it is hardly surprising that linkage studies should have been attempted. This should perhaps rank as example of the 'displacement phenomena' so well described by psychodynamic theorists.

GENES RELATED TO BRAIN FUNCTION

Linkage studies can only be expected to yield results if the disorder is the consequence of one or very few loci, even if, singly or severally, they are not strong enough to express the phenotype in more than a minority of those with a sufficient genotype. It seems very unlikely that anything so complicated as the brain or particularly its functional disturbances, which differ from the norm in degree rather than kind, should be dissociated from the wider aspects of its evolution, and not be dispersed throughout the genome. It hardly seems likely that what we like to think of as the crowning achievement of evolution, the human mind, should need, for its major variants, a coding framework of less than a thousandth of the genome. If the determinants are numerous and dispersed there is no point in looking for straws in a haystack. Can the diapason really close fully in a few bars? This is an *a priori* view, and while it seems to me so self-evident that I cannot understand why such massive resources should be diverted to linkage, it could be wrong, as it would be if applied to the immune system.

On the other hand, disease resistance is complicated. The defence system of the body occupies a volume and handles an energy budget equal to that of the brain, with which its capacity for storage and processing of information may also be comparable. It is dominated by a single DNA segment representing a thousandth of the genome, the HLA complex, within which multiple loci are represented. These include loci involved in the judgment and execution of foreign, sickly or mutinous cells. Its many allelic variants, spread over many loci, some apparently irrelevant to defence, can hardly fail to be *associated* with resistance, impaired resistance or inappropriate response to attack. Although allelic association with disease is not linkage, it can masquerade as linkage so that linkage analysis can lead to the detection of such loci. If such a phenomenon underlies the psychoses, then one extensive set of families studied by the numerous highly informative probes available should be sufficient for the world. If no such locus exists, then its non-existence will be an expensive demonstration. Even if there were enough gold it is not clear if there would be enough blood from adequately informative schizophrenic families. Lander (1989), a major exponent of Mendelian studies of non-Mendelian disorders, stated recently: 'If the trait is more complicated than assumed, linkage will not be detected. A negative result to a complete genome search will at least prove that the disease is more complex than had been assumed.' An assumption needs an assumer.

THE NATURE OF LINKAGE

Linkage is the procedure for making a locus map, that is, of positioning the loci on the chromosomes. As maps go, this has the distinctive features of extreme simplicity in its nature and extreme complexity in its decipherment. It is a one-dimensional map and no map can be simpler. However, the methods used for its decipherment in man require observations on families not compounded to assist in map-making. The members only survive for two or three generations and, in the psychoses, usually become affected about mid-life. The investigator has an active professional life of less than two generations. The map-makers are further handicapped by working in various self-induced fogs and by various very complicated methods of analysis which, undisturbed by the limitations of the data, produce results to many places of decimals. With codominant loci, such as the DNA markers, and a complete set of grandparents (as in the reference set of families collected by the Centre des Etudes Polymorphisms

Humanes), simple methods suffice, but such families are rare in adult disorders. The sheer complexity of these methods imposes the need to collaborate. This risks imposing unseen barriers of mutual ignorance, and of using computer programs as alternatives, rather than as ancillaries, to detailed scrutiny of the data. Such complex approaches often befog the sandy nature of their foundations and the ease with which simple logical shortcomings are overlooked. It is no criticism to build on sand if there is no alternative: it is merely necessary to invest in simple buildings or secure foundations. One example, which has had serious consequences both in diverting studies of mania and in devaluing the power of appropriate linkage studies, has followed an apparent linkage due to cosegregation of segments of DNA on chromosome 11. Any screening for these, as in the Amish study (Egeland *et al.*, 1987), with the following up of apparent linkage with more probes selected for laying on these segments, introduces serious and difficult problems (Edwards and Watt, 1989). Lander (1989) appears to recommend this, stating, 'Once the pedigrees under study have been genotyped for each of these loci . . . any interval showing evidence for linkage will then be studied with a higher density of RFLPs . . .' (restriction fragment length polymorphisms).

THE BASIS OF LINKAGE ANALYSIS

Each individual is compounded from two gametes, one from each parent, and each chromosome passed on to any child may be derived from either one grandparent or may be a hybrid derived from two through the cut-and-join event of recombination at gamete formation. Recombination occurs after the chromosomes have paired and divided and involves two of the four strands, so that the number of hybrid chromosomes cannot be more than half the number of crossovers or cut-and-join events. In the human male there are about 60 crossovers, so that most of the chromosomes in sperm will be hybrid: the limited data from the female suggest a higher proportion of hybrid chromosomes. While human chromosomes vary in size, all have at least one crossover, so that in each gamete every chromosome has a chance of at least 50% of being hybrid; the larger chromosomes are usually hybrid through more than one recombination, so that two segments from one grandparental chromosome may be separated by a segment from the other grandparent, a double crossover. Small, interspersed segments are probably rare and are easily inferred in error from diagnostic, technical or labelling errors.

If two loci are on the same chromosome and separated by less than half the length of a small chromosome, which is about a fifth the length of a large chromosome, then the tendency for their alleles to cosegregate will usually be manifest in a few dozen informative meioses. By an informative meiosis is meant one in which there is sufficient parental allelic variety to deduce the alleles conveyed in the gametes derived from the grandparents.

This can always be done if the parents have four distinct alleles at both loci and the grandparents have been typed. In practice this is rare: recombinants must be inferred by finding the most likely recombination fraction by trial and error and assessing the strength of the evidence by Morton's z scores (Morton, 1955), either from his tables or from one of the various programs available (e.g. LIPED (Ott, 1974) or LINKAGE (Lathrop and Lalouel, 1984)). The basic procedure is that, where there is not a complete set of grandparents, a complete set of foursomes of ghost grandparents is fabricated, with proportions defined by the gene frequencies. After rejecting any set inconsistent with the phenotypes of their children, the remaining sets are used to estimate the likelihood of a linkage for various recombination fractions, the resulting likelihoods are weighted by the relative probability of the grandparental foursomes, and the likelihoods (not the log-likelihoods) are added.

The simplest approach to a study of the resolving power of linkage is to consider hypothetical families that convey the maximum information. The resolving power in real families will always be worse, usually very much worse, and the numbers needed for the same degree of confidence necessarily greater, usually by a factor of between 2 and 10.

As a simple model consider an organism with 20 chromosomes which never recombine, a dominant disorder of sufficient rarity to ignore homozygosity in the affected parent, a locus with numerous rare alleles so that all four parental alleles differ, and information on the affected grandparent, the affected parent and one child. If we had 20 such families with 20 loci defined by letters A–T, and if we defined the recombinants being so defined by upper case letters, the non-recombinants remaining in lower case, we would expect a pattern of the general form shown in Table 4.1, except that all alleles from the locus on chromosome E would be lower case.

The linked locus will have no recombinants by necessity but unlinked loci may also have no recombinants by chance. In such a set of families the locus must lie somewhere. If we only had a few of the 20 chromosomes under examination, fortuitous cosegregation could mislead and the weight of evidence is most simply assessed by a simple, chi-square test comparing expected and observed. For any unlinked chromosome, half the chromosomes are expected to be recombinant under the null hypothesis of no linkage; when there are r recombinants and n non-recombinants, the expected value of chi square equals:

$$(n - r)^2 / (n + r) \tag{1}$$

or, with allowance for continuity,

$$(n - r - 1)^2 / (n + r) \tag{2}$$

when, as expected, n exceeds r.

The chance of no recombinants out of 10, which gives a chi-square value

Table 4.1

								Loci											
A	*B*	*C*	*D*	*E*	*F*	*G*	*H*	*I*	*J*	*K*	*L*	*M*	*N*	*O*	*P*	*Q*	*R*	*S*	*T*
								Alleles											
A	B	C	d	e	f	g	H	i	J	k	L	M	N	O	P	q	R	s	T
A	B	C	D	e	F	G	H	I	j	K	l	M	N	o	P	q	R	S	T
a	b	C	D	E	f	g	h	i	J	K	L	m	N	O	P	Q	R	s	T
A	B	c	d	E	F	g	h	i	J	K	l	m	N	O	P	q	R	S	t
a	b	C	D	e	F	g	h	i	J	K	l	M	n	o	P	q	R	S	T
a	B	C	d	e	f	g	h	I	J	k	L	m	n	o	P	q	r	s	T
A	B	c	d	E	f	G	H	i	j	k	L	M	n	O	p	Q	r	S	t
A	B	c	D	e	F	g	H	I	J	k	L	M	N	O	P	q	r	s	t
a	b	c	D	e	f	g	h	I	j	K	L	M	n	O	p	Q	r	s	T
a	b	c	d	e	F	g	h	i	J	k	L	M	n	O	P	p	r	s	t
a	B	c	d	e	F	G	h	i	J	k	L	m	N	O	P	q	R	S	t
A	B	c	d	e	f	g	H	i	j	k	L	m	N	O	P	q	r	s	T
a	b	c	d	E	F	G	h	I	j	k	L	M	N	O	P	Q	r	s	t
a	b	c	d	e	f	G	H	I	j	K	l	M	n	O	p	Q	r	s	T
A	B	c	D	e	f	g	H	I	j	k	L	m	n	o	P	q	R	s	t
A	B	c	D	e	f	g	H	I	j	k	L	m	n	o	P	q	R	s	t
A	B	C	d	e	f	g	H	I	j	k	L	m	n	o	P	q	R	s	t
A	B	C	D	e	f	G	h	i	j	K	l	m	N	O	P	q	R	S	T
a	b	c	d	e	f	G	h	i	j	K	l	m	n	O	P	q	R	S	t
10	12	7	9	4	8	9	8	8	8	11	11	8	13	14	9	9	10	6	10

An example of twenty hypothetical gametes conveying a known abnormal allele on chromosome E from an individual who had all lower case alleles from the affected parent and all upper case alleles from the other. The model has 20 chromosomes labelled A-T with a recombination fraction of 0.15. The number of recombinants is given on the bottom line. Linkage with locus E is clearly suggested.

of (100/10) or 10, has a related probability of 1/1600 for a one-tailed test; for 1/10 or 9:1 it is just under 1/1000. As there are almost 20 unlinked chromosomes, the chance of a false linkage is about 20/1000 or 1 in 50.

In terms of likelihoods the chance of a series of non-recombinants is a half to the power of 10 and the likelihood ratio, or odds ratio, 1:1024. In this case the likelihood ratio is identical to the exact probability, which is 1/1024. In man, as there are 22 autosomes of varying length and at least half are hybrid, the chance of a false linkage with an odds ratio of 1000:1 for linkage is about 1000/50 or 1/20 (Morton, 1955). The logarithm of an odds ratio of 1000:1, known as a LOD (colloquially, lod—see Chapter 3), will be 3.0. Likelihoods are related to pairs of hypotheses and are exact if the hypotheses are defined before examining the data. In practice this is never done, leading to a non-conservative but tolerable bias in the maximum likelihood estimate. This bias, while small if only one parameter is estimated on the same data, may be substantial and highly misleading if several parameters are estimated. Probabilities relate to a wide range of hypotheses and there can be no simple exchange rate between likelihood and probability except in various extreme cases, such as zero recombination.

Under these ideal conditions of 10 informative children with an affected parent and grandparent, we could usually define a linkage with a 20:1 or so surety. If schizophrenia were due to an allele at one locus that had a 1 in 10 chance of being manifest (which is consistent with the sib and child risk), we would only get substantial evidence from affected individuals, the unaffected only being of value in defining the phase of a parent. By phase is meant the relationship of the marker allele to the disease allele: the phase of two alleles is defined as being in coupling if they are on the same chromosome or in repulsion if one is on each of the paired chromosomes.

In practice, linkage will rarely be complete and, excepting for candidate loci, most linkages will be defined through loci with recombination fractions of 5 to 25%. This introduces even greater problems. Tables 4.1 and 4.2 show an example based on 15% recombination from 20 hypothetical sets of 20 families.

If penetrance were 1/10, then only a tenth of one-child families would show parent–child affliction, and 10 times as large a sample of schizophrenics would be needed to define this: if two affected children with an affected parent were selected then, in a population of two-child families, about one affected parent in a thousand would provide suitable families. This, while reducing the number of families available, would not reduce the information from ascertained families and would be feasible in so common a disorder.

If, due to a shortage of families, we use affected sib-pairs without reference to parentage, then in most such families (over 80%) there will be no affected parent and we will need to assume that one or the other is a carrier. This greatly reduces the power of linkage and increases several fold the number of families needed to define a linkage with a defined degree of surety.

Given parental alleles a,b from the father and c,d from the mother, and arbitrarily assuming a or c are the schizophrenic alleles, then the chance of paternal or maternal identity in two affected siblings will be a half in the presence of linkage and a quarter in its absence, so that the most likely value of chi-square in n sib-pairs in the presence of close linkage will be:

$$(n/2 - n/4)^2/(n/2) \text{ or } n/8 \tag{3}$$

and we would need about 80 such families to reach an uncorrected chi-square value of 10. If, as is usual, we have probes with only two alleles, even the most efficient probe with a gene frequency of a half for each allele would only be fully informative in a quarter of families, so that some 300 families would be needed even if the linkage were complete with no recombination. Families with three sibs would be more efficient but even rarer. If the chance of defining a true linkage were to be at least 20-fold that of defining a false linkage, very large numbers would be needed, even on the unlikely hypothesis of a single locus being involved in the great

Table 4.2

A	B	C	D	E	F	G	H	I	J	K	L	M	N	O	P	Q	R	S	T
13	10	5	11	5	11	10	12	10	9	10	13	10	12	13	10	11	13	10	9
8	8	11	10	4	10	9	9	10	9	9	8	14	11	16	8	9	9	9	8
8	12	10	13	2	9	11	12	12	9	9	9	11	10	10	8	15	9	8	8
12	9	10	6	1	8	13	10	12	11	12	12	12	10	7	13	9	12	9	10
10	7	9	9	3	10	10	9	10	10	11	6	12	11	14	9	12	9	12	10
11	11	5	10	2	11	13	9	9	9	11	9	14	10	9	10	11	10	13	17
12	10	8	7	5	9	13	11	11	12	9	8	11	7	9	11	11	7	9	7
13	13	12	11	4	8	11	7	15	14	8	5	13	13	11	8	12	13	8	13
14	9	7	8	2	9	9	9	11	10	6	12	13	6	9	6	9	9	10	3
8	12	13	12	3	10	12	10	13	9	10	9	12	9	7	8	8	8	10	9
12	10	10	10	3	11	8	10	13	11	10	11	10	8	11	6	13	10	13	11
8	11	5	8	0	10	8	8	8	10	9	11	13	10	11	11	7	13	11	8
8	7	11	8	4	9	10	11	11	13	10	13	12	11	10	11	9	8	8	9
12	8	8	11	5	9	11	9	14	7	13	7	12	9	11	8	13	11	13	12
9	11	11	9	4	15	11	11	6	8	9	8	11	10	9	8	12	9	9	10
9	9	10	8	3	7	6	12	15	8	10	8	12	10	10	6	8	10	9	11
13	10	6	9	4	7	8	11	11	8	9	8	10	13	11	8	9	8	12	10
4	9	7	10	3	6	14	14	11	8	7	9	11	10	13	5	14	11	10	7
8	10	9	4	2	7	9	12	8	11	12	7	13	7	3	7	9	12	10	15
				59															

Recombinants	Non-recombinants	z
1	19	3.86
2	18	3.10
3	17	2.35
4	16	1.60
5	15	0.84

The result of twenty sets of twenty families exposed to a recombination fraction of 0.15 on chromosome E as in table 4.1. Above average numbers of recombinants on chromosome E are shown in bold type as are fortuitously low numbers of recombinants on other chromosomes. The figures below give the z scores for various numbers of recombinants. It will be noted that while there were 59 recombinants out of 400 meioses, which is very close to the 60 expected. If only the families with a z score exceeding 3.0 were counted there would be 9 recombinants in 120 families, giving a seriously biased recombination fraction of 0.82.

majority of cases. As the limiting factor is the amount of segmentation imposed by recombination, a multiple locus analysis will have little to offer, except complexity, until a linkage had been established. It has little place in the presence of the highly informative probes now available, except to define in more detail an established linkage.

PROCEDURES FOR INCREASING THE YIELD OF LINKAGE DATA

Enrichment by selection for large families

One approach to an increase in efficiency, in terms of information per test, is to find exceptional families with numerous affected individuals—families with a very unusual density of affected members, such as those with manic-depression in the Amish community in the USA (Egeland *et al.*, 1987) and with schizophrenia and other disorders in Iceland (Hodgkinson *et al.*, 1987) (see Chapters 7 and 11). In both cases there are problems in analysis. Even if these could be fully satisfied, the problem remains that families with a concentration of disease beyond the experience of most psychiatrists are being used to make inferences about the common disorder as seen in the consulting room. Such families are, of course, of major interest and may suggest various candidate loci. However, their rarity makes it impossible to come down to a resolution of less than tens of megabases, as well as casting doubt on the relevance of such families to the disorder in its usual setting. In so common a disorder, with limited penetrance, if several loci are implicated in the population, then the larger the family the greater the chance of confusion from the presence of predisposing alleles from more than one locus.

Unfortunately the tolerance of both *Nature* and *Science* to publish pedigrees altered in the interests of anonymity makes it difficult to check any analysis. The use of sexless symbols, such as diamonds, with disordered sibships, and with an assumption of an equal recombination rate by sex in the published analyses should allow referees and other readers to attempt their own evaluation in this notoriously difficult field. Meanwhile, a simple test is to ignore the 'unaffecteds' and, assuming the interpretation most favourable to linkage, count the number of recombinants and non-recombinants, subtracting one non-recombinant from each family as a simple ascertainment correction. If this crude, simple and biased test fails to find clearcut linkage, any more complicated method making a similar claim should be doubted.

Criteria of credulity

If, as seems plausible, more than one locus is involved, far larger numbers will be needed if apparent linkages are to be more than apparent, especially if we allow for the prior probability of a model with only a very few, strongly determining loci. This probability, unlike that derived from chromosome numbers and shapes, is necessarily subjective: it is also necessarily less than one. It would be appropriate to add the logarithm of the reciprocal of this likelihood to the z score accepted as achieving the threshold of credulity.

If several loci are involved, then the numbers needed are even larger. If we pick out the results most favourable to linkage with any of four loci, with 20 loci on non-recombining chromosomes, there will be: $20 \times 19 \times 18 \times 17/(2 \times 3 \times 4)$ or over 4000 ways this could happen.

In practice the human data are equivalent to about 50 'solid' chromosomes, giving some 230 000 ways of selecting four loci, and allowance must be made for this.

The feasibility of linkage as an aid to the understanding of schizophrenia is largely dependent on *a priori* views of the nature of cerebral development and function: the view that the brain is too complicated to be disordered in such simple ways in psychosis is plausible but may be wrong. But those who pursue such studies may also be wrong: at least it is clear that adequately informative families are rare; that unaffected individuals have little to offer except information on phase; and that the plasma may be at least as informative as the DNA. It is not acceptable to fail to store both. The DNA from unaffected at-risk patients has little to offer unless they become psychotic, because it is invariant by nature, but changes in plasma constituents may give guidance on the candidate loci without which family studies would seem doomed to a continuing and expensive sterility.

Candidate loci

While a blind search through the genome is unlikely to provide evidence from which an offending locus could be inferred with acceptable reliability and precision, there is another approach within the necessary resolving power. Where there is evidence of some locus being associated with schizophrenia, confirmation by comparing affected relatives should be possible. Selecting a small number of suitable candidates is clearly difficult, but the undoubted efficacy of some drugs, the occasional manifestation of schizophrenia in response to amphetamines, and the association of schizophrenia-like syndromes with a wide variety of metabolic disorders may suggest various loci whose products lie on or near the relevant biochemical pathways. Although it will not usually be expressed, such a candidate locus will, by definition, never recombine, and the analysis is simple. When these loci can be defined by DNA variants within or very close to the gene, they will show a different distribution of allelic variants in affected and unaffected individuals and these disproportions will be relatively robust to diagnostic difficulty or technical error (Arnason, 1977). This is the method of allelic association, sometimes called linkage disequilibrium.

Allelic association

There are necessarily fewer ancestors than descendants as not everyone leaves descendants. Any sampling of alleles at pairs of closely linked loci will therefore lead to a lack of independence, a phenomenon first studied by Robbins (1918), who termed it linkage inequality. It has since been confused by various names, including linkage equilibrium (Fisher, 1930) and linkage disequilibrium (Kojimo and Lewontin, 1970), but it is simpler to use the descriptive term 'allelic association' (Edwards, 1980). Data from the HLA region suggest that in Western societies the breeding structure was such that a recombination fraction of about 1% will lead to demonstrable allelic association in less than 100 individuals and in far less if their haplotypes have been defined from an affected sib, parent or child. A segment of chromosome with a 1% recombination fraction between its ends will have a 99% chance of surviving intact through each meiosis and a 50% chance of surviving 70 meioses; 70 generations is equivalent to about 2000 years. As there are about 60 chiasmata in male meiosis and about three thousand million base pairs, the chance of one of the thirty recombinant events per gamete cutting a segment of a megabase is about 1%, so that, very roughly, any pair of loci lying within a megabase should show some allelic association and vice versa. As most genes are shorter than a megabase, any DNA variants within a gene would be expected to show allelic association. This provides a powerful and simple method of screening for candidate loci by using affected members, even without family data. The information is related to the number of independent segments in the very close linkage defined by allelic association, as opposed to the looser linkages better detected by studies of large families, so multiple, small families with at least two affected members provide the most efficient approach because each family will usually provide only one predisposing haplotype. Unaffected members, excepting those needed to define phase, provide little information. The problem is discussed in detail by Sturt and McGuffin (1985).

Fortunately, studies on candidate loci require similar techniques. Apart from smaller families being relatively more informative, the same procedures for the ascertainment of families apply, with the overriding necessity of the highest standards of psychiatry. DNA and plasma keep and can be shared. Patients change, move and die.

REFERENCES

Arnason S., Larsen B., Marshall W. H. *et al.* (1977). Very close linkage between HLA-B and Bf inferred from allelic association. *Nature*; **268**: 527–8.

Botstein D., White R. L., Skolnick M., Davis R. W. (1980). Construction of a genetic linkage map in man using restriction fragment length polymorphisms. *American Journal of Human Genetics*; **32**: 314–31.

Comings D. E. (1980). Editorial. *American Journal of Human Genetics*; **32**: 453–4.

Edwards J. H. (1980). Allelic association in man. In: *Population Structure and Genetic Disorders* (Eriksson A. W., ed.), pp. 239–55. London: Academic Press.

Edwards J. H. (1989). The locus positioning problem. *Annals of Human Genetics*; **53**: 271–5.

Edwards J. H., Watt D. C. (1989). Caution in locating the gene(s) for affective disorder (Editorial). *Psychological Medicine*; **19**: 273–5.

Egeland J. A., Gerhard D. S., Pauls D. L. *et al.* (1987). Bipolar affective disorders linked to DNA markers on chromosome 11. *Nature*; **325**: 783–7.

Emery A. E. H. (1985). *An Introduction to Recombinant DNA*. Chichester: Wiley Medical.

Fisher R. A. (1922). The systematic location of genes by means of crossover observations. *American Naturalist*; **56**: 406–11.

Fisher R. A. (1930). *The Genetical Theory of Natural Selection.* Edinburgh: Oliver and Boyd.

Gottesman I. I., Shields J. (1982). *Schizophrenia: the Epigenetic Puzzle.* Cambridge: Cambridge University Press.

Haldane, J. B. S. (1919). The combination of linkage values and the calculation of distances between the loci of linked factors. *Journal of Genetics*; 8: 299–309.

Hodgkinson S., Sherrington R., Gurling H. *et al.* (1987). Molecular genetic evidence for heterogeneity in manic depression. *Nature*; 325: 805–6.

Kojimo K., Lewontin R. C. (1970). Evolutionary significance of linkage and epistasis. In: *Mathematical Topics in Population Genetics* (Kojima K., ed.), vol. 1 (*Biomathematics*), pp. 367–88. Berlin: Springer-Verlag.

Kerem B. S., Rommens J. M., Buchanan J. A. (1989). Identification of cystic fibrosis gene: genetic analysis. *Science*; 245: 1073–80.

Lander E. S. (1989). In: *Genome Analysis.* Oxford: IRL Press.

Lathrop G. M., Lalouel J. M. (1984). Easy calculations of lod scores and genetic risks on small computers. *American Journal of Human Genetics*; 36: 460–5.

Morton N. E. (1955). Sequential tests for the detection of linkage. *American Journal of Human Genetics*; 7: 277–318.

Ott J. (1974). Estimation of the recombination fraction in human pedigrees: efficient computation of the likelihood for human linkage studies. *American Journal of Human Genetics*; 26: 588–97.

Robbins R. B. (1918). Some applications of mathematics to breeding problems. III. *Genetics*; 3: 375–89.

Smith C. A. B. (1989). Some simple methods of linkage analysis. *Annals of Human Genetics*; 53: 277–83.

Sturt E., McGuffin P. (1985). Can linkage and marker association resolve the genetic aetiology of psychiatric disorders? Review and argument. *Psychological Medicine*; 15: 455–62.

Sturtevant A. H. (1913). The linear arrangement of six sex-linked factors in *Drosophila*, as shown by their mode of association. *Journal of Experimental Zoology*; 14: 43–59.

Weatherall D. J. (1982). *The New Genetics and Clinical Practice.* London: Nuffield Provincial Hospitals Trust.

Weatherall D. J. (1985). *The New Genetics and Clinical Practice.* Oxford: Oxford University Press.

5 Schizophrenia: How far can we go in defining the phenotype?

ANNE E. FARMER, PETER McGUFFIN, IAN HARVEY AND
MAUREEN WILLIAMS

In a chapter on phenomenology in an earlier volume in this series, we drew attention to the view of Luxenburger (quoted in Jaspers, 1963) that for genetic research, 'schizophrenia is no more than a working hypothesis' (Farmer et al., 1988). In the 60 years or so since the pioneering work of Luxenburger and others in the late 1920s and early 1930s, much effort has been expended on refining the hypothesis and in defining ever more explicit and reliable ways of identifying schizophrenia and allied disorders. Most recent work has focused on the application of operational diagnostic criteria, such that it has now become virtually mandatory to use an operational definition for schizophrenia in any paper aimed for publication in a peer-reviewed journal. An operational concept is one defined in terms of the set of operations that are performed in order to determine its applicability. This sounds like a somewhat circular approach but it is by no means peculiar to psychiatry and is derived not from medical or behavioural sciences but from physics (Bridgman, 1927). The idea that operational definitions can be applied in psychiatry requires that the clinician can elicit certain signs and symptoms, which are 'inter-subjectively verifiable', and that these are taken as an approximate equivalent to the physicist performing a series of experiments (Hempel, 1961). It then becomes a comparatively straightforward exercise to group the required clinical features in some agreed way to provide an explicit definition of a certain disorder.

This general approach became widely accepted in psychiatric research in the 1970s, following the introduction of the St. Louis criteria (Feighner et al., 1972), and appeared to be reaching its culmination in 1980 with the publication of the third edition of the *Diagnostic and Statistical Manual* (DSM-III; American Psychiatric Association, 1980). However, this was subsequently replaced by a revised edition, DSM-IIIR (American Psychiatric Association, 1987), and along the way many other systems of operational diagnosis were proposed, particularly for schizophrenia and other forms of 'functional' psychosis (see Berner et al., 1983 for review and compilation).

In general, operational definitions enhance inter-rater agreement and, particularly if some standard method of eliciting and recording clinical information is used, excellent reliability coefficients can be achieved. The main difficulty for schizophrenia research is that we now have not just one reliable and explicit working hypothesis but many, and there is no certain way of choosing between them for the purposes of genetic research studies. An associated problem, which goes beyond the valid definition of the core syndrome, is that we now also have seemingly precise ways of defining other psychotic or psychotic-like states and personality types that may have some relationship to schizophrenia, and we face the problem of which of these can be legitimately included within an extended schizophrenia phenotype. This is particularly pertinent to current interests in linkage studies where for most purposes a clearcut separation of individuals into 'affected' and 'unaffected' is desirable.

In this chapter we will begin with consideration of how to capture the 'most valid' phenotype in genetic research. In general we will suggest that this can only be achieved by adopting an open-minded, polydiagnostic approach to defining schizophrenia, and we will briefly outline the advantage of this and the practicalities of how it can be achieved. We will then go on to discuss how we might 'optimize' the definition of schizophrenia by varying the breadth of criteria in classical genetic studies, and we will suggest how this strategy might be used in studies using DNA polymorphisms as markers of genetic linkage.

WHICH CRITERIA ARE THE 'MOST VALID' FOR GENETIC RESEARCH?

As we have outlined, the geneticist is now presented with a bewildering array of operational definitions of schizophrenia, most of which have proven reliability but unproven validity. While it is tempting merely to settle for the most recently developed criteria, the most familiar or those most earnestly recommended by colleagues, this is to risk the possibility that the definition of schizophrenia with the greatest 'biological validity' will be overlooked. Thus, rather than choosing a single diagnostic system, an alternative solution is to adopt a polydiagnostic approach where multiple sets of criteria are applied to each subject (Kendell, 1975b). The different definitions are then set up, as it were in competition with each other, allowing a choice of the one that provides the most satisfactory validity. Although this seems to be a commonsense, pragmatic approach it poses several problems. The first is a familiar practical difficulty concerning multiple statistical testing. Thus, if some biological variable is measured and compared in individuals with and without the disorder and the disorder is defined in multiple ways, then statistical significance levels need to be corrected for the increased probability that differences between the affected and unaffected groups have arisen by chance. The second problem is of a more theoretical nature and relates to the intrinsic limitations of operational diagnostic criteria and whether these can do justice to the complexities of psychiatric diagnosis. The third problem is again a practical one and concerns the procedural difficulties in actually applying multiple definitions of disorder in the same group of patients. The multiple testing problem occurs again in relation to genetic linkage studies. We will delay further consideration of it until later in the chapter and we will now discuss the limitations of operational criteria, following this with a description of an application of a polydiagnostic approach and the pattern of results that derive from this.

THE LIMITATIONS OF OPERATIONAL CRITERIA

Although in most senses the introduction of operationalized criteria can be regarded as a change for the better of almost revolutionary proportions in terms of improved reliability, this improvement is not without cost. Operational definitions are inevitably constrained and 'two-dimensional' in form. Clinicians in practice use many sources of information when making a diagnosis which may be excluded when applying operational definitions. For example, operational definitions are often heavily dependent on subjective accounts of symptoms and may leave little room for an informant history, or assessment of the social context or the cultural background. A further problem is of the subject who just fails to fulfil criteria but where the clinician feels that this truly is 'a case' of the disorder. One suspects that there is frequently a tendency for clinicians to follow intuition and to make the diagnosis first and to fit the criteria second. This we can call the Procrustean approach to diagnosis after the Greek innkeeper of legend who always made sure that his guests exactly fitted their bed.

Most operational systems operate on a 'top-down' principle where the rules for diagnosis are predetermined and hence the information which is collected is also determined by these rules. For example, in its original form, the research interview called the Schedule for Affective Disorders and Schizophrenia (SADS) was designed to arrive at a diagnosis according to the research diagnostic criteria (RDC) of Spitzer *et al.* (1978). Hence the questions asked when carrying out a SADS interview are explicitly directed towards determining whether the RDC rules for each diagnostic category apply. An alternative is to proceed in a 'bottom-up' fashion in which the symptoms and signs are defined first. This is the approach adopted by the authors of the Present State Examination (PSE; Wing *et al.*, 1974) and contained in the associated method of classification using the CATEGO computer program. The program carries out a complex grouping and regrouping of syndromes, finally arriving at a most likely diagnostic category. Thus, in some ways the CATEGO program more closely approximates to the probabilistic reasoning and sometimes 'fuzzy logic' of normal clinical practice and is less likely to result in many subjects being placed in a residual 'not yet diagnosed' or 'not elsewhere classified' category, as tends often to occur with top-down systems.

A further contentious area concerns diagnostic hierarchies. Most clinicians in practice aim to achieve a single diagnosis upon which management plans are based. By contrast, in applying operational criteria, it is possible for one subject to fulfil several definitions simultaneously (i.e. to use the current jargon there may be 'co-morbidity') and there may be no built-in guidance on how to decide which diagnosis is primary. Although earlier operational criteria imposed a sort of hierarchy by specifying exclusion items (e.g. syndrome X cannot be superimposed upon affective disorder or be due to organic mental disorder), the authors of DSM-IIIR have stated that their intention is to remove such exclusion criteria because 'studies have shown that research and clinical practice would improve by eliminating many of the diagnostic hierarchies that prevent multiple diagnosis when different syndromes occur together in the same episode of illness' (American Psychiatric Association, 1987). This may not be problematical in certain types of research where, if necessary, the investigator can impose a hierarchy that is appropriate to the nature of the study being undertaken. But where operational criteria are a required procedure for clinical diagnosis, as in the United States, real practical problems are posed. In the absence of hierarchical rules, the clinician is presumably left to his or her own decision regarding which of several criteria fulfilled by a patient is the main current diagnosis. However, if this decision is made without the explicit rules, the process of diagnosis again becomes highly subjective, leading to problems of inter-clinician agreement and defeating the original purpose for which operational definitions were introduced.

In addition, allowing the coexistence of multiple categories of diagnosis runs counter to the usual logical rules applied in classification, which assume that 'abstract classes should be mutually exclusive and jointly exhaustive: i.e. that each class member possesses the defining attributes of one class only and possesses none of the attributes of any other class' (Kendell, 1975a). While classification in psychiatry can almost never achieve this ideal, because of overlapping symptoms between diagnostic groups, a hierarchical approach does at least allow the assignment of a single diagnostic category for each subject.

Abandoning diagnostic hierarchies has a particularly important effect on the diagnosis of psychotic disorders. For example, most British psychiatrists would place schizophrenia above affective psychosis in the diagnostic hierarchy. Hence 'nuclear' features of schizophrenia such as Schneiderian first-rank symptoms usually take precedence over other symptoms and result in a diagnosis of schizophrenia, irrespective of whether symptoms of other disorders are present. In DSM-IIIR and indeed in the most recent draft of the 10th Edition of the *International Classification of Diseases* (ICD-10; World Health Organization, 1989), some nuclear symptoms of schizophrenia, such as thought insertion and thought broadcast, are allowed in affective disorder, so that a patient in whom depressive features coexist with these symptoms may be placed in the DSM-IIIR category of major depression with mood incongruent delusions. Therefore, once again, in subjects who have an admixture of symptoms the final arbiter is the clinician, who is left to his or her own inclination to decide whether the subject 'really' has schizophrenia or affective illness.

A POLYDIAGNOSTIC APPROACH TO THE CLASSIFICATION OF PSYCHOTIC ILLNESS

We have pointed out that in the absence of any clear evidence concerning validity it makes sense to collect diagnostic information for biological research in such a way that multiple definitions of schizophrenia or other psychoses can be applied. Unfortunately, this can be a cumbersome exercise, and so, in order to try and facilitate the simultaneous application of multiple sets of operational criteria, we have devised a package consisting of an Operational Criteria checklist for psychotic illness and associated computer scoring programs (OPCRIT). The checklist contains 73 items, mainly relating to psychopathology and premorbid functioning. The computer programs (a) allow entering of the items on the computer; (b) provide definitions of the items; and (c) use algorithms based upon published criteria to provide a classification of subjects. The checklist is derived from the constituent items in five sets of criteria covering schizophrenia, affective illness and other forms of psychosis (Feighner *et al.*, 1972; Spitzer *et al.*, 1978; Taylor and Abrams, 1978; American Psychiatric Association, 1980, 1987), two commonly applied definitions of schizophrenia (Schneider, 1959; Carpenter *et al.*, 1973), and a version of the French criteria for non-affective psychosis based upon the writings of Pull *et al.* (1987) and Pichot (1984). In addition, three explicit methods of subtyping schizophrenia are included: the criteria of Tsuang and Winokur (1974), Farmer's (1984) criteria, and an operationalized version of Crow's (1980) concepts of type 1, type 2 and 'mixed' schizophrenia. A reliability study of the OPCRIT checklist gave satisfactory item-by-item agreement between three independent raters and highly significant levels of agreement for diagnostic categories (McGuffin *et al.*, in press).

The checklist has been applied to 144 consecutive cases of psychotic illness admitted to the King's College Hospital (Dulwich North) Psychiatric Unit, London (Harvey *et al.*, 1990) and an earlier version of the checklist has been used on a reassessment of Gottesman and Shields' (1972) series of schizophrenic twins (McGuffin *et al.*, 1984; Farmer *et al.*, 1987). We will compare the results from these two studies and use these as a means of focusing on the relationship between different operational diagnostic criteria for schizophrenia.

Figure 5.1 shows the frequency of operational definitions fulfilled in the two data sets (only the 60 probands from the twin series are included). As

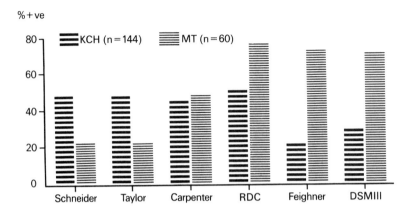

Fig. 5.1 *Operational criteria for schizophrenia: Frequencies from the King's College Hospital (KCH) consecutive series of patients and the probands in the Maudsley Twin (MT) series of schizophrenia (after Gottesman and Shields, 1972). The named criteria are explained and referenced in the text*

we can see, the relationship between the different criteria for schizophrenia is complicated and appears to be variable for different data sets. For the King's College Hospital (KCH) series, the majority of subjects were considered to be schizophrenic on the basis of having one or more first-rank symptoms, whereas in the Maudsley twin (MT) series far fewer subjects fulfilled this definition. With the exception of the RDC of Spitzer *et al.* (1978), which provide the broadest definition of schizophrenia in both samples, there is almost a reversal of order of the frequencies of the different criteria fulfilled in each data set. Thus the KCH series is mainly positive for the Schneider (1959), and Taylor and Abrams (1978) criteria, and the criteria of Carpenter *et al.* (1973), whereas in the MT series, the RDC, DSM-III criteria and those of Feighner *et al.* (1972) are the most commonly fulfilled. Rater variation cannot explain these differences, as two out of three raters were the same in both studies (AEF and PMcG). One more obvious difference is that the KCH series was selected on the basis of broadly defined psychotic illness whereas the MT series was selected by more specifically concentrating on schizophrenia. On the other hand, this would not account for the low frequency of schizophrenics according to first-rank symptom (FRS) criteria in the MT series. We therefore think that the main differences derive from two sources. These are, first, from the ways in which the diagnostic information was collected and recorded and, second, from intrinsic differences in the clinical composition of the two series. Thus, in the MT series, information was collected in a standard way but this was carried out before the days of structured interviews and by researchers who did not have a particularly 'Schneider-orientated' view of psychopathology. By contrast the KCH series was studied by a 'Schneider-orientated' group of researchers and, moreover, two of the psychiatrists in the group (PMcG and IH) between them interviewed all of the patients using the PSE, in which a Schneiderian view of psychopathology is evident. The information used to score the OPCRIT checklist derived both from the hospital case notes and from the PSE interviews. Therefore, it is probably not surprising that the proportion of patients who were found to have first-rank symptoms is high, because questions on such symptoms are mandatory in the full version of the PSE.

The second important difference between the two samples concerns the method of selection. The probands in the MT series were ascertained via the Maudsley twin register, which was started in its present form in 1948. However, the study was not carried out until the mid-1960s, so that many of the subjects included in the series had psychiatric histories extending back over several, and in some cases many, years. By contrast, the KCH series consisted of consecutive acute admissions, including some first admissions, and hence on average had a much shorter previous history than the MT series. It might be expected, therefore, that the MT series would show a higher proportion of 'hits' on those definitions of schizophrenia, such as in DSM-IIIR, that require an illness of specified duration without return to the premorbid level of functioning, together with the accumulation of a specified number of various types of symptoms. This is indeed the pattern of results we obtained, so that in the MT series most probands fulfilled DSM-III criteria for schizophrenia whereas only a minority did so in the KCH series. In the light of these findings we need to question the commonly held view that certain definitions of schizophrenia are particularly 'narrow' and 'strict' while others are 'broad' and 'liberal'. In our two samples, two quite different patterns occur for all criteria other than the RDC, so that, for the MT series, a definition of schizophrenia based on Schneider's first-rank symptoms is 'narrow' while the DSM-III definition is 'broad'. Just the opposite occurs in the KCH series, where the Schneider definition is fairly 'broad' and the DSM-III definition is 'narrow' by comparison. Hence the results obtained appear to be crucially dependent upon the way in which clinical information is collected and recorded and on the way the sample is collected.

Another interesting way of examining the KCH series is to take those 70 patients who had one or more first-rank symptoms and find out which diagnosis they were assigned by DSM-III or DSM-IIIR. The results of this are shown in Fig. 5.2 and it is noteworthy that a majority of subjects who are Schneider-positive are classified as not having either schizophrenia or schizophreniform disorder according to DSM-III and DSM-IIIR. Moreover, using the DSM-III classification, it is somewhat paradoxical that the commonest category of psychosis among Schneider-positive subjects is called 'atypical'. Both DSM-III and -IIIR classify some first-rank symptom-positive subjects as having affective disorder: indeed, with DSM-IIIR there is quite a substantial proportion of such cases, amounting

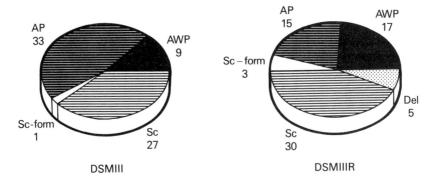

Fig. 5.2   *DSM-III and DSM-IIIR diagnoses in 70 'Schneider-positive' patients. AP = atypical psychosis; AWP = affective disorder with psychosis; Sc = schizophrenia; Sc-form = schizophreniform disorder; Del = delusional disorder*

to almost a quarter. Our results are in keeping with the interesting phenomenon, commented upon by others (Wing, 1983), which consists of the expansion of the concept of affective disorder in North America so that it encroaches considerably on the territory previously regarded by most British psychiatrists as definitely schizophrenic. As we have earlier discussed, much of this encroachment probably results from the fact that hierarchies have been abandoned.

HOW BROAD A PHENOTYPE?

Another major issue in genetic research is how broadly to define schizophrenia and what other related disorders, if any, should be included within the phenotype. Even if we restrict ourselves to one operational diagnostic system, such as DSM-III, a number of different disorders can be considered as legitimate candidates for inclusion within an expanded hypothesis of schizophrenia. Some of these disorders differ from schizophrenia largely on the basis of only one or two items, for example, duration (schizophreniform disorder and brief reactive psychosis), age of onset (paranoid or delusional disorder), or on the presence or absence of prominent affective symptoms (affective disorder with psychosis and mood-incongruent delusions). In addition, some personality types have been proposed to have a biological relationship to schizophrenia; in particular, schizotypal personality disorder, as formulated in DSM-III, is a more restricted and explicit version of some earlier varieties of schizophrenia 'spectrum disorders'. Lastly, there is atypical psychosis or psychosis not otherwise specified, which, as we have mentioned above, often includes a large proportion of patients and forms a sort of residual or 'rag-bag' category that defies any other attempt at classification in a 'top-down' scheme. Therefore, it could be argued that all of these categories are phenomenologically similar to schizophrenia and so the question for the geneticist is whether they can be considered as a variant of the same phenotype.

We have explored the problem of defining the phenotype using the twin method to arrive at the 'most genetic' combination of diagnoses from DSM criteria (Farmer *et al.*, 1987). By applying the full range of possible DSM-III diagnoses to the probands and co-twins from the MT series, we calculated the effects of various combinations of diagnosis on the monozygotic to dizygotic (MZ/DZ) concordance ratio. A disadvantage of this approach is that this ratio is a fairly crude index of the size of the genetic contribution, which does not take into account the population base rates. In many respects it is preferable to apply a liability/threshold model and to estimate heritability (Chapter 2). In order to do this, base rates of the disorder in the population must be known, and we have shown (Farmer *et al.*, 1987) that an estimate of the population frequency of DSM-III schizophrenia can easily be obtained, given the proportion of a systematic series of probands who fulfil this diagnosis and the morbid risk of hospital-diagnosed schizophrenia for the general population. (We used an estimate derived from the Camberwell psychiatric case register.) We found that the heritability of schizophrenia using the DSM-III definition is about 85%. However, once we start broadening the definition to include other types of DSM-III disorders, the population base rates can no longer be calculated in a straightforward fashion. Hence the MZ/DZ concordance ratio has to be used as an alternative. This approach has been criticized on methodological grounds (Kendler, 1989), but if we take our results from an earlier examination of the MT series (McGuffin *et al.*, 1984), where we applied multiple operational definitions of schizophrenia and were able to calculate heritabilities, we find that there is a simple linear relationship between MZ/DZ concordance ratio and heritability, with a highly significant correlation between the two (Spearman's $\rho = 0.84$, $p = 0.001$). In view of this, we suggest that our data, as summarized in Fig. 5.3, provide a rational starting point for a general methodology to explore how schizophrenia may be optimally defined in genetic research.

Broadening the phenotype to include affective disorder with mood-incongruent delusions produces a rise in the MZ/DZ concordance ratio from 4.7 to over 6, and there is a further rise to almost 8 when schizotypy and atypical psychosis are added. By contrast, the addition of paranoid disorder produces a reduction in the MZ/DZ concordance ratio, and a very broad definition, where twins are considered concordant if the co-twin has any axis-1 DSM-III diagnosis, results in a marked lowering of the MZ/DZ ratio. It must be pointed out that our sample size was small here and no definite conclusions can be drawn about what we should consider as the 'most valid' phenotype for schizophrenia research but we do have some general indications. Thus the original DSM-III definition of schizophrenia on its own describes a highly heritable disorder, so that from the

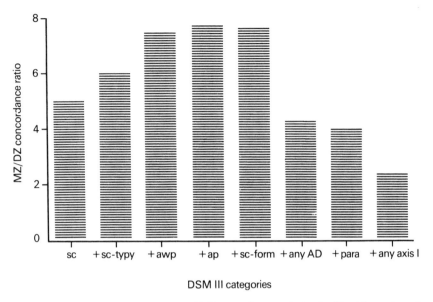

Fig. 5.3 *DSM-III categories and MZ/DZ concordance ratio in the Maudsley twin series reanalysis (Farmer et al., 1987): sc = schizophrenia; sc-typy = schizotypal personality; awp = affective disorder with (mood-incongruent) psychosis; ap = atypical psychosis; sc-form = schizophreniform disorder; any AD = any form of affective disorder; para = paranoid disorder; any axis 1 = any axis-1 DSM-III category*

viewpoint of genetics it has validity as well as high reliability. However, it is capable of being 'improved' by broadening the concept to include other types of disorder and schizotypal personality. Moreover, it is possible to arrive at an optimal broadening of the phenotype after which the addition of further disorders results in a decrease in the MZ/DZ ratio.

It would obviously be of great interest to repeat this exercise on a larger and more up-to-date twin series which has been studied with the specific objective of refining diagnostic issues. However, we suggest that the approach has a more general applicability to other types of genetic studies. In particular, an exploration of the schizophrenia phenotype within the context of linkage studies seems sensible. Indeed, most recent attempts to search for linkage between genetic markers and schizophrenia have included an examination of alternative definitions of the disorder (e.g. McGuffin *et al.*, 1983; Sherrington *et al.*, 1988; St. Clair *et al.*, 1989). In most cases the exploration of the phenotype has not been as extensive or as systematic as the approach we have taken with twins, and again this is probably sensible as extensive exploration of phenotypic boundaries only becomes feasible once a clear validating criterion is available. Means of validation are obviously already available in twin studies (i.e. examination of MZ/DZ ratio or estimation of heritability) but will not be definitely provided by linkage studies until a well-replicated linkage is discovered. The linkage-study findings that perhaps provoked the greatest recent interest are those of Sherrington *et al.* (1988), where strong evidence of linkage arose between a putative schizophrenia susceptibility gene and markers on the long arm of chromosome 5 (see also Chapter 7). Sherrington *et al.* applied a range of 'diagnostic models' in their families, who were multiply affected by schizophrenia and other psychiatric conditions, and found that the most impressive evidence for linkage, as reflected in a maximum lod score (see Chapter 3), occurred with a very broadly defined phenotype that included various non-psychotic conditions. This appears surprising because, by analogy with our twin results, we might have expected the strongest evidence for linkage to have occurred with some definition of the phenotype that was intermediate in breadth between schizophrenia alone and the very wide grouping of psychopathologies included by Sherrington *et al.* However, it is noteworthy that the findings on chromosome 5 linkage have not been replicated by other groups and so might just possibly have reflected a chance positive finding (Kennedy *et al.*, 1988; Detera-Wadleigh *et al.*, 1989; St. Clair *et al.*, 1989; McGuffin *et al.*, 1990).

Despite the obvious attractions of an attempt to define diagnostic boundaries by 'optimizing' an operational definition against genetic criteria, there is an important drawback to be considered. Earlier in the chapter we mentioned that one of the overall difficulties of adopting a polydiagnostic outlook on schizophrenia is that it introduces the statistical problem of multiple testing. This is of particular relevance in linkage studies but has tended to be overlooked in recent work. It has been pointed out by Ott (1990) that conventional calculation of lod scores starts off from the premise that there is a clear and explicit definition of the disease phenotype, which is not subsequently altered. Conventionally, a lod score of 3 is taken as acceptable in evidence in favour of linkage; on the face of it, this is conservative and reflects odds on linkage of 1000 to 1, as the prior probability of linkage is low at about 1 in 50. Hence a lod score of 3 corresponds to a 1 in 20 posterior probability that the apparent 'linkage' has arisen by chance (see Chapters 3 and 4). Once multiple definitions of the disease phenotype are applied, the picture becomes even more complicated. Effectively, N different definitions of the phenotype mean an N-fold increase in the number of tests for linkage which will be performed. Hence the probability of achieving the conventional lod score level of 3 by chance alone increases. Ott (1990) has shown that it is possible to correct for the effects of optimizing on the phenotype at the same time as carrying out a more conventional optimization on the recombination fraction. The details are complicated but, in essence, such double optimization requires that there is an increase in the level of lod scores that should be taken as acceptable evidence in favour of linkage.

CONCLUSIONS

Operational definitions for schizophrenia have been a boon to the genetic researcher in facilitating greater reliability in family, twin and adoption studies. There is therefore greater confidence in the findings from genetic studies and these can often be interpreted with greater clarity than can earlier studies when only descriptive clinical definitions of disorder were used. However, despite the ascendency of DSM-III and more recently DSM-IIIR, we have not just one but many competing operational definitions of schizophrenia and allied disorders, and there is no clear indication which of these is most valid from a genetic perspective. For the time being we suggest that researchers should try and preserve an open-minded polydiagnostic approach in their studies. Although at first sight this is cumbersome, it is possible to devise methods, such as the OPCRIT system which we have described, to accomplish a polydiagnostic study reliably and without being unnecessarily time-consuming. Again in their placement of the boundaries of a schizophrenia phenotype, researchers need to be open-minded. There is still no certain way of delineating the legitimate range of the schizophrenia spectrum but genetic studies can provide some pointers. Twin studies may be particularly of use in this respect and the same general approach of attempting to 'optimize' the phenotype against genetic criteria has a more general applicability in studies of linkage markers.

REFERENCES

American Psychiatric Association (1980). *DSMIII: Diagnostic and Statistical Manual of Mental Disorders*. Washington DC: APA.

American Psychiatric Association (1987). *DSM-IIIR Diagnostic and Statistical Manual of Mental Disorders*. Washington DC: APA.

Berner P., Gabriel E., Katschnig H., *et al.* (1983). Diagnostic Criteria for Schizophrenic and Affective Psychoses. World Psychiatric Association, Distributed by American Psychiatric Press. Inc, Washington D.C.

Bridgman P. W. (1927). *The Logic of Modern Physics*. New York: Macmillan.

Carpenter W. T., Strauss J. P., Bartko J. J. (1973). Flexible system for the diagnosis of schizophrenia: report from the WHO pilot study of schizophrenia. *Science*; 182: 1275–8.

Crow T. J. (1980). Molecular pathology of schizophrenia: more than one disease process? *British Medical Journal*; 280: 66–8.

Detera-Wadleigh S. D., Goldin L. R., Sherrington R. *et al.* (1989). Exclusion of linkage to 5q11–13 in families with schizophrenia and other psychiatric disorders. *Nature*; 339: 391–3.

Farmer A. E. (1984). Searching for the split in schizophrenia: a twin study perspective. *Psychiatry Research*; 13: 109–18.

Farmer A. E., McGuffin P., Bebbington P. (1988). The phenomena of schizophrenia. In: *Schizophrenia: The Major Issues* (Bebbington P., McGuffin P., eds.). London: Heinemann.

Farmer A. E., McGuffin P., Gottesman I. I. (1987). Twin concordance for DSM-III schizophrenia: scrutinising the validity of the definition. *Archives of General Psychiatry*; **44**: 634–41.

Feighner J. P., Robins E., Guze S. B. *et al.* (1972). Diagnostic criteria for use in psychiatric research. *Archives of General Psychiatry*; **26**: 57–62.

Gottesman I. I., Shields J. (1972). *Schizophrenia and Genetics: a Twin Vantage Point*. New York: Academic Press.

Harvey I., Williams M., Toone B. K. *et al.* (1990). The ventricular-brain ratio (VBR) in functional psychoses: the relationship of lateral ventricular and total intracranial area. *Psychological Medicine*; **20**: 55–62.

Hempel C. G. (1961). Introduction to problems of taxonomy. In: *Field Studies in the Mental Disorders* (Zubin J., ed.), pp. 3–22. New York: Grune and Stratton.

Jaspers K. (1963). *General Psychopathology*. Manchester: Manchester University Press.

Kendell R. E. (1975a). *The Role of Diagnosis in Psychiatry*. Oxford: Blackwell Scientific.

Kendell R. E. (1975b). Schizophrenia: the remedy for diagnostic confusion. In: *Contemporary Psychiatry. British Journal of Psychiatry* Special Publication No. 9 (Silverstone T., Barraclough B., eds.), pp. 11–17. Ashford: Headley.

Kendler K. S. (1989). Limitations of the ratio of concordance rates in monozygotic and dizygotic twins. (Letter). *Archives of General Psychiatry*; **46**: 477–8.

Kennedy J. L., Guiffra L. A., Moises H. W. *et al.* (1988). Evidence against linkage of schizophrenia to markers on chromosome 5 in a northern Swedish pedigree. *Nature*; **336**: 3443–6.

McGuffin P., Farmer A. E., Gottesman I. I. *et al.* (1984). Twin concordance for operationally defined schizophrenia. Confirmation of familiality and heritability. *Archives of General Psychiatry*; **41**: 541–5.

McGuffin P., Festenstein H., Murray R. M. (1983). A family study of HLA antigens and other genetic markers in schizophrenia. *Psychological Medicine*; **13**: 31–43.

McGuffin P., Sargeant M. P., Hett G. *et al.* (1990). Exclusion of a schizophrenia susceptibility gene from the chromosome 5q11–q13 region: new data and a re-analysis of previous reports. *American Journal of Human Genetics*, **47**: 524–35.

McGuffin P., Farmer A. E., Harvey I. (1991). A polydiagnostic application of operational criteria in studies of psychotic illness: Development and reliability of the OPCRIT system. *Archives of General Psychiatry* (in press).

Ott J. (1990). Paper presented in the *German Society of Human Genetics* Symposium (March).

Pichot P. J. (1984). The French approach to psychiatric classification. *British Journal of Psychiatry*; **144**: 113–18.

Pull M. C., Pull C. B., Pichot P. (1987). Des critères empiriques français pour les psychoses. *L'Encephale*; **XIII**: 53–66.

St. Clair D., Blackwood D., Muir W. *et al.* (1989). No linkage of 5q11–q13 markers to schizophrenia in Scottish families. *Nature*; **339**: 305–9.

Schneider K. (1959). *Clinical Psychopathology* (Hamilton M. W., trans.). London, New York: Grune and Stratton.

Sherrington R., Brynjolffson J., Petersson H. *et al.* (1988). Localization of a susceptibility locus for schizophrenia on chromosome 5. *Nature*; **336**: 164–7.

Spitzer R. L., Endicott J., Robins E. (1978). Research diagnostic criteria rationale and reliability. *Archives of General Psychiatry*; **35**: 773–82.

Taylor M. A., Abrams R. (1978). The prevalence of schizophrenia: A reassessment using modern diagnostic criteria. *American Journal of Psychiatry*; **135**: 945–8.

Tsuang M. T., Winokur G. (1974). Criteria for sub-typing schizophrenia. *Archives of General Psychiatry*; **31**: 43–7.

Wing J. K. (1983). Use and misuse of the PSE. *British Journal of Psychiatry*; **143**: 111–17.

Wing J. K., Cooper J. E., Sartorius N. (1974). *The Measurement and Classification of Psychiatric Symptoms*. Cambridge: Cambridge University Press.

World Health Organization (1989). *International Classification of Diseases* 10th edn. (Draft) Geneva: WHO.

6 Schizophrenia: Classical approaches with new twists and provocative results

IRVING I. GOTTESMAN AND AKSEL BERTELSEN

HISTORICAL DEMOGRAPHY AND CONTEMPORARY EPIDEMIOLOGY

Age-corrected or lifetime morbid risks for current definitions of schizophrenia in the general population range from 0.2% in Iowa to 1.39% in southern Sweden and even higher in some inbred isolates (Gottesman and Shields, 1982; Häfner, 1987; Jablensky, 1988). With use of the semi-structured interview, Present State Examination (PSE), and the CATEGO computer program, the World Health Organization (Sartorius *et al.*, 1986) report a range of morbid risks for a broad CATEGO definition of schizophrenia ranging from 1.74% in rural India to 0.56% in urban Denmark, values not too far from the textbook bench-mark of 1%. Such risk figures provide important points of departure for evaluating the meaning of 'familiality' of schizophrenia and remind us that genetic studies of families require *local* control values and not just textbook values. However, the point we wish to make here is that whatever value is preferred it places schizophrenia among the common as opposed to the rare genetic disorders such as Huntington's disease, which has a population risk of only 0.005%. Common genetic disorders require a different frame of reference from that used for determining the aetiology of rare ones (Vogel and Motulsky, 1986).

Given that schizophrenia is now regarded as a common disorder, how is it that it appears to be so rare before 1800 and only seems to rise to an appreciable level toward the end of the nineteenth century? Scholars have debated such a 'recency hypothesis' for schizophrenia and it is an important issue (Hare, 1983, 1988; Scull, 1984; Torrey, 1989). It is an empirical fact that the Board of Control for England and Wales reported a prevalence of 36 480 'lunatics, idiots, and persons of unsound mind' in 1859, when the total population, including children, was about 20 million; by 1899 the population had grown to 32 million while the prevalence of a deranged population had increased to 103 247, a huge jump. As the concepts of dementia praecox or schizophrenia did not yet exist in that period, the data are very difficult to use in support of theories about acute changes in the incidence, or in formulating theories about the aetiology of this disorder. However, even if only a portion of the rise in lunacy in the nineteenth century can be attributed to schizophrenia (Hare [ibid.] estimates some 40%), it begs for some kind of explanation. Speculation has centred on a mutated virus or gene, the effects of the industrial revolution, treatment of 'pauper lunatics', policies for handling the poor in work-houses, increasing availability of alcohol, an over-supply of beds in the asylum-building programme of the new Lunacy Commission (after 1845, cf. Hervey, 1985, and Walton, 1985), increasing urbanization, and different diagnostic practices. Another problem is that the sharp national increase in lunacy between 1890 and 1910 was mainly due to increases in London (Cochrane, 1988). We are persuaded that there was a real increase in the incidence and prevalence of schizophrenia but would like to add to the speculations by invoking demographic changes in Western Europe asso-ciated with increases in longevity and population size (Hollingsworth, 1969; Cox, 1970) as competitive, partial explanations.

The correct answer to the riddle of the origins of the putative increases over the course of the nineteenth century is important as a clue to aetiology. Most people interested in public health know the story (apocry-phal or not) of how understanding the cause of cholera was furthered by John Snow's observation, in 1854, of a decreased incidence of disease after removing the pump handle from the Broadstreet well, which supplied water to a heavily affected neighbourhood of London. This circumstantial evidence had to await the use of the microscope and advances in the culture of bacteria by Robert Koch in 1883 before the culprit bacillus could actually be isolated and identified. In the same vein, but more directly relevant to our purpose here, is the example of the observed patterning/ epidemiology of a mental disease in the United States in the 1930s that appeared differentially to affect black paupers in the southern states. Although it mainly resembled an organic psychosis, it could imitate catatonic or paranoid schizophrenia. Careful detective work by Joseph Goldberger in 1915 had identified the disease as nutritionally caused pellagra; however, it was not until 1938 that Tom Spies traced the cause of the psychosis to the dietary deficiency in the B vitamin niacin in *anyone* dependent on unprocessed maize (corn) for a major part of their diet. In the interim, explanations that involved genetic inferiority of races or social classes were invoked for the observed patterns. The geographical and sociopsychological epidemiology of acquired immune deficiency syndrome (AIDS) as a clue to its aetiology are too recent for us to require a reminder of yet another instance where the facts of first appearance and subsequent spread provided vital information.

Returning to schizophrenia, its median age of onset in Norway is reported (Saugstad, 1989) to be 27 years for males and 33 years for females, and the median age for first hospitalization with schizophrenia in England and Wales for the same time period was 30 years for males and 32 years for females (Slater and Cowie, 1971). If everyone were to die by the age of 31 years or so—an apocalyptic conjecture—the number of schizophrenics in the population would drop by half.

Fig. 6.1 shows the average length of life expected at birth from ancient times to the present; estimates come from historical demographers, often using crude data such as the estimated ages of skulls from graveyards. The management of infectious disease and improved nutrition may be the major causes of the leaps in longevity depicted from the Bronze Age to nineteenth century Britain and the United States, that is from an average age at death of 18 to 49 years. Many people, of course, survived into their 50s and 60s throughout this historical interval, but they were the exceptions.

We can then look at the actual number of persons in a cohort of age-mates alive at each age who survive up to each succeeding age under the conditions prevailing at the time of their birth. Fig. 6.2 presents such survival curves for cohorts of 100 000 males, one for the rural England of 1700 (Cox, 1970), and two for cohorts in the United States born in 1940 and 1967. The contrast between the England of 1700 and the pre- and post-war curves for the USA is striking; by age 30, 52% of the English cohort of males had died (30% of them by the age of 5 years) compared with only 6% of the 1967 birth cohort. It should be remembered that populations with very high birth-rates and very high neonatal and infant

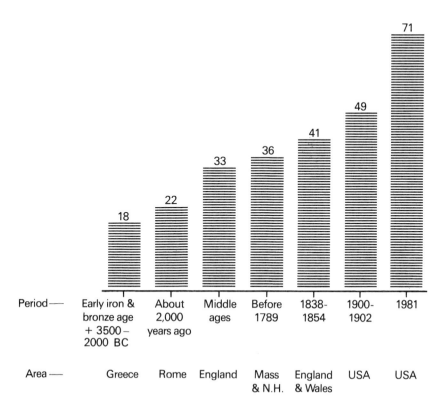

Fig. 6.1   *Average expected length of life from ancient to modern times (after Gottesman, 1991)*

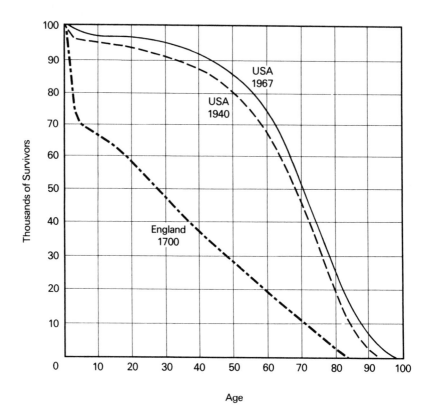

Fig. 6.2 *Number of survivors per 100 000 live-born males at each age since birth for three cohorts: English males born 1700, US males born 1940 and 1967 (after Gottesman, 1991)*

mortality rates produce population 'pyramids' with a large proportion of persons under the age of 15 years (about 40%), further decreasing the chance of observing schizophrenics in these 'developing' nations. Another fact to add to this pot of observations is that only a dozen cities in Europe had more than 100 000 inhabitants by the year 1700, and only two, London and Paris, had more than half a million. By 1800, the population of London was 959 000, with the next largest city in England being Liverpool with only 82 000 inhabitants (Barraclough, 1986). By stringing these observations together, we can feed the speculation that the rarity of schizophrenia before 1800 and its growing prevalence after the middle of the nineteenth century was in part due to changes in the demography of the European population related to age structure and population density, which provided the opportunity for schizophrenia to develop in an ageing and growing population. No one has raised a 'recency hypothesis' to account for the changes in prevalence of Alzheimer's disease over the past hundred years!

In sum, in this instance the apparent sharp rise in incidence of psychosis in the nineteenth century probably provides information about sharp changes in population structure and public health but no clues about the aetiology of psychoses.

FAMILIAR FAMILIAL RISKS AS CLUES TO MODE OF TRANSMISSION

As we currently lack definitive experimental evidence to resolve the uncertainty surrounding the mode of transmission of schizophrenia or any other major mental disorder, theoretical arguments, including computer simulations, that weigh various alternatives can help to advance the search for truth. Western European family studies conducted since 1920 are summarized in Fig. 6.3 (with a few exceptions; cf. Gottesman and Shields, 1982). The results can be used to fit various models from genetic epidemiology and thus provide clues that may inform 'new genetic' strategies. It is immediately clear that the pattern of risks is not consistent with any simple pattern of Mendelian inheritance. The risks presented are

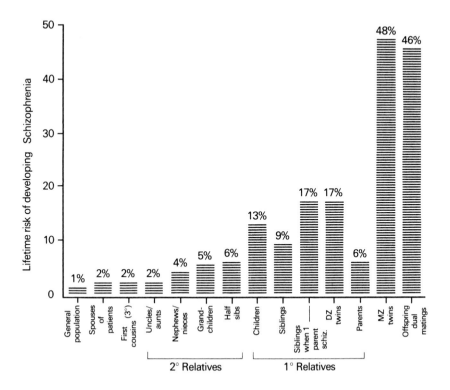

Fig. 6.3 *Pooled Western European lifetime morbid risks for definite plus probable schizophrenia in systematic family and twin studies, 1920–1987 (after Gottesman, 1991)*

for definite-plus-probable schizophrenia and only the twin data are not age-corrected.

A distinctive feature of the pattern of familial risks is the very high risk for identical twins and for the offspring of two schizophrenic parents, some five times that in first-degree relatives. The exponential decline is a strong suggestion, if heterogeneity can be ignored, of multifactorial polygenic inheritance (Vogel and Motulsky, 1986); such a pattern does not fit any generalized single locus (GSL) model, even with assumptions allowing for incomplete penetrance. Unlike the GSL model, a multifactorial threshold (MFT) model provides for both familial and non-familial environmental influences on the liability for developing schizophrenia. GSL models with low penetrance and MFT models with low heritability cannot be distinguished from each other, as they generate similar patterns of familial risk. However, SML transmission with moderate to high penetrance—an ideal situation for linkage approaches—can be distinguished from MFT transmission with moderate to high heritability, largely due to the figures for risk of monozygotic twins (MZ) and dual matings; thus, strategies using only lifetime risk data on first-, second-, and third-degree relatives are not enough to resolve models of transmission.

Under the influence of the *Zeitgeist* prevailing at the Washington University Departments of Psychiatry and Biostatistics (Morton and MacLean and Lalouel *in absentia*, Rao, Reich, Cloninger, Rice, and Suarez) McGue and myself (McGue and Gottesman, 1989; Gottesman and McGue, 1991) were motivated to fill the gap left by the above findings in regard to the fit of yet another family of models, mixed model analysis (MMA), which allows for the identification of a major gene against a multifactorial background. We again used the old data shown in Fig. 6.3 (but only for definite cases) and proceeded to two different simulation 'experiments'. Without belabouring the details, we first ran 275 combinations of various degrees of penetrance for a putative major gene, various degrees of heritability, and various proportions of phenocopies, that is, schizophrenics who did not have a copy of the major gene. With Rao, we had earlier shown (McGue *et al.*, 1985) that the familial risks were consistent with an MFT model with high heritability. The new simulations added two further models consistent with the risks: (1) a mixed model with a major gene with high penetrance (greater than 0.40), but with a very high proportion of phenocopies (greater than 0.60), and a large residual heritability (greater than 0.60), and, frustrating for single-minded linkage searchers, a low derived gene frequency of 0.003, implying that most schizophrenics do not have the major gene but are affected because of their high multifactorial loading; (2) a mixed model with a major gene with low penetrance (less than 0.20), a high residual heritability (greater than 0.60), and not sensitive to the proportion of phenocopies. Although with the latter mixed model most schizophrenics will have the gene, its low penetrance will make it intractable for the usual linkage strategies.

Building on these simulations we then proceeded to ask how often the consistent models would generate two-generation, multiply affected pedigrees in the general population, and, to what extent would multiplex sampling strategies lead to enriching a sample of pedigrees with the major gene. Our use of 50 000 families for each of four consistent models, and allowing for expected marriage rates and expected sibship sizes from US census data, resulted in paradoxical findings. Only 2 families in 200 000 contained five or more affected members and only 11 families in 200 000 contained four or more affected members. Multiplex ascertainment for one of the consistent mixed models did result in most sampled families carrying the major gene, but it had a low penetrance (0.10) and generated a high false-positive rate, i.e. individuals without the disease but with the gene (52% of normals). Of course, these are only simulations or 'thought experiments'; their value depends on the validity of the assumptions and the reader's attitude toward modelling exercises. A major advantage is that they are cheap.

Single-gene major effects may exist for schizophrenia. The simulations suggest that if they do, they are likely to be the result of either a highly prevalent gene with a very low penetrance or a highly penetrant gene with a very low frequency. An analogy with Huntington's disease may be useful. This, in the older published record at least, was often diagnosed as paranoid schizophrenia with some 20% of Huntington phenotypes reported as presenting with symptoms characteristic for the phenotype of schizophrenia. Table 6.1 illustrates the analogy. Huntington's disease is rare in the general population, with a lifetime risk of 5 per 100 000. From the total population study of Essen-Möller *et al.* (1956) in Lundby (southern Sweden), which used in-depth interviews by experienced clinical psychiatrists, we can obtain a conservative lifetime risk for clinical schizophrenia of 139 per 10 000 inhabitants. We can now answer the question: what proportion of schizophrenia-like psychoses are actually caused by what we now know to be a mutated dominant gene on the distal tip of chromosome 4 leading to Huntington's disease? Dividing the two population values and then taking 20% to be the approximate proportion of Huntington cases with an initial presentation imitating schizophrenia reveals that 7 of 10 000 schizophrenic phenotypes are attributable to this 'major gene for a schizophrenia-like psychosis'. That gene would be identified by studying multiplex families with the appropriate probes and a lucky choice of chromosome 4 as a starting point for a linkage research

Table 6.1 What proportion of schizophreniform psychoses is caused by Huntington's disease?

$$\frac{5/100\,000}{139/10\,000} \times 0.20 = 0.0007$$

or, 7 cases per 10 000

One swallow doesn't make a summer

programme. By pursuing the pathophysiology and neuropathology involved in cases of Huntington's disease that mimic schizophrenia, important leads to the pathophysiology of many of the remaining cases of 'proper' schizophrenia may be discovered (cf. Lantos, 1988 and Slater *et al.*, 1963 on epilepsy). Fig. 6.4 is submitted as a speculative summary of the kinds and amounts of aetiological heterogeneity that may underlie the phenotype of schizophrenia; it is a 'combined model' that allows for the various, published suggestions including purely environmental ones, but it allocates rough proportions of causes according to the results of the simulations above. It would be no surprise if similar efforts to sketch combined models for coronary heart disease and diabetes yielded roughly similar sketches.

UNEXPRESSED GENOTYPES, PATHOPLASTIC PHENOTYPES, AND COMPLEXITY

The American curmudgeon H. L. Mencken has bequeathed researchers into psychopathology the following epigram: 'For every complex problem there is an easy answer, and it is wrong.' We may find that thought comforting when we re-examine two further classical approaches in psychiatric genetics. Identical twins discordant for schizophrenia and for affective psychoses at the time of initial evaluation are now old enough in some studies to have developed the disorders (they are through the risk periods) and to have produced offspring old enough to assess their risk for their parents' disorders. Table 6.2 summarizes the results from our (Gottesman and Bertelsen, 1989) following up the offspring of Margit Fischer's (1971, 1973) Danish twin study of schizophrenia. As schizo-

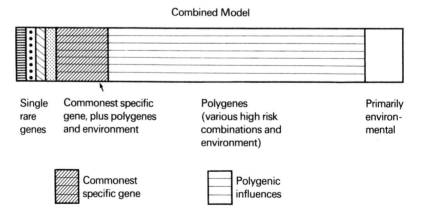

Fig. 6.4 *Combined model for the aetiologies of schizophrenia; speculations showing the proportion of phenotypes that might be allocated to different causes and modes of transmission (after Gottesman, 1991)*

Table 6.2 Schizophrenia (Sch) and schizophrenia-like psychosis in offspring of schizophrenic twins (after Gottesman and Bertelsen, 1989)

Monozygotic sample

	Offspring		
Index parents	*No.*	*Sch + Sch-like*	*MR (%)*
Schizophrenic twins (N=11)	47	6	16.8
'Normal' co-twins (N=6)	24	4	17.4*

Dizygotic sample

	Offspring		
Index parents	*No.*	*Sch + Sch-like*	*MR (%)*
Schizophrenic twins (N=10)	27	4	17.4
'Normal' co-twins (N=20)	52	1	2.1*

* Difference significant, $p < 0.05$, by unidirectional log-rank test.

phrenia is accompanied by lowered rates of marriage and reproduction, our sample of offspring of such twins is necessarily small. Despite the large standard errors on the morbid risk figures, the high rate of schizophrenia among the offspring of normal co-twins of MZ schizophrenics is significantly higher than the rate among the normal co-twins of dizygotic (DZ) schizophrenics—17.4% versus 2.1%. The former risk does not differ from the risks observed among the offspring of the MZ and DZ twins who were schizophrenic, 16.8% and 17.4%. All of our follow-up information came from the Danish National Psychiatric Register, death certificates, and other public records acquired since Fischer last studied the sample of twins and their offspring. As the normal co-twins were quite old at the last collection of information, median age 64 years for the MZ normals and 69 years for the DZ normals, the results suggest to us that discordance for schizophrenia in identical twins past the risk period may primarily be explained by the capacity of the schizophrenic genotype or diathesis to remain unexpressed unless it is released by non-familial and/or familial stressors. If our findings can be generalized, it would lead to a decrease in emphasis on sporadic cases and phenocopies of schizophrenia caused by cerebral abnormalities or putative viruses. Infrequent phenocopies should encourage linkage researchers, but the unexpression of genotypes will generate false negatives in pedigrees (i.e. having the marker but not the disease) and frustrate them. Unexpressed genotypes revealed by disease transmission from normal co-twins are not unique to schizophrenia. The normal co-twins of Danish MZ manic-depressives had offspring with a risk of 24.7% compared to 20.7% in the offspring of the affected MZ proband; the corresponding risks among the affected DZ probands were 14.0% and for their normal co-twins' offspring, 2.1% (Bertelsen and Gottesman, 1986).

In an effort to probe the nature of the phenotypic boundaries between affective psychoses and schizophrenia as a clue to their genetic distinctiveness, we, together with our late colleague Margit Fischer, ascertained all psychiatric patients in the Danish Register who had had children by other in-patients. We were following the trail opened by such pioneers as Schulz, Kahn, and Elsässer, but our interests were more focused on taxonomic or nosological validity than genetic transmission *per se*. Our findings are only preliminary. From the beginning of the registration system until the mid 1960s, we ascertained 139 couples not constrained to be homotypic who had offspring surviving to at least the age of 15 years, of whom there were 378. Table 6.3 shows the initial results for one of our 'best cells' in an 8×8 variation of the diallele cross method used with plants and animals, 17 homotypic manic-depressive couples (International Classification of Diseases [ICD] 8 definitions) with 55 offspring well into or through various risk periods by the time of final follow-up in 1988.

The very high risk (68%) in offspring for manic-depressive diagnoses approaches the value expected for a dominant gene with complete penetrance (75%), at least for this sample, and should encourage those of our colleagues who prefer that model. The results do not support the view of a continuum of psychopathology between affective and schizophrenic psychoses because the risk of schizophrenia from such dual-mating manic-

Table 6.3 Danish dual mating study: morbid risk in offspring of parent combinations with both parents having manic-depressive psychosis

		Offspring			
		No. affected		Risk (%)	
Offspring diagnoses	No. at risk	Definite	Probable	Definite	Total
Manic-depressive psychosis	41.5	18	8	43.4	62.7
Manic-depression related	41.5	0	2		4.8
Schizo-affective	44.0	1		2.3	
Schizophrenia	46.5	2		4.3	
Reactive psychosis	55.0	1		1.8	

depressives is close to the base rate for the general population. We are dependent for our information on various excellent registers, without benefit of interviews; so far we have found no excess of either affective or schizophrenic 'spectrum' disorders but we are in the process of gathering data from the general practitioners of the offspring. In one of our smaller cells, 11 couples with one schizophrenic and one manic-depressive patent who had 25 offspring, seven were manic-depressive (MR 32%), one was schizophrenic (MR 4%), and one was schizoaffective (ICD 8, 296.8/ 295.7; MR 4%). Such preliminary results are consistent with those reported by Elsässer (1952): for 20 M × M couples with 47 offspring at risk, ten were manic-depressive but only one was schizophrenic; for 19 S × M couples with 68 offspring at risk, eight were schizophrenic and eight were manic-depressive, as would be expected with genetic independence. The state of uncertainty surrounding diagnosis or phenotype specification for genetic research has been the topic of intense scrutiny by Crow (1987), Farmer *et al.* (1987, 1988), and Kendler (1988) among others (see Chapter 5) and will not go away so long as we are dependent upon our judgements of such clinical phenomena as feelings, will, insight, and non-understandability. Our initial results from the dual-mating strategy do not resolve the uncertainty but serve to remind us that tolerance of ambiguity is an advantageous trait for researchers in psychiatric genetics.

CONCLUSIONS

There need be no unhealthy tension or conflict in goals between the welcome reductionism of the new genetics and the *Gestalt* or macro approach of the classical genetics. It is the wise researcher in the field of mental illness who knows enough about the ontogeny of the firm facts and received wisdom about 'functional (i.e. with unknown aetiology) psychoses' to guide their formulation of new hypotheses and innovative research designs. Both sets of strategies are interdependent as they search for still-to-be-discovered endophenotypes that mediate their interests in the *entire* gene-to-behaviour pathway.

REFERENCES

Barraclough G., ed. (1986). *The Times Concise Atlas of World History*, revised edn. Maplewood, NJ: Hammond.

Bertelsen A., Gottesman I. I. (1986). Offspring of twin pairs discordant for psychiatric illness. *Acta Geneticae Medicae et Gemellogiae*; 35: 310 (abstract).

Cochrane D. (1988). 'Humane, economical, and medically wise': The LCC as administrators of Victorian lunacy policy. In: *The Anatomy of Madness Vol. III, The Asylum and its Psychiatry* (Bynum W. F., Porter R., Shepherd M., eds.), pp. 247–72. London: Routledge.

Cox P. R. (1970). *Demography*. Cambridge: Cambridge University Press.

Crow T. J. (1987). Psychosis as a continuum and the virogene concept. *British Medical Bulletin*; 43: 754–67.

Elsässer G. (1952). *Die Nachkommen Geisteskranker Elternpaare*. Stuttgart: Thieme.

Essen-Möller E., Larsson H., Uddenberg C. E., White G. (1956). Individual traits and morbidity in a Swedish rural population. *Acta Psychiatrica et Neurologica Scandinavica* (supplement 100).

Farmer A. E., McGuffin P., Bebbington P. (1988). The phenomena of schizophrenia. In: *Schizophrenia: The Major Issues* (Bebbington P., McGuffin P., eds.), pp. 36–50. Oxford: Heinemann.

Farmer A. E., McGuffin P., Gottesman I. I. (1987). Twin concordance for DSM-III schizophrenia: scrutinizing the validity of the definition. *Archives of General Psychiatry*; 44: 634–41.

Fischer M. (1971). Psychoses in the offspring of schizophrenic monozygotic twins and their normal co-twins. *British Journal of Psychiatry*; 118: 43–52.

Fischer M. (1973). Genetic and environmental factors in schizophrenia. *Acta Psychiatrica Scandinavica* (supplement 283).

Gottesman I. I. (1991). *Schizophrenia Genesis: The Origins of Madness*. New York: W. H. Freeman.

Gottesman I. I., Bertelsen A. (1989). Confirming unexpressed genotypes for schizophrenia—risks in the offspring of Fischer's Danish identical and fraternal discordant twins. *Archives of General Psychiatry*; 46: 867–72.

Gottesman I. I., Bertelsen A. (1989). Dual mating studies in psychiatry— offspring of inpatients with examples from reactive (psychogenic) psychoses. *International Review of Psychiatry*; 1: 287–96.

Gottesman I. I., McGue M. (1991). Mixed and mixed-up models for the transmission of schizophrenia. In: *Thinking Clearly About Psychology: Essays in Honor of P. E. Meehl* (Grove W., Cichetti D., eds.), Minneapolis: University of Minnesota Press.

Gottesman I. I., Shields J. (with the assistance of Hanson D. R.) (1982). *Schizophrenia—The Epigenetic Puzzle*. Cambridge: Cambridge University Press.

Häfner H. (1987). Epidemiology of schizophrenia. In: *Search for the Causes of Schizophrenia* (Häfner H., Gattaz W. F., Janzarik W., eds.), pp. 47–74. Berlin: Springer-Verlag.

Hare E. (1983). Was insanity on the increase? *British Journal of Psychiatry*; 142: 439–55.

Hare E. (1988). Schizophrenia as a recent disease. *British Journal of Psychiatry*; 153: 521–31.

Hervey N. (1985). A slavish bowing down: the Lunacy Commission and the psychiatric profession 1845–1860. In: *The Anatomy of Madness Vol. II, Institutions and Society* (Bynum W. F., Porter R., Shepherd M., eds.), pp. 98–131. London: Routledge.

Hollingsworth T. H. (1969). *Historical Demography*. Ithaca, NY: Cornell University Press.

Jablensky A. (1988). Epidemiology of schizophrenia. In: *Schizophrenia: The Major Issues* (Bebbington P., McGuffin P., eds.), pp. 19–35. Oxford: Heinemann.

Kendler K. S. (1988). Familial aggregation of schizophrenia and schizophrenia spectrum disorders. *Archives of General Psychiatry*; **45**: 377–83.

Lantos P. L. (1988). The neuropathology of schizophrenia: a critical review of recent work. In: *Schizophrenia: The Major Issues* (Bebbington P., McGuffin P., eds.), pp. 73–89. Oxford: Heinemann.

McGue M., Gottesman I. I., Rao D. C. (1985). Resolving genetic models for the transmission of schizophrenia. *Genetic Epidemiology*; **2**: 99–110.

McGue M., Gottesman I. I. (1989). Genetic linkage in schizophrenia: perspectives from genetic epidemiology. *Schizophrenia Bulletin*; **15**: 281–92.

Sartorius N., Jablensky A., Korten A. *et al.* (1986). Early manifestations and first contact incidence of schizophrenia in different cultures. *Psychological Medicine*; **16**: 909–28.

Saugstad L. (1989). Social class, marriage, and fertility in schizophrenia. *Schizophrenia Bulletin*; **15**: 9–43.

Scull A. (1984). Was insanity increasing? A response to Edward Hare. *British Journal of Psychiatry*; **144**: 432–6.

Slater E., Beard A. W., Glithero E. (1963). The schizophrenia-like psychoses of epilepsy. *British Journal of Psychiatry*; **109**: 95–150.

Slater E., Cowie V. (1971). *The Genetics of Mental Disorders.* Oxford: Oxford University Press.

Torrey E. F. (1989). Schizophrenia: fixed incidence or fixed thinking? *Psychological Medicine*; **19**: 285–7.

Vogel F., Motulsky A. G. (1986). *Human Genetics: Problems and Approaches* 2nd edn. Berlin: Springer-Verlag.

Walton J. K. (1985). Casting out and bringing back in Victorian England: pauper lunatics, 1840–70. In: *The Anatomy of Madness Vol. II, Institutions and Society* (Bynum W. F., Porter R., Shepherd M., eds.), pp. 132–46. London: Routledge.

7 Genetic linkage studies of schizophrenia

H. M. D. GURLING, T. READ AND M. POTTER

INTRODUCTION

Advances in recombinant DNA technology have stimulated a rapid increase in the amount of research aimed at identifying genetic markers linked to schizophrenia susceptibility loci. However, the first reported linkage to a schizophrenia susceptibility gene on chromosome 5 has not been replicated and the significance of this finding is uncertain. The likely presence of heterogeneity of linkage where there are multiple single-gene predispositions to schizophrenia localized to distinct chromosomal regions in different families complicates the outlook for future linkage studies because large samples will be needed. If the extent of heterogeneity of linkage can be understood, then refined diagnosis based on genetic aetiology should enable more accurate prognosis as well as improved treatment and prevention. If recombinant DNA research succeeds in identifying a disease pathway by the cloning and sequencing of a mutation that confers susceptibility to schizophrenia, then this will enable new treatments to be designed that act on the disease pathway.

GENETICS AND SCHIZOPHRENIA

The observation that schizophrenia often affects more than one member of the same family is evidence that familial factors must be involved in its development. Such factors might be genetic or environmental. Genetic methods for analysing human behavioural characteristics that have usually been thought to have a polygenic, multifactorial (i.e. complex) origin have traditionally consisted of family, twin, adoption and half sib studies. These approaches can be subsumed under the titles of either *variance component* or *path analysis* (Fulker, 1978; Wright, 1983). Such analyses must always incorporate various assumptions that may be unjustified and as a result there are limitations as to how accurately the proportions of genetic and environmental variance that contribute to a disease can be measured (Henderson, 1982; Feldman and Cavalli-Sforza, 1977; 1979). However, a general impression of the relative contributions of genetic and environmental effects can be gained if all the traditional genetic methods for behaviour are used in a variety of different environments at different points in time.

Methods that attempt to identify the specific mode of transmission of any genetic effect can be incorporated into the variance component or path analysis. The principal methods for identifying a mode of transmission are known as *segregation analysis* and *genetic linkage analysis*. Segregation analysis can, theoretically at least, attempt to identify whether there may be many or a few genes (polygenic or oligogenic transmission) conferring liability to the disease. A third possibility which can be tested by segregation analysis is that there is a single, abnormal gene providing most of the genetic effect; this is known as transmission by a single major locus (Morton *et al.*, 1983). Such an effect may be recessive, when two disease alleles, one from each parent, must be inherited, dominant when only one disease allele is transmitted to an affected person, or 'intermediate' when all homozygotes and a proportion of heterozygotes are affected (see Chapter 2). Morton and Maclean (1974) have proposed a 'mixed' model that combines a single major locus, a polygenic background and environmental effects.

Quantitative estimates of the genetic component of schizophrenia range from 70 to 80% (Fulker, 1973; Kendler, 1983; McGue *et al.*, 1985). These estimates are based on combined family, twin and adoption data. There have been a number of attempts to determine a mode of transmission by the use of segregation analysis or the mixed model, when combined single-gene effects are studied in relation to familial and cultural transmission. Baron (1986) has comprehensively reviewed these past studies and comments that there was considerable variation between them, and conflicting results. The single, major locus model was compatible with the data in seven out of the twelve analyses but was rejected by five. In contrast, the multifactorial, polygenic model was rejected in only one of five studies, while two studies rejected both the single, major locus and polygenic models. Finally, two studies that used the mixed model concluded that single, major locus transmission with polygenic background was compatible with the data. Mention should also be made of the work of Karlsson in Iceland, who provided arguments for a single, major gene effect in schizophrenia (Karlsson, 1986; 1988). This work did not use modern methods of segregation analysis or of psychiatric diagnosis but did suggest that some forms of schizophrenia were confined to certain large, Icelandic, multigenerational kindreds. Extensive pedigree studies of schizophrenia in a northern Swedish population have also led to the conclusion that, at least in some specific families, schizophrenia may be transmitted as an autosomal-dominant gene disorder (Book, 1953; Book *et al.*, 1978).

Population differences may have contributed to the conflicting results but it is clear that schizophrenia is a complex trait which does not always show simple Mendelian inheritance. This is perhaps not surprising, considering its association with reduced fertility and social isolation. Other potential sources of error include reduced penetrance (i.e. the incomplete manifestation of a trait in individuals who carry the pathogenic genotype); the existence of phenocopies (i.e. cases that do not carry the genotype but who nevertheless manifest the disorder); and genetic heterogeneity, diagnostic difficulties, sampling bias, ascertainment bias, mortality and variable age of onset. All these factors may make segregation analysis inexact (Kendler, 1986).

Genetic linkage analysis is potentially more powerful than segregation analysis for identifying single, major gene transmission in schizophrenia. If various single, major loci can be established as having a widespread role in subtypes of schizophrenia, then future recombinant DNA research will eventually create new treatments and preventive strategies based on a knowledge of exactly which genes are involved. At the present time, considerable effort is being focused on genetic linkage analysis of schizophrenia, and this review is itself focused on such recent work.

Genetic linkage analysis

Genetic linkage analysis specifies regions of a chromosome by the use of polymorphic DNA markers that are unambiguously associated with the illness. This region of genetic material will tend to be inherited by all other affected individuals within a specific family. For disorders in which a single-gene effect can be strongly hypothesized, genetic linkage analysis is an attractive approach because, if successful, it provides confirmation and clarification of a mode of transmission, unlike segregation analysis. Moreover, the successful finding of a linkage on a particular chromosome can lead on to the cloning and sequencing of the mutant gene itself. Here, use may be made of the phenomenon of linkage disequilibrium to identify regions of DNA that are very close to the disease mutation.

Linkage disequilibrium refers to the fact that genetic variations close to each other on the same chromosome may be inherited together over many generations without becoming separated at gametogenesis when recombination (crossing over) between homologous chromosomes takes place. This tends to result in allelic association in the population (see Chapter 4). One million base pairs of DNA in the human genome is equivalent to about 1% recombination. Over this distance, this means that only one crossover or recombinant will occur every 100 times a gamete is formed. Over smaller distances there is likely to be cosegregation at meiosis and therefore association at the population level between two adjacent polymorphisms or between a polymorphism and a disease mutation.

Most linkage markers are at a great enough distance from the disease mutation for there to be no population association between the marker polymorphism and the disease. In this case it is random as to which marker allele segregates with the disease in a given family. The closer the marker is to the disease mutation, the more likely it will be that there is one specific allele rather than another which is associated with the disease mutation. However, even if a marker polymorphism is very close to a disease mutation, linkage disequilibrium is not necessarily observed, at the population level, as an association. The reason for this is that a variety of different mutations may have occurred at the disease locus at different times during evolution or that a number of different alleles at the marker locus originated after the disease mutation.

The use of linkage disequilibrium in genetics has brought about the successful cloning of the cystic fibrosis gene (Rommens *et al.*, 1989). The fine mapping of genes in the region and the eventual cloning of the disease gene was done by calculating the strength of linkage disequilibrium for a series of polymorphisms. That is, when the polymorphisms were close to the disease mutation, then the coefficient of disequilibrium was strong; when the polymorphisms were further away, the observed linkage disequilibrium was weaker.

Lastly, it should be mentioned that cytogenetic abnormalities which are localized in people suffering from schizophrenia can give valuable clues as to where abnormal genes may be localized in families where there are no cytogenetic abnormalities. The fact that recombinant DNA technology has created markers that span most of the human genome means that any favoured locus identified by having a cytogenetic abnormality can be readily investigated in many samples of families.

Despite the fact that a mode of genetic transmission has not been very precisely defined, or that polygenic/multifactorial models are in some respects more statistically satisfactory, one cannot exclude the possibility of a major gene contributing to the liability for developing specific subtypes of schizophrenia (McGue *et al.*, 1985). Reviewers of this topic (Sturt and McGuffin, 1985; Kendler, 1986; McGuffin and Sturt, 1986) have therefore supported the search for genetic susceptibility through the study of biological vulnerability traits and genetic markers.

Genetic linkage studies of schizophrenia

Genetic markers correspond to loci with known chromosomal assignments and have simple Mendelian modes of inheritance. They may be variant proteins, such as the blood groups, which are encoded by specific genes, or they may be specific DNA sequences as identified by restriction enzymes. In order to obtain information for genetic linkage analysis within a given family, there must be at least two or more alleles or alternative versions of the DNA sequence or restriction site with which to distinguish homologous parental chromosomes. It then becomes possible to observe or infer which of the two out of four possible alleles (i.e. at marker and disease loci) the offspring have inherited from their parents. The more polymorphic a locus, the more useful it becomes in linkage studies. With the complication of incomplete penetrance, as found in schizophrenia, there is a strong argument for obtaining highly polymorphic markers in order to maximize the information obtained from affected rather than unaffected individuals.

The use of DNA sequences as linkage markers in the investigation of genetic disease has been revolutionized by the use of restriction fragment length polymorphisms (RFLPs). Restriction enzymes are bacterial products that cut double-stranded DNA at special sequences of nucleotide base pairs. DNA variation can only occur between homologous chromosomes and some of these variations may create or destroy a restriction enzyme-cutting site. This produces changes in the fragment lengths produced by specific enzymes. The variation in fragment lengths so produced is observed by transferring restricted DNA fragments to a suitable membrane and hybridizing those fragments to a cloned radioactive gene or DNA segment (known as a probe) so that any fragments containing the same sequence as the probe will become visible (Gurling, 1986; see also Chapter 1).

With the increasing numbers of RFLPs (Donis-Keller *et al.*, 1987), it should eventually be possible to cover the entire genome. However, this may involve in excess of 200 markers (Lange and Boehnke, 1982) and thus 'blind' linkage studies will require formidable resources. A slightly easier strategy is to concentrate on areas where there is an *a priori* reason for suspecting involvement between marker and disease. Investigation, by linkage, of loci implicated by cytogenetic abnormalities or by previous association studies both offer potentially fruitful approaches.

Linkage analysis consists of finding polymorphic genetic markers that are close enough to the disease on the same chromosome for them to be inherited together with the disease mutation from one generation to the next. In such cases the marker and disease are said to be linked. The distance between the illness gene and the marker gene can be calculated by observing the number of recombinations that occur. The closer the disease locus is to the marker, the less likely is recombination. Recombination is measured by the recombination fraction θ. This is the proportion of meioses within a pedigree in which the disease and the marker are not inherited together. A value of 0.5 (50%) indicates independent assortment of the alleles; a value approaching zero indicates that linkage may be present.

The presence and strength of linkage is usually expressed as the lod score (logarithm to the base 10 of the odds), calculated by using likelihood methods and incorporating a variety of parameters such as penetrance and the presence of phenocopies. At any specific value of θ a lod score exceeding 3.0 is said to confirm linkage and a value less than -2.0 allows rejection of linkage. If penetrance is jointly estimated with the recombination fraction, then the slightly higher lod of 3.85 is accepted as evidence of linkage (Sherrington *et al.*, 1988). A lod of 3.00 is approximately equivalent to a posterior probability of rejecting the null hypothesis of $p < 0.05$, although it is an odds ratio of 1:1000 (see Chapter 3).

Early attempts at linkage studies in schizophrenia were hampered by the small number of potential (usually protein) markers available and their relatively low degree of polymorphism. This made most studies largely uninformative. There have been nine linkage studies of schizophrenia published to date (Elston *et al.*, 1973; Turner, 1979; McGuffin *et al.*, 1983; Andrew *et al.*, 1987; DeLisi *et al.*, 1988; Gurling *et al.*, 1988; Kennedy *et al.*, 1988; Detera-Wadleigh *et al.*, 1989; St. Clair *et al.*, 1989). Positive lod scores have been reported for the immunoglobulin proteins, Gm and Bc (Elston *et al.*, 1973) and phosphoglucomutase (Andrew *et al.*, 1987). There have been reports that the polymorphic alleles of serum protein Gc are associated with, rather than linked to, schizophrenia (Book *et al.*, 1978; Lange, 1982; Papiha *et al.*, 1982), but these are not consistent (Beckman *et al.*, 1980; Rudduck *et al.*, 1985). Extensive association studies and some of linkage between the HLA genes and schizophrenia have also not produced consistent results (Baron, 1986; Kendler, 1986).

Cytogenetic abnormalities reported in combination with schizophrenic psychoses include fragile sites (Chodirker *et al.*, 1987), deletions and pericentric inversions (Hong, 1986; Axelsson, 1981), trisomies (Turner and Jennings, 1961; Sperber, 1975), acentric fragments (Kaplan, 1970; Das-gupta *et al.*, 1973), translocations or sex chromosome abnormalities (Kaplan, 1970; Crow, 1988). However, these lesions are found only in a very small proportion of those suffering from schizophrenia. They might, however, sometimes be indicative of a subtype of schizophrenia normally caused by other abnormalities at the same genomic site. The cosegregation of schizophrenia with a genetic disease could also point to a chromosomal localization. An example of such cosegregation between schizophrenia and albinism within a family has been reported by Baron (1976). The first evidence for a genetic basis to schizophrenia using linkage markers has been obtained by investigating a chromosomal region implicated by a cytogenetic abnormality. This followed a report from Canada of a chromosomal abnormality in a Chinese man and his nephew, both suffering from schizophrenia, facial dysmorphism and other abnormalities such as renal dysgenesis. At cytogenetic examination an area of trisomy on chromosome 5 (5q11–q13) was found (Bassett *et al.*, 1988; Bassett, 1989). Later, Wahlstrom (1989) reported a translocation involving 5q13 in a single schizophrenic in Sweden. Further investigation of this individual's family is being made in order to identify other possible cases of schizo-phrenia with the translocation.

Linkage studies using probes localized to the chromosomal area 5q11–5q13 have been made in five Icelandic and two British families. The results were analysed using a variety of diagnostic classifications for schizophrenia and its associated disorders. The initial lod scores ranged from 2.45 to 6.45, depending on the model used, and provided strong evidence for the segregation of a dominant schizophrenia susceptibility allele on chromosome 5 (Sherrington *et al.*, 1988). Subsequently, lod scores incorporating a third marker (M4), localized between the two marker loci originally found to be linked to schizophrenia, confirmed the information obtained from one of the original probes but showed up two cases of either incomplete penetrance or recombination not previously identified. The revised lod scores ranged from 2.9 for the analysis involving affected cases only, to 5.9 for the model in which all possible cases of schizophrenia as well as unaffected individuals were included. This implies that the highest score for linkage was with the broadest definition of caseness (Sherrington *et al.*, 1988; Gurling *et al.*, 1989). The following sampling criteria were employed in the study.

1. Medium to large pedigrees with schizophrenia in at least three generations were sampled. This allowed computation of lod scores suggestive of linkage within single families. It was hoped this would facilitate the use of statistical tests that would permit establishment of the extent that susceptibility genes at different loci might be causing schizophrenia within specific families (i.e. tests of homogeneity could be carried out).
2. High-density pedigrees were sampled so that it would be possible to test for linkage by considering affected cases alone. This approach offers a method of circumventing the problems of incomplete penetrance, which can easily confound the detection of the presence of linkage.
3. Families in which manic-depression was present were excluded. This was made possible by extensive tracing of pedigrees. Three families were encountered in which both schizophrenia and manic-depression were present but in each family there were clearly bilineal sources for the two disorders, suggesting that they were caused by distinct genes inherited from different sides of each family.
4. Families were obtained where it was likely that there was only one possible source for a schizophrenia susceptibility allele segregating into a kindred.
5. The bulk of the sample was obtained from a population (Iceland) that has some of the characteristics of a genetic isolate, thus increasing the chance of obtaining a homogeneous sample.

As mentioned above, the highest concordance for linkage was with the broadest definition of psychiatric disorder, which included the so-called 'fringe' phenotypes. An example of one such patient was someone who appeared chronically and atypically depressed and who had received a research diagnostic criteria (RDC) diagnosis of major depressive disorder. For this person there was a history of 'schizophrenia simplex' diagnosed at the age of 17 years, but no evidence of psychosis was recorded in medical notes at this time or at any time later. It may be surmised that such a patient might have been suffering from the effect of a schizophrenia genotype which had manifested itself in the blunted affect, withdrawal, anhedonia and poverty of thought/speech found in the negative or type 2 schizophrenic (Crow, 1980). Further evidence that these fringe phenotypes are indeed variant expressions of the same underlying mutation is required, as the elevation of the lod that occurred when they were included as 'cases' for linkage analysis was only about 2.00 and this could have arisen by chance. The initial lod score for schizophrenia, schizoid personality and schizotypal disorders was also significantly in favour of linkage (lod = 5.20) independent of the fringe cases, so that the evidence for linkage did not depend on the atypical cases alone.

The Icelandic/UK study found that all the traditional subtypes of schizophrenia, i.e. paranoid, hebephrenic, catatonic, undifferentiated and unspecified psychosis, were present in the same families within the sample. The standardized diagnostic interview used (the RDC/SADS-L: Spitzer *et al.*, 1978) was also used in the other recent linkage studies of schizophrenia, making these studies comparable. The findings in the Iceland/UK study suggest that one genotype can give rise to clinical diversity. They also indicate that clinical heterogeneity does not necessarily imply genetic heterogeneity. This aspect of the study confirms family and twin studies (DeLisi *et al.*, 1987; Kendler *et al.*, 1988) where no evidence of homotypia was found. Other studies have suggested a mild tendency towards homotypia in families with the paranoid and hebephrenic subtypes (Tsuang and Winokur, 1974; Tsuang *et al.*, 1974; Scharfetter and Nusperli, 1980; McGuffin *et al.*, 1987) as well as for the catatonic subtype (Scharfetter, 1981a,b). The hebephrenic form of schizophrenia may be more heritable than the paranoid variety (Winokur *et al.*, 1974; McGuffin *et al.*, 1984), which lends some support to Tsuang and Winokur's (1974) concept of a hebephrenic–paranoid continuum of illness, with the hebephrenic type being the most advanced and severe form.

In general, the proportion of schizophrenia that is related to an underlying single-gene susceptibility is unknown. The proportion that is attributable to the chromosome 5 mutation is also unknown. Already it seems likely that only a minority of cases will be caused by the chromosome 5 abnormality. Other studies (Kennedy *et al.*, 1988; Detera-Wadleigh *et al.*, 1989; St. Clair *et al.*, 1989; McGuffin *et al.*, 1990) have failed to demonstrate chromosome 5 linkage.

However, perhaps some of the apparently negative results reported for chromosome 5 markers and schizophrenia should be treated with caution. The study by Kennedy *et al.* (1988) used a single large multiplex Swedish pedigree and produced good evidence that the chromosome 5q11–13 locus was not responsible. A statistical test of homogeneity rejected the null hypothesis and thus provided evidence that the two samples had heterogeneity of linkage (Kennedy *et al.*, 1989). However, this sample is not comparable with the UK/Icelandic sample for rates and types of the non-psychotic, schizophrenia-related disorders. This is because sampling of affected cases in the Swedish pedigree was deliberately biased away from phenotypes that were difficult to diagnose. This approach has particular merit for linkage studies of schizophrenia but somewhat restricts the full exploration of genetic caseness at an early stage of a linkage study.

The studies of Detera-Wadleigh *et al.* (1989) and St. Clair *et al.* (1989) used families containing both bipolar disorder and schizophrenia. A substantial proportion of the cases for genetic analysis were bipolar or schizoaffective rather than schizophrenic, and such a number of false-positive cases could obscure a finding of positive linkage. However, in both cases, an analysis excluding the pedigrees containing bipolar disorder also failed to confirm linkage on chromosome 5.

In the UK/Iceland study (Sherrington *et al.*, 1988), the best estimate of penetrance was 71% for schizophrenia, rising to 76% when including the spectrum disorders, and to 86% when counting the fringe diagnoses; only approximately 14% of those individuals who had inherited the disease genotype were clinically normal and about 29% did not develop the full syndrome. The Icelandic families studied were genetically isolated and had an unusually high density of illness, indicating that this may be an unusual variant of schizophrenia. Fischer (1971) showed that monozygotic twins discordant for schizophrenia had the same incidence of the illness (16%) among their respective offspring. This illustrates that the schizophrenia genotype is not always expressed phenotypically and that penetrance is often incomplete. Fischer's study suggested a penetrance of 32%. Others have different figures: Karlsson (1988) suggested 25% while Eliot Slater thought the overall figure was in the region of 20% (Slater and Cowie, 1972).

The factors influencing penetrance are likely to be a productive research area in the future, with implications for preventive psychiatry. The effects of interaction between genotype and life events, expressed emotion and organic variables such as head injury, obstetric complications or substance abuse are likely to be important. If high-risk individuals in genetically vulnerable families can be identified by DNA testing, research will be able to focus on which interventions minimize psychiatric morbidity.

New understanding of schizophrenia will also come from comparing aetiological subtypes, as defined by genetic linkage markers, with clinical variables, especially those which also seem to have a genetic basis. Brain ventricular size is known to be abnormal in some schizophrenics (Johnstone *et al.*, 1976; Turner *et al.*, 1986). Although there is no firm concensus, this may be a marker for a less genetic form of the illness (Reveley *et al.*, 1984), especially when associated with perinatal complications (Turner *et al.*, 1986; Murray *et al.*, 1988). This relationship also seems to hold for some familial cases, suggesting that the two aetiological factors can operate in a cumulative way (Murray *et al.*, 1988) and providing an example of how penetrance might be affected by environmental factors. Negative features and lack of response to neuroleptics are also said to be characteristic of the more genetic forms of schizophrenia (Dworkin and Lenzenweger, 1984; Keefe *et al.*, 1987; Silverman *et al.*, 1987).

CONCLUSIONS

Schizophrenia is perhaps best conceptualized as being similar to diabetes with which it shares a similar population prevalence. It is known that one subtype of diabetes is caused by a single, point mutation in the insulin gene (hyperinsulinaemic diabetes; Haneda *et al.*, 1983), another is strongly genetic and has a late age of onset. A third type is less strongly genetic, has an early age of onset and appears to be associated with the HLA genes that affect immunological susceptibility (Green *et al.*, 1985). Eventually, through the use of genetic linkage markers, we may learn that schizophrenia is composed of different genetic and biological subtypes. Both recessive and dominant modes of transmission of major gene effects may be present. The genes responsible may encode for neurotransmitter receptors, enzymes, neuromodulators or genes responsible for brain development. Although there are limits to the ease with which a complex disease such as schizophrenia can be studied by the use of genetic linkage markers there is no reason why large samples (Ott, 1986) cannot be used in order to resolve the issues of complex aetiology and genetic heterogeneity. The molecular genetic techniques for moving closer to the schizophrenia susceptibility genes and finally cloning and sequencing them are constantly being improved and should eventually produce knowledge about the precise pathogenesis of schizophrenia.

ACKNOWLEDGEMENTS

The research in Iceland and the UK has been funded by the Wellcome Trust and the Rothschild Schizophrenia Research Fund. The work of Dr. H. Petursson, Dr. J. Brynjolfsson and Dr. Thordor Sigmundsson is acknowledged.

REFERENCES

Andrew B., Watt D. C., Gillespie C., Chapel H. (1987). A study of genetic linkage in schizophrenia. *Psychological Medicine*; **17**: 363–70.

Axelsson R., Wahlstrom J. (1981). Mental disorder and inversion on chromosome 9. *Hereditas*; **95**: 337.

Baron M. (1976). Albinism and schizophreniform psychosis: a pedigree study. *American Journal of Psychiatry*; **133**: 1070–2.

Baron M. (1986). Genetics of schizophrenia. II. Vulnerability traits and gene markers. *Biological Psychiatry*; **21**: 1189–211.

Bassett A. S. (1989). Chromosome 5 and schizophrenia: implications for genetic linkage studies. *Schizophrenia Bulletin*; **15**: 393–402.

Bassett A. S., McGillivray B. C., Jones B. *et al.* (1988). Partial trisomy chromosome 5 co-segregating with schizophrenia. *Lancet*; i: 799–800.

Beckman L., Beckman G., Perris C. (1980). Gc serum groups and schizophrenia. *Clinical Genetics*; **17**: 149–52.

Book J. A. (1953). A genetic and neuropsychiatric investigation of a North Swedish population. *Acta Genetica*; **4**: 189–249.

Book J. A., Wetterberg L., Modrzewska, K. (1978). Schizophrenia in a North Swedish geographical isolate 1900–1977. Epidemiology genetics and biochemistry. *Clinical Genetics*; **14**: 373–94.

Chodirker B., Chudley A., Ray M. *et al.* (1987). Fragile 19p13 in a family with mental illness. *Clinical Genetics*; 31: 1–6.

Crow T. J. (1980). Molecular pathology of schizophrenia; more than one disease process. *British Medical Journal*; 1: 66–8.

Crow T. J. (1988). Sex chromosomes and psychosis. *British Journal of Psychiatry*; 153: 675–83.

Dasgupta J., Dasgupta D., Balasubrahmanyan M. (1973). XXY syndrome XY/XO mosaicisms and acentric chromosomal fragments in male schizophrenics. *Indian Journal of Medical Research*; 61: 62–70.

DeLisi L. E., Goldin L. R., Maxwell L. W. *et al.* (1987). Clinical features of illness in siblings with schizophrenia or schizoaffective disorder. *Archives of General Psychiatry*; 44: 891–7.

Detera-Wadleigh S. D., Goldin L. R., Sherrington R. *et al.* (1989). Exclusion of linkage to 5q11–13 in families with schizophrenia and other psychiatric disorders. *Nature*; 340: 391–3.

Donis-Keller H., Green P., Helms C., Cartinhour S. (1987). A genetic linkage map of the human genome. *Cell*; 51: 319–37.

Dworkin R. H., Lenzenweger M. F. (1984). Symptoms and genetics of schizophrenia, implications for diagnosis. *American Journal of Psychiatry*; 141: 1541–5.

Elston R. C., Kringlen E., Namboodiri K. K. (1973). Possible linkage relationship between certain blood groups and schizophrenia. *Behavioral Genetics*; 3: 101–6.

Feldman M. W., Cavalli-Sforza L. L. (1977). The evolution of continuous variation. II. Complex transmission and assortative mating. *Theoretical Population Biology*; 11: 161–81.

Feldman M. W., Cavalli-Sforza L. L. (1979). Aspects of variance and covariance analysis with cultural inheritance. *Theoretical Population Biology*; 15: 276–307.

Fischer M. (1971). Psychoses in the offspring of schizophrenic monozygotic twins and their normal co-twins. *British Journal of Psychiatry*; 118: 43–52.

Fulker D. W. (1973). A biometrical genetic approach to intelligence and schizophrenia. *Social Biology*; 20: 266–75.

Fulker D. W. (1978). Multivariate extensions of a biometric model of twin data. In: *Twin Research: Psychology and Methodology* (Nance W. E., ed.), pp. 217–36. New York: Alan Liss.

Green A., Svejgaard A., Platz P. *et al.* (1985). The genetic susceptibility to insulin-dependent diabetes mellitus: combined segregation and linkage analysis. *Genetic Epidemiology*; 2: 1–5.

Gurling H. M. D. (1986). Candidate genes and favoured loci. *Psychiatric Developments*; 4: 289–309.

Gurling H. M. D., Sherrington R., Brynjolfsson J. *et al.* (1988). Genetic linkage studies of schizophrenia using the M13, 33.15 and 33.6 hypervariable DNA polymorphisms. In: *A Genetic Perspective for Schizophrenia and Related Disorders* (Smeraldi E., Kidd K., eds.), pp. 43–8. Milan: Edi-Hermes.

Gurling H. M. D., Sherrington R. P., Brynjolfsson J., Petursson H. (1989). Multipoint map of the 5q11–5q13 schizophrenia susceptibility locus. Human gene mapping 10. *Cytogenetics and Cell Genetics*; 51: 1077.

Haneda M., Chan S. J., Kwok S. C. M. *et al.* (1983). Studies on mutant human insulin genes: identification and sequence analysis of a gene encoding

[SerB24] insulin. *Proceedings of the National Academy of Sciences (USA)*; **80**: 6366–70.

Henderson N. (1982). Behaviour genetics. *Annual Review of Psychology*; **33**: 403–40.

Hone M. L. (1986). *Clinical Journal of Neurological Psychiatry*; **19**: 188–91.

Johnstone E. C., Crow T. J., Frith C. D. *et al.* (1976). Cerebral ventricle size and cognitive impairment in chronic schizophrenia. *Lancet*; **ii**: 924–6.

Kaplan A. (1970). Chromosomal mosaicisms and occasional acentric chromosomal fragments in schizophrenic patients. *Biological Psychiatry*; **2**: 89–94.

Karlsson J. L. (1986). Variable penetrance in partly dominant human disorders. *Biologisches Zentralblatt*; **105**: 599–603.

Karlsson J. L. (1988). Partly dominant transmission of schizophrenia in Iceland. *British Journal of Psychiatry*; **152**: 324–9.

Keefe R. S. E., Mohs R. C., Losonczy M. F. *et al.* (1987). Characteristics of very poor outcome schizophrenia. *American Journal of Psychiatry*; **144**: 889–94.

Kendler K. S. (1983). Overview: a current perspective on twin studies of schizophrenia. *American Journal of Psychiatry*; **140**: 1413–25.

Kendler K. (1986). The feasibility of linkage studies in schizophrenia. In: *Dahlem Konferenzen, Biological Perspectives in Schizophrenia*, Berlin: Dahlem Foundation.

Kendler K. S., Gruenberg A. M., Tsuang M. T. (1988). A family study of the subtypes of schizophrenia. *American Journal of Psychiatry*; **145**: 57–62.

Kennedy J. L., Giuffra L. A., Moises H. W. *et al.* (1988). Evidence against linkage of schizophrenia to markers on chromosome 5 in a northern Swedish pedigree. *Nature*; **336**: 167–70.

Kennedy J. L., Giuffra L. A., Moises H. W. *et al.* (1989). Molecular genetic studies in schizophrenia. *Schizophrenia Bulletin*; **15**: 383–91.

Lange V. (1982). Genetic markers for schizophrenia subgroups. *Psychiatric Clinics*; **15**: 133–44.

Lange K., Boehnke M. (1982). How many polymorphic genes will it take to span the human genome? *American Journal of Human Genetics*; **34**: 842–5.

McGue M., Gottesman I. I., Rao D. C. (1985). Resolving genetic models for the transmission of schizophrenia. *Genetic Epidemiology*; **46**: 44–55.

McGuffin P., Sturt E. (1986). Genetic markers in schizophrenia. *Human Heredity*; **36**: 65–8.

McGuffin P., Farmer A. E., Gottesman I. I. *et al.* (1984). Twin concordance for operationally defined schizophrenia. *Archives of General Psychiatry*; **41**: 541–7.

McGuffin P., Farmer A. E., Gottesman I. I. (1987). Is there really a split in schizophrenia? The genetic evidence. *British Journal of Psychiatry*; **150**: 581–92.

McGuffin P., Festenstein H., Murray R. (1983). A family study of HLA antigens and other genetic markers in schizophrenia. *Psychological Medicine*; **13**: 31–43.

McGuffin P., Sargeant M. P., Hett G. *et al.* (1990). Exclusion of a schizophrenia susceptibility gene from the chromosome 5q11–q13 region: New data and a reanalysis of previous reports. *American Journal of Human Genetics*, **47**: 524–35.

Morton N. E., Maclean C. J. (1974). Analysis of family resemblance III. Complex segregation analysis. *American Journal of Human Genetics*; **26**: 489–503.

Morton N. E., Rao D. C., Lalouel J. M. (1983). *Methods in Genetic Epidemiology*. Basel: Karger.

Murray R. M., Lewis S. W., Owen M. J., Foerster A. (1988). The neurodevelopmental origins of dementia praecox. In: *Schizophrenia: The Major Issues* (Bebbington P., McGuffin P., eds.), pp. 90–107. Oxford: Heinemann.

Ott J. (1986). The number of families required to detect or exclude linkage heterogeneity. *American Journal of Human Genetics*; **39**: 159–65.

Papiha C. S., Roberts D. F., McLeigh L. (1982). Group specific component (Gc) subtypes and schizophrenia. *Clinical Genetics*; **22**: 321–6.

Reveley A. M., Reveley M. A., Murray R. M. (1984). Cerebral ventricular enlargement in non genetic schizophrenia: a controlled twin study. *British Journal of Psychiatry*; **144**: 89–93.

Rommens J. H., Tannuzzi J. C., Karem B. S. *et al.* (1989). Identification of the cystic fibrosis gene: chromosome walking and jumping. *Science*; **245**: 1059–65.

Rudduck C., Franzen G., Hansson A. (1985). Gc serum groups in schizophrenia. *Human Heredity*; **35**: 11–14.

St. Clair D., Blackwood D., Muir W. *et al.* (1989). No linkage of chromosome 5 markers to schizophrenia in Scottish families. *Nature*; **339**: 305–9.

Scharfetter C. (1981a). Subdividing the functional psychoses; a family hereditary approach. *Psychological Medicine*; **11**: 637–40.

Scharfetter C. (1981b). Schizophrenias—family heredity data of subtypes. *Clinical Genetics*; **20**: 388.

Scharfetter C., Nusperli M. (1980). The group of schizophrenias, schizo-affective psychoses and affective disorders. *Schizophrenia Bulletin*; **6**: 586–91.

Sherrington R., Brynjolfsson J., Petursson H. *et al.* (1988). The localization of a susceptibility locus for schizophrenia on chromosome 5. *Nature*; **336**: 164–7.

Silverman J. M., Mohs R. C., Davidson M., Losonczy M. F. (1987). Familial schizophrenia and treatment response. *American Journal of Psychiatry*; **144**: 1271–6.

Slater E., Cowie V. (1972). *The Genetics of Mental Disorders*. Oxford: Oxford University Press.

Sperber M. A. (1975). Schizophrenia and organic brain syndrome with trisomy 8 (group C—trisomy 8 [47xx, 8 +] *Biological Psychiatry*; **10**: 27–43.

Spitzer R. L., Endicott J., Robins E. (1978). *Research Diagnostic Criteria for a Selected Group of Functional Disorders* 3rd edn. New York: New York State Psychiatric Institute.

Sturt E., McGuffin P. (1985). Can linkage and marker association resolve the genetic aetiology of psychiatric disorders? Review and argument. *Psychological Medicine*; **15**: 455–62.

Tsuang M. T., Winokur G. (1974). Criteria for subtyping schizophrenia. Clinical differentiation of hebephrenic and paranoid schizophrenia. *Archives of General Psychiatry*; **31**: 43–7.

Tsuang M. T., Fowler R. C., Cadoret R. J., Monnelly E. (1974). Schizophrenia among relatives of paranoid and non paranoid schizophrenics. *Comprehensive Psychiatry*; **15**: 295–302.

Turner B., Jennings A. N. (1961). Trisomy for chromosome 22. *Lancet*; **ii**: 49–50.

Turner S. W., Toone B. K., Brett-Jones J. R. (1986). Computerised tomography scan changes in early schizophrenia preliminary findings. *Psychological Medicine*; **16**: 219–25.

Turner W. J. (1979). Genetic markers for schizotaxia. *Biological Psychiatry*; **14**: 177–206.

Wahlstrom J. (1989). Verbal communication to the European Science Foundation meeting of the Network for the Molecular Neurobiology of Mental Illness, Madrid.

Winokur G., Morrison J., Clancy J., Crowe R. (1974). The Iowa 500. The clinical and genetic distinction of hebephrenic and paranoid schizophrenia. *Journal of Nervous and Mental Disorders*; **159**: 12–19.

Wright S. (1983). On 'Path Analysis in Genetic Epiemiology': a critique. *American Journal of Human Genetics*; **35**: 757–68.

8 *Aberrant neurodevelopment as the expression of the schizophrenia genotype*

PETER JONES AND ROBIN M. MURRAY

There have been remarkable advances over the past 15 years in the biological understanding of schizophrenia, particularly in neuro-imaging and neuropathology. However, genetic theorizing concerning schizophrenia has remained largely oblivious to these advances, and genetically orientated researchers have continued to be preoccupied with, and perplexed by, the vagaries of the adult clinical phenotype (reviewed by Murray *et al.*, 1986; McGuffin *et al.*, 1987). For example, many studies have examined relatives of schizophrenics or twin pairs diagnosed according to a variety of different operational definitions of schizophrenia, and then attempted to use the clinical presentation in adult life to derive the most genetically valid definition (see Chapter 5). Similarly, the application of linkage analysis to families multiply affected with schizophrenia has resulted in controversy over what exactly are the clinical borders of the adult phenotype (see Chapter 7). Not only does such research ignore the vast published record that has arisen in recent years on the brain abnormalities found in schizophrenia, it also ignores the lesson of the history of medicine that aetiology and clinical syndrome do not necessarily coincide. Instead, a variety of causes can give rise to a single syndrome while a single cause may give rise to a variety of syndromes.

In our view, it is no longer enough just to fit genetic models to adult clinical data. Any adequate model of the transmission of schizophrenia must be compatible with what we have learned regarding the abnormalities of brain structure that are seen in schizophrenia, and that are now regarded as consequent upon defective neurodevelopment rather than as a result of the disease process or its treatment (Murray *et al.*, 1985; Murray and Lewis, 1987; Weinberger, 1987). Brain development involves an intricate programme of gene expression that leads to the establishment of many neuronal phenotypes and a wonderfully complex pattern of connections between them. It seems increasingly likely that the genetics of schizophrenia will ultimately be reduced to an understanding of what goes wrong in the genetic specification of this morphological network. This chapter will therefore briefly review the structural abnormalities found in the brains of some schizophrenics and the evidence that these are developmental in origin. Then it will discuss what is known about the normal process of brain development in the light of the post-mortem findings in schizophrenia. Finally it will put forward a few speculations concerning the possible role of mutant genes in producing the aberrant neuronal phenotype that underlies the clinical presentation of schizophrenia.

NEURO-IMAGING STUDIES

Many schizophrenic patients have enlargement of the cerebral ventricles on computed tomography (CT) scanning, although the exact proportion of cases and the extent of the enlargement is still disputed. Ventricular enlargement is present at the onset of positive symptoms (Schulz *et al.*, 1983; Turner *et al.*, 1986), is not related to length of illness, and shows no evidence of progression on follow-up for up to eight years (Illowsky *et al.*, 1988; Vita *et al.*, 1988). Indeed, the changes seem to precede the onset of the adult syndrome of delusions and hallucinations (Murray *et al.*, 1988; O'Callaghan *et al.*, 1988).

Recently, magnetic resonance imaging (MRI) has been applied to schizophrenic patients. This has confirmed the finding of increased ventricular size in a proportion of schizophrenics (DeLisi *et al.*, 1990), and has also shown a reduced volume of temporal lobe structures, and of the hippocampus in particular (Suddath *et al.*, 1989; Bogerts *et al.*, 1990a). The size of the hippocampus in schizophrenic patients appears to be inversely related to lateral ventricular volume (Nasrallah *et al.*, 1990). Barta *et al.* (1990) have also reported a decreased volume of the superior temporal gyrus, particularly on the left side; the reduction in this region, which is an auditory association area, correlated with the severity of hallucinations.

Considerable effort has been expended in comparing the findings from CT scans in familial and non-familial schizophrenics. A number of studies have shown that patients with a family history of serious mental illness are less likely to have enlarged ventricles than those without (Reveley *et al.*, 1984; Reveley, 1985; Turner *et al.*, 1986; Sacchetti *et al.*, 1987; Owen *et al.*, 1988; Cannon *et al.*, 1989); however, other studies, including two from our own group (Nimgaonkar *et al.*, 1988; Owen *et al.*, 1989) have not concurred. That of Owen *et al.* found that among schizophrenics, those with a family history of affective disorder were least likely to show ventricular enlargement. This suggests that the inclusion of such patients in 'familial' groups may partly account for the reports of smaller ventricles in this group. Only one substantial MRI study has so far addressed the familial/sporadic issue. Schwarzkopf *et al.* (1990a), who examined 72 schizophrenic and schizo-affective patients, concluded that lateral ventricular enlargement was indeed more common among those patients without a first- or second-degree relative affected with psychosis.

Monozygotic (MZ) twins discordant for schizophrenia have been examined as another means of ascertaining the relative importance of genetic and environmental factors in the causation of structural brain abnormalities. Thus, Reveley *et al.* (1982) showed that schizophrenic twins have larger ventricles on CT scan than their non–schizophrenic MZ co-twins. More recently, Suddath *et al.* (1990) examined 15 pairs of discordant MZ twins and confirmed that the illness is associated with enlarged lateral and third ventricles, and smaller hippocampi. In 13 out of 15 pairs, the total volume of grey matter in the left temporal lobe was smaller in the schizophrenic twin than in the normal MZ co-twin.

EARLY DEVELOPMENTAL FACTORS

The originators of various twin studies consider that the structural abnormalities are, at least in part, non–genetic. Thus, Casanova *et al.* (1990) concluded that their MRI study of discordant twins showed 'ventriculomegaly is the result of an environmental lesion'. The environmental factors most consistently associated with schizophrenia are obstetric complications. The histories of schizophrenic patients are characterized by an excess of pre- and perinatal problems when compared to controls and to patients suffering from other psychiatric disorders (McNeil and Kaij, 1978; Lewis and Murray, 1987; Eagles *et al.*, 1990).

Almost all adequate studies of schizophrenic patients have found a history of pre- and perinatal hazards to be associated with ventricular enlargement (Cannon *et al.*, 1989; reviewed by Lewis *et al.*, 1989). Therefore, obstetric complications could be acting with, or even substituting for, mutant genes to cause the structural abnormalities associated with the subsequent development of schizophrenia (Murray *et al.*, 1985; 1988). However, it has also been suggested that late (and detectable) obstetric complications may be an indirect indicator of some earlier (and undetectable) insult to the nervous system, or even be a secondary consequence of a genetic defect in neural development (Owen *et al.*, 1988; Goodman, 1989). The first of these alternatives seems quite possible but the latter is less likely, given the evidence that a history of obstetric complications is less common in those schizophrenics with a similarly affected relative (Lewis and Murray, 1987; O'Callaghan *et al.*, 1990b).

Minor physical anomalies or MPAs (e.g. malformed ears or palate) are trivial abnormalities in ectodermal development which are of little consequence in themselves. However, ectodermal development during fetal life closely parallels that of the central nervous system and MPAs are known to occur in excess in patients with developmental disorders (Smith, 1976). The three studies that have examined schizophrenic patients for such abnormalities have all reported more MPAs than in controls (Gualtieri *et al.*, 1982; Guy *et al.*, 1983; Green *et al.*, 1987). Like obstetric complications, MPAs implicate a pathological process operating very early in life, but unlike them they are found more frequently in familial schizophrenics (Waddington *et al.*, 1990).

As is well known, schizophrenics are born slightly more often (7–15%) in the late winter and spring. This excess is largely confined to those without a family history of psychiatric disorder (Shur, 1982; Sacchetti *et al.*, 1989; Schwarzkopf *et al.*, 1990b). For example, in a study of 105 'familial' and 185 non-familial cases, O'Callaghan *et al.* (1990a) found no increase in winter births in the former, but an excess of 34% in the latter. Furthermore, ventricular size varies with season of birth in non-familial cases but not familial cases (Sacchetti *et al.*, 1987; Jones *et al.*, 1990). Together, these data suggest the operation of some seasonal factor that has disrupted fetal or neonatal brain development in non-familial cases.

Several lines of evidence, therefore, suggest that the pathogenic processes, both genetic and environmental, of schizophrenia are active many years before the onset of the florid psychotic illness. The findings concerning obstetric complications and season of birth indicate that the crucial factors operate during the vulnerable period when the brain is still developing. It is, therefore, necessary to understand the epigenetic processes that determine the development of the human brain in order to understand how some of the abnormalities seen in schizophrenia may have arisen.

NEURODEVELOPMENT AND NEUROPATHOLOGY

In the human cerebral cortex alone there are around 10^{10} neurones and perhaps 10 times as many glial cells (Blinkov and Glezer, 1968). The neurones constitute the neural networks that process incoming information and compute the necessary responses. Glial cells have a variety of supportive functions in the adult central nervous system (CNS) and play a primary role in neurodevelopment (Kuffler *et al.*, 1984).

Before networks can form, neurones must be produced. In the human embryo, at around 14 days, chemical signals cause ectodermal cells to divide and form a sheet known as the neural plate. This invaginates along the length of the embryo, folding in on itself to form the neural tube. This elongates, and three swellings appear during the fourth week to form the primitive forebrain, midbrain, and hindbrain. Circumferential growth occurs contemporaneously and these structures subdivide over the next week to create the anatomical parts of the adult brain. Interference at this early stage causes profound CNS abnormality (e.g. spina bifida), which is rarely seen in schizophrenia. Indeed, intuitively one would expect a disorder characterized mainly by psychological dysfunctions to be the result of more subtle change. Development in the radial dimension, the thickness of the tube, is more likely to be relevant to schizophrenia. Proliferation, migration and differentiation occur in the radial plane, and give rise to the laminated structures so characteristic of the regions thought to be abnormal in schizophrenia.

Neuropathological studies show that, compared to controls, schizophrenics have reduced brain weight and length; furthermore, Bruton *et al.* (1990) have shown that the poorer the premorbid function, the lighter and shorter the brain. They also confirmed the increased ventricular size found in CT and MRI studies, and revealed that the left temporal horn was especially enlarged. It has been known for many years that schizophrenia-like symptoms occur with unexpected frequency in temporal lobe epilepsy (Slater *et al.*, 1963). Much interest has therefore focused on the temporal lobe in the search for structural abnormalities in non-epileptic schizophrenics.

Bogerts *et al.* (1985) showed a decrease of 20 to 30% in the volume of the limbic temporal lobe (amygdala, hippocampus, parahippocampal gyrus), and later confirmed the smaller volume of the hippocampal formation in a second series of schizophrenic brains (Bogerts *et al.*, 1990b). Together with the results of MRI studies, these findings pose the question of whether schizophrenia could arise from some defect in the development of the medial temporal lobe.

Cell proliferation

Both neurones and glia are generated by the proliferative zones that appear adjacent to the inner wall of the neural tube. The nuclei of cells lining the prototypical cerebral ventricles move radially with the cell cycle, and mitosis always occurs away from the ventricular surface so that postmitotic cells accumulate outside the ventricular zone in centrifugal fashion. The basic structure of the spinal cord (Nornes and Das, 1974) and the CA1, CA2 and CA3 regions of the hippocampus (Nowakowski and Rakic, 1981) develop in this way, with the original young neurones being displaced away from the ventricular surface as more are produced by the ventricular zone. Thus, neurones and glia are produced as clones from a small number of autonomous progenitor cells (Wetts and Herrup, 1982; Temple and Raff, 1986).

We noted earlier that MRI and neuropathological studies have shown a decreased volume of the hippocampi in schizophrenics. Falkai and Bogerts (1986) found lower cell counts in the hippocampus, as did Jeste and Lohr (1989); McLardy (1974) reported that one-third of schizophrenics had a more shallow granular layer in the dentate gyrus of the hippocampal formation than normal. Gliosis is the usual glial cell reaction to neuronal damage (except in the fetus) and its absence in most but not all schizophrenics (Falkai and Bogerts, 1986; Bruton *et al.*, 1990), raises the question of a defect in cell proliferation in the developing brain, particularly affecting the hippocampal formation. The hippocampus has received great attention from developmental neurobiologists as it is a relatively clearly defined structure and can be followed during neurogenesis. It is a phylogenetically ancient structure, which develops exclusively from the ventricular zone (see Nowakowski and Rakic, 1981), and is unusual in that development continues after birth and into the second year of life. The smaller cell numbers in the hippocampi of schizophrenics (see above) could, therefore, be a consequence of abnormal control of proliferation in the ventricular zone, either generally or affecting cells destined for a specific site.

Cell migration

Young cortical neurones migrate across the intermediate zone to produce the cortical plate from which the mature cerebral cortex develops. The cells forming the cortical plate are arranged in such a way that the first to be generated remain nearest to the proliferative zone and subsequent generations are to be found progressively further away. This 'inside out' pattern of neurogenesis is characteristic of the development of laminated structures (Hickey and Hitchcock, 1984), and clearly comes from a more complex migratory process than the passive displacement of cells destined for the spinal cord.

How is the migration so carefully controlled, sometimes over relatively long distances? Neurones destined for the cortex and cerebellum are intimately associated with elongated glial cells throughout migration (Rakic, 1971). These cells are known as radial glia because of the way in which their processes stretch from the ventricular to the pial surfaces like the spokes of a wheel. Radial glia act as guides for young neurones, providing both support and directional information (Eckenhoff and Rakic, 1984), and their interaction with neurones involves several stages. Initially, the young neurone becomes apposed to the glial fibre. This is followed by its migration along the fibre, always away from the proliferative zone through the intermediate zone to the cortical plate. Finally, contact between the two cells is severed at the correct time and, therefore, position. Once this has occurred, another young neurone from the proliferative zone becomes attached to the fibre and remains so until it has passed the position of its predecessor, thus establishing the columnal character of the cortex.

If neuronal migration is disrupted, then an abnormality in cell position results. Kovelman and Scheibel (1984) claimed to find such positional disarray of the normally regimented ranks of pyramidal neurones in the CA1/CA2 regions of the hippocampus in schizophrenia. However, two subsequent studies failed to find a statistical difference in neuronal disorganization between schizophrenics and controls, though one of these did report greater cellular disarray among those schizophrenics with a more severe psychosis (Altschuler, 1987; Christison *et al.*, 1989).

Jakob and Beckmann (1986) found that in the brains of some adult schizophrenics, particularly those with an early onset, pre-alpha neurones normally located in the superficial layers of the entorhinal cortex are displaced deep to their expected position. Falkai *et al.* (1988) replicated this finding by calculating the distance between the pial surface of the entorhinal cortex and the centre of the pre-alpha cell clusters and showing this to be relatively increased in schizophrenia. Some defect in control of embryonic neuronal migration is an appealing explanation of this, particularly as a variety of rare migrational disorders have been associated with schizophrenia. These include porencephalic and arachnoid cysts (Lewis, 1986; Blackshaw and Bowen, 1987), cavities of the septum pellucidum (Lewis and Mezey, 1985), and aqueduct stenosis (Reveley and Reveley, 1983). According to Barth (1987), these are manifestations of neuronal migration disorders, and are usually accompanied by pervasive neuronal abnormalities.

It is not inconceivable that the primary defect in schizophrenia could arise in the radial glia, and that the neuronal abnormalities could be secondary. As it is the interaction between neurones and glia that determines migration, it is also possible that the defect could lie in their interface. Adhesion between cells is mediated by cell surface glycoproteins; a specific class of these cell adhesion molecules is found in neurones (N-CAMs), and developing neurones adhere to each other when N-CAM on their surface binds together (Edelman, 1985). One type of N-CAM, Ng-CAM (neurone–glia) appears to mediate the variable cell–cell adhesion during the initial alignment of the neurone on the glial fibre, its subsequent migration, and eventual uncoupling (Chuong and Edelman, 1984). In mouse mutations involving defects of cellular migration into the hippo-campus and cerebellum, heterotopic neurones are found for which abnor-malities of N-CAMs may be responsible (Edelman and Chuong, 1982; Pinto-Lord *et al.*, 1982). It has been suggested that similar processes may be affected in schizophrenia (Conrad and Scheibel, 1987; Nowakowski, 1987). One study (Lyons *et al.*, 1988) claimed to find raised serum N-CAM levels in adult schizophrenics but the significance of this is unclear.

Differentiation and cell death

Differentiation of cells in the nervous system is extraordinarily complex. Neurones communicate with each other firstly via efferent pathways, the axons, which grow out, often over long distances, and secondly via the afferent structures, the dendrites on to which the axons terminate. Growing axons have specialized structures at their tips known as growth cones, which are highly dynamic (Raper *et al.*, 1988), and axonal growth is dependent upon the stabilization of the structural microtubules, probably by regulatory proteins that undergo changes in expression during develop-ment (Matus, 1988). Several factors are involved in guiding the growth cone towards the correct target, the body or dendritic tree of another neurone. These include mechanical constraints, growth over preformed glial structures, electromechanical forces, interactions with N-CAMs, and attraction towards sources of specific chemicals. The growing axons seem to feel or sniff their way along to their targets (Raper *et al.*, 1988; Stirling and Summerbel, 1988).

It was formerly thought that all these factors combine with great economy to produce the desired connections between cells but this appears not to be the case. Developing axons form many transient connections with targets that they do not innervate in the adult. During development, these exuberant connections are eliminated by several types of regressive processes. Indeed, varying estimates suggest that between 30 and 75% of all cells generated in the nervous system die by the time it is mature (Cowan *et al.*, 1984). This process appears to be dependent upon trophic factors such as nerve growth factor produced by target cells, as well as by the formation of functioning connections (Oppenheim, 1981; Henderson *et al.*, 1986). Thus, like birds competing for food in the winter, those neurones which lose out in the race to target cells die. Similarly, some axon collaterals are pruned (O'Leary and Stanfield, 1985) and terminal arborizations of axons or dendritic trees shrink (Wiesel, 1982) with consequent decreases in synaptic densities (Oppenheim, 1981; Rakic *et al.*, 1986).

Benes *et al.* (1986) found that the neuronal density was less in schizophrenics in layer VI of the prefrontal cortex, layer V of the cingulate gyrus and layer III of the motor cortex. They suggest that this could have arisen from 'an accelerated process of neuronal drop-out early in life, perhaps related to a perinatal insult'. Later Benes and Bird (1987) found increased numbers of vertical axons in the cingulate cortex of schizophrenics, a finding compatible with less death among primitive neurones as a compensatory phenomenon. Similarly, Deakin *et al.* (1989) attribute what they suggest is an abnormally dense glutamatergic innervation in the frontal cortex of schizophrenics to 'an arrest or failure of the process by which transient callosal projections normally are eliminated during development'.

Connectivity

Patterns of connections are further honed after birth by the function of the network itself. For example, in the visual system, the detailed connections of axon terminals in the lateral geniculate nuclei and visual cortex depend upon the quality of visual experience during a critical neonatal period (Hubel and Wiesel, 1970; Greenough *et al.*, 1987). Randall (1983) and Goodman (1989) have suggested that abnormal neuronal connections may cause some of the symptoms of schizophrenia. Abnormalities in a wide spectrum of developmental events could give rise to misconnections; these abnormalities could primarily affect the formation of connections or be associated with neuronal heterotopia.

The association between schizophrenia and temporal lobe epilepsy may throw some light on the relationship between the timing and the nature of possibly causal misconnections. While only 5% of epileptics with mesial temporal sclerosis have concurrent psychosis, 23% of those with temporal lobe gangliogliomas (also called hamartomas) have psychotic symptoms (Taylor, 1975). Goodman (1989) has pointed out that gangliogliomas contain wildly abnormal neurones, and arise early in fetal development while axonal connections are still forming. By contrast, mesial temporal sclerosis occurs in infancy, probably post-dating the phase when most axonal connections are formed. As a result, gangliogliomas may be more likely than mesial temporal sclerosis to initiate misconnections within the limbic system (Murray *et al.*, 1990).

Glia have an important role in the maturation of connections. Myelination of axons, a function of mature oligodendroglia, continues well into adolescence (Yakovlev and Lecours, 1967). The ongoing process of myelination provides one way of explaining the late behavioural consequences of an early brain lesion in schizophrenia (Randall, 1983; Weinberger, 1987). For example, Benes (1989) has shown the appearance of strikingly increased myelination of the subicular and presubicular regions during the late adolescent period. She notes that these structures have a strategic location within the corticolimbic circuitry of the brain; the subiculum, for example, receives its principal input from the CA1 sector of the hippocampus, a sector which, as we noted above, may contain abnormally positioned cells in schizophrenia. The presubiculum sends efferents to many sites and, via the perforant pathway, provides one of the most extensive inputs to the hippocampus. Could myelination of one or two links in this circuitry in some way allow a pre-existing but latent defect in the hippocampus to become manifest clinically?

GENETIC SPECIFICATION OF NEURODEVELOPMENT

At least 30% of human genes are expressed exclusively in the brain (Sutcliffe *et al.*, 1984). However, as there are far more cells in the human CNS than there are genes, even this massive commitment is not enough for the nervous system to be organized in a point-to-point fashion under direct genetic control. Instead, the genetic specification of neuronal architecture is executed via epigenetic mechanisms that keep the necessary 'instructions' to manageable proportions. Thus, brain development involves a cascade of signals between genes that regulate each others' expression, and interact with local environmental factors to activate an array of regulatory proteins.

Relatively little is known about the control of the early stages in the process whereby cells of the ectoderm become committed to forming the different parts of the human CNS. However, work with drosophila has identified several genes whose inactivation leads to a striking hyperplasia of the CNS (Glysen and Dambly-Chaudierre, 1989). Thus, these 'neurogenic' genes appear to allow a subset of ventral ectodermal cells to become neuroblasts, and then, through some form of lateral inhibition, impose a different fate on the neighbours of the committed cells by preventing them from also becoming neuroblasts. As such genes are highly conserved throughout species, it seems quite possible that some similar sequence of cell specification will operate in the human embryo.

Homeobox (Hox) genes comprise a multigene family, whose members have been shown to play an important controlling role in the specification of regional differences in the CNS of organisms as diverse as drosophila and the mouse. For example, in the mouse, homeobox genes determine the pattern of anterior–posterior differentiation in the CNS; different homeobox genes have different limits of expression along the anterior–posterior axis which reflect their position within the homeobox gene clusters, e.g. certain homeobox genes specify the subdivisions of the primitive hindbrain. Homeobox mutations appear to be implicated in neural crest abnormalities and craniofacial defects in the mouse. As vertebrates appear to have a common molecular programme for early embryological development, it seems likely that homeobox genes will have a role in modulating particular patterns of gene expression, and therefore regional differentiation, in the human brain (Schugart *et al.*, 1989). Rakic (1988) suggests that in primates a set of regulatory genes, analogous to homeobox genes, may parcellate proliferative units within the ventricular zone into a protomap of basic cytoarchitectonic areas. Then, Rakic postulates, the radial glial scaffolding simply translates the map from the ventricular zone to the expanding cortical plate. After the number of proliferative units is established, homeotic selector genes may turn on another set of genes that determines the individual cellular phenotypes within that unit.

He *et al.* (1989) describe a family of homeobox-like genes, the POU-domain genes, which have distinct temporal and spatial patterns of expression during brain development in the rat. Certain of these genes (Brn-2 and Tst-1) are widely expressed in the proliferative zone and early cortical plate but later their expression is restricted to different layers that reflect the mature laminar patterns. Thus, these genes appear to be involved both in the generation of neurones from the proliferative zone and then in their subsequent migration to the superficial layers, where they subsequently reside.

Already researchers are examining the role of homeobox genes in schizophrenia; J. Kennedy *et al.* (personal communication), for example, have excluded linkage of the homeobox 2 gene cluster, located on chromosome 17, to schizophrenia. This is not surprising as one might suspect that a homeobox mutation would produce more pervasive CNS defects rather than the relatively circumscribed abnormalities characteristic of schizophrenia. Many other types of genes are now being implicated in mammalian embryonic development; these include zinc finger-containing genes and oncogenes. As befits genes implicated in tumour formation, most oncogenes are involved in cell proliferation; others may be involved in cell differentiation. For example, Greenberg *et al.* (1990) have identified a T-cell oncogene on chromosome 11p which is expressed segmentally in the mouse hindbrain early in embryonic development, and subsequently in other tissues including certain cell layers of the hippocampus. We should be particularly interested in genes that are expressed in the hippocampal formation in view of the evidence from post-mortem studies of schizophrenic brains suggesting a premature arrest of neuronal migration into the hippocampus and parahippocampal gyrus (Jakob and Beckmann, 1986; Falkai *et al.*, 1988). For example, the pathological picture seen in schizophrenia could be a consequence of a defect in the genetic control of the proliferation and/or migration of the pre-alpha cells or their glial guides.

There is some knowledge of the genetic control of hippocampal development in mice because its structure is predictably affected by four, well-characterized, single-gene defects which cause abnormal migration into the hippocampus (Caviness and Rakic, 1978; Nowakowski, 1987). In the NZB/BINJ mutation, abnormally positioned neurones have migrated too far; in the Hld, dreher, and reeler mice, the abnormally positioned cells have not migrated far enough. Conrad and Scheibel (1987) were struck by the similarities in the pattern of laminar organization produced by these defects and the pattern they claimed to find in schizophrenia, and suggested that they may 'serve as a conceptual model, or perhaps a caricature of a more subtle developmental anomaly in the schizophrenias'.

Thus, the genes controlling neuronal proliferation and migration into the medial temporal lobe could be considered as possible 'candidate genes' for schizophrenia. However, Herndon *et al.* (1971) and Nowakowski (1987) have shown that identical neuronal phenotypes to those that result in the mutant mice can be produced by environmental hazards such as ionizing radiation, excessive alcohol, or maternal viral infection, provided these operate at the critical period of fetal brain development. Mednick *et al.* (1990) have reported that Helsinki residents who were in their second trimester of fetal development during the 1957 influenza epidemic had a significantly increased risk of later schizophrenia. Conrad and Scheibel (1987) particularly suspect neuraminidase-bearing viruses, such as for influenza, which can interfere with the adhesive actions of N-CAMs and perturb the migration of hippocampal cells. Finally, one should not forget that the pyramidal cells of the hippocampus are among the most vulnerable in the brain to mild anoxia-ischaemia in both humans and experimental animals (Brown and Brierley, 1973; Jørgensen and Diemer, 1982). Thus, hypoxic-ischaemic damage to the fetal brain could conceivably produce a similar picture.

CONCLUSION

It will be evident from the foregoing that in seeking to understand the genetics of schizophrenia, we should not expect to find a gene that codes directly for first-rank or negative symptoms. Instead, we may find a defect in the control of neurodevelopment which produces some structural change that predisposes to later schizophrenia. The process of brain development is so complex that a variety of mutations affecting glia or the proliferation and migration of neurones could produce a similar morphological and clinical phenotype; indeed, environmental interference with the same developmental processes may mimic the pathological and psychopathological picture. Such a hypothesis implies that schizophrenia is aetiologically heterogeneous (Murray *et al.*, 1985). However, developmental processes in the brain may, like nuclear power-stations, have built-in safety margins so that breakdown only results if a succession of errors occurs. Thus schizophrenia may result only when an individual inherits several contributory genes or when an individual with the abnormal genotype also suffers fetal adversity. This view is compatible with suggestions that familial data in schizophrenia are best explained by some gene–gene or gene–environmental interaction (Risch, 1990). It remains to be seen whether such an aetiological model is correct. What is no longer in doubt is that psychiatric geneticists need to focus more of their effort on understanding the molecular rules governing neurodevelopment, and how they may be transgressed in schizophrenia.

ACKNOWLEDGEMENTS

We are grateful to the Mental Health Foundation and the Leverhulme Trust for their support of this work.

REFERENCES

Altschuler L. (1987). CT scan and MRI findings in a child with schizophrenia. *Journal of Child Neurology*; **2**: 105–10.

Barta P. E., Pearlson G. D., Powers R. D. *et al.* (1990). MRI of superior temporal gyrus and hallucinations. *Proceedings of the American Psychiatric Association (Annual Meeting)* p. 301. New York: APA.

Barth P. G. (1987). Disorders of neuronal migration. *Canadian Journal of Neurological Science*; **14**: 1–16.

Benes F. M. (1989). Myelination of cortical-hippocampal relays during late adolescence. *Schizophrenia Bulletin*; **15**: 585–93.

Benes F. M., Bird E. D. (1987). An analysis of the arrangement of neurons in the cingulate cortex of schizophrenic patients. *Archives of General Psychiatry*; **44**: 608–16.

Benes F. M., Davidson J., Bird E. D. (1986). Quantitative cyto-architectural studies of the cerebral cortex of schizophrenics. *Archives of General Psychiatry*; **43**: 31–5.

Blackshaw S., Bowen R. C. (1987). A case of atypical psychosis associated with alexithymia and a left fronto-temporal lesion. *Canadian Journal of Psychiatry*; 32: 688–92.

Blinkov S. M., Glezer I. I. (1968). *The Human Brain in Figures and Tables: A Quantitative Handbook*. New York: Plenum.

Bogerts B., Ashtari M., Degreef G. *et al.* (1990a). Reduced temporal limbic structure volumes on magnetic resonance images in first episode schizophrenia. *Psychiatry Research Neuroimaging*; 35: 1–13.

Bogerts B., Falkai P., Haupts M. *et al.* (1990b). Postmortem volume measurements of limbic systems and basal ganglia structures in chronic schizophrenics. *Schizophrenia Research* (in press).

Bogerts B., Meertz E., Schonfeldt-Bausch R. (1985). Basal ganglia and limbic system pathology in schizophrenia: a morphometric study of brain volume and shrinkage. *Archives of General Psychiatry*; 42: 784–91.

Brown A. W., Brierley J. B. (1973). The earliest alterations in rat neurons and astrocytes after anoxia-ischaemia. *Acta Neuropathologica (Berlin)*; 23: 9–22.

Bruton C. J., Crow T. J., Frith C. D. *et al.* (1990). Schizophrenia and the brain. *Psychological Medicine*; 20: 285–304.

Cannon T., Mednick S. A., Parnas J. (1989). Genetic and perinatal determinants of structural brain deficits in schizophrenia. *Archives of General Psychiatry*; 46: 883–9.

Casanova M., King M. L., Atkinson D. *et al.* (1990). Morphometry of brain structures in schizophrenia. *Proceedings of the American Psychiatric Association (Annual Meeting)* p. 300. New York: APA.

Caviness V. S., Rakic P. (1978). Mechanisms of cortical development. A view from mutations in mice. *Annual Review of Neuroscience*; 1: 297–326.

Christison G. W., Casanova M. F., Rawlings R., Kleinman J. E. (1989). A quantitative investigation of pyramidal cells in schizophrenia. *Archives of General Psychiatry*; 46: 1027–32.

Chuong C. M., Edelman G. M. (1984). Alterations in neuronal cell adhesion molecules during development of different regions of the nervous system. *Journal of Neuroscience*; 4: 2354–68.

Conrad A. J., Scheibel A. B. (1987). Schizophrenia and the hippocampus. The embryological hypothesis extended. *Schizophrenia Bulletin*; 13: 577–87.

Cowan W. M., Fawcett J. W., O'Leary D. D., Stanfield B. B. (1984). Regressive events in neurogenesis. *Science*; 225: 1258–65.

Deakin J. F. W., Simpson M. D. C., Gilchrist A. C. *et al.* (1989). Changes in aspartate and kainate binding in schizophrenic post mortem brains. *Journal of Neurochemistry*; 52: 1781–6.

DeLisi L. E., Hoff A. L., Schwartz J. *et al.* (1990). Brain morphology at the onset of schizophrenics. *Proceedings of the American Psychiatric Association (Annual Meeting)* p. 301. New York: APA.

Eagles J. M., Gibson I., Bremner M. H. *et al.* (1990). Obstetric complications in DSM III schizophrenics and their siblings. *Lancet*; 335: 1139–41.

Eckenhoff M. F., Rakic P. (1984). Radial organisation of the hippocampal dentate gyrus. A golgi, ultrastructural and immunocytochemical analysis in the developing rhesus monkey. *Journal of Comparative Neurology*; 223: 1–21.

Edelman G. M. (1985). Cell adhesion and the molecular processes of morphogenesis. *Annual Review of Biochemistry*; 54: 135–69.

Edelman G. M., Chuong C. M. (1982). Embryonic to adult conversion of neural cell adhesion molecules in normal and staggerer mice. *Proceedings of the National Academy of Sciences (USA)*; **79**: 7036–40.

Falkai P., Bogerts B. (1986). Cell loss in the hippocampus of schizophrenics. *European Archives of Psychiatry and Neurological Science*; **236**: 154–61.

Falkai P., Bogerts B., Rozumek M. (1988). Limbic pathology in schizophrenia. The entorhinal region—a morphometric study. *Biological Psychiatry*; **24**: 515–21.

Glysen A., Dambly-Chaudierre C. (1989). Genesis of the drosophila peripheral nervous system. *Trends in Genetics*; **5**: 251–5.

Goodman R. (1989). Neuronal misconnections and psychiatric disorder. *British Journal of Psychiatry*; **154**: 292–9.

Green M. F., Satz P., Soper H. V., Kharabi F. (1987). Relationship between physical anomalies and age of onset of schizophrenia. *American Journal of Psychiatry*; **144**: 666–7.

Greenberg J. M., Boehm T., Sofroniew M. V. *et al.* (1990). Segmental and developmental regulation of a presumptive T-cell oncogene in the central nervous system. *Nature*; **344**: 158–60.

Greenough W. T., Black J. E., Wallace C. S. (1987). Experience and brain development. *Child Development*; **58**: 539–59.

Gualtieri C. T., Adams A., Shen C. D., Loiselle D. (1982). Minor physical anomalies in alcoholic and schizophrenic adults and hyperactive and autistic children. *American Journal of Psychiatry*; **139**: 640–3.

Guy J. D., Majorski L. V., Wallace C. J., Guy M. P. (1983). The incidence of minor physical anomalies in adult male schizophrenics. *Schizophrenia Bulletin*; **9**: 571–82.

He X., Treacy M. N., Simmons D. M. *et al.* (1989). Expression of a large family of POU-domain regulatory genes in mammalian brain development. *Nature*; **340**: 35–42.

Henderson C. E., Benoit P., Huchet M. *et al.* (1986). Increase of neurite-promoting activity for spinal neurons in muscles of 'paralysed' mice and tenotomised rats. *Brain Research*; **390**: 65–70.

Herndon R. M., Margolis G., Kilham L. (1971). The synaptic organisation of the malformed cerebellum induced by perinatal infection with feline panleukopenia virus (PLV): I. Elements forming the cerebellar glomeruli. *Journal of Neuropathology and Experimental Neurology*; **30**: 196–205.

Hickey T. L., Hitchcock P. F. (1984). Genesis of neurons in the dorsal lateral geniculate nucleus of the cat: a ³H-thymidine study. *Journal of Comparative Neurology*; **228**: 186–99.

Hubel D. H., Wiesel T. N. (1970). The period of susceptibility to the physiological effects of unilateral eye closure in kittens. *Journal of Physiology*; **206**: 419–36.

Illowsky B., Juliano D. M., Bigelow L. B., Weinberger D. R. (1988). Stability of CT scan findings in schizophrenia. *Journal of Neurology, Neurosurgery and Psychiatry*; **51**: 209–13.

Jakob H., Beckmann H. (1986). Prenatal development disturbances in the limbic allocortex in schizophrenics. *Journal of Neural Transmission*; **65**: 303–26.

Jeste D. V., Lohr J. B. (1989). Hippocampal pathologic findings in schizophrenia: a morphometric study. *Archives of General Psychiatry*; **46**: 1019–24.

Jones P., Owen M. J., Goodman R. *et al.* (1990). Neurodevelopment and the chronological curiosities of schizophrenia. In: *Proceedings of NATO Conference on Fetal Neurodevelopment in Schizophrenia.* New York: Plenum Press.

Jørgensen B. J., Diemer N. H. (1982). Selective neuron loss after cerebral ischaemia in the rat: possible role of transmitter glutamate. *Acta Neurologica Scandinavica*; **66**: 536–46.

Kovelman J. A., Scheibel A. B. (1984). A neurohistological correlate of schizophrenia. *Biological Psychiatry*; **19**: 1601–21.

Kuffler S. W., Nicholls J. G., Martin A. R. (1984). *From Neuron to Brain: A Cellular Approach to the Function of the Neuronal System* 2nd edn. Sunderland: M. A. Sinauer.

Lewis S. W. (1986). Schizophrenics with and without intracranial abnormalities on CT. Unpublished M Phil. thesis, University of London.

Lewis S. W., Mezey G. C. (1985). Clinical correlates of septum pellucidum cavities. *Psychological Medicine*; **15**: 43–54.

Lewis S. W., Murray R. M. (1987). Obstetric complications, neurodevelopmental deviance and risk of schizophrenia. *Journal of Psychiatric Research*; **21**: 413–21.

Lewis S. W., Murray R. M., Owen M. J. (1989). Obstetric complications in schizophrenia. Methodology and mechanisms. In: *Schizophrenia: Scientific Progress* (Schultz S. C., Tamminga C. A., eds.). Oxford: Oxford University Press.

Lyons F., Martin M. L., Maguire C. *et al.* (1988). The expression of an N-CAM serum fragment is positively correlated with severity of negative features in type II schizophrenia. *Biological Psychiatry*; **23**: 769–75.

Matus A. (1988). Microtubule-associated proteins and neuronal morphogenesis. In: *The Making of the Nervous System* (Parnavalas J. G., Stern C. D., Stirling R. V., eds.), pp. 421–33. Oxford: Oxford University Press.

McGuffin P., Murray R. M., Reveley A. M. (1987). Genetic influence on the psychoses. *British Medical Bulletin*; **43**: 531–56.

McLardy T. (1974). Hippocampal size and structural deficit in brains from chronic alcoholics and some schizophrenics. *Journal of Orthomolecular Psychiatry*; **4**: 32–6.

McNeil T. F., Kaij L. (1978). Obstetric factors in the development of schizophrenia. In: *The Nature of Schizophrenia* (Wynne L. C., Cromwell R. L., Matthysse S., eds.). New York: Wiley.

Mednick S. A., Machon R. A., Huttunen M. O. (1990). An update on the Helsinki influenza project. *Archives of General Psychiatry*; **47**: 292.

Murray R. M., Lewis S. W. (1987). Is schizophrenia a neurodevelopmental disorder? *British Medical Journal*; **295**: 681–2.

Murray R. M., Lewis S. W., Owen M. J., Foerster A. (1988). The neurodevelopmental origins of dementia praecox. In: *Schizophrenia: The Major Issues* (Bebbington P., McGuffin P., eds.), pp. 90–107. Oxford: Heinemann.

Murray R. M., Lewis S. W., Reveley A. M. (1985). Towards an aetiological classification of schizophrenia. *Lancet*; i: 1023–6.

Murray R. M., Owen M. J., Goodman R., Lewis S. W. (1990). A neurodevelopmental perspective on some epiphenomena of schizophrenia. In: *Plasticity and Morphology of the Central Nervous System* (Cazzullo C. L., Invernizzi G., Sacchetti E., Vita A., eds.). London: MTP Press.

Murray R. M., Reveley A. M., McGuffin P. (1986). Genetic vulnerability to schizophrenia. In: *Schizophrenia* (Roy A., ed.). *Psychiatric Clinics of North America*; **9**: 3–16.

Nasrallah H. A., Bogerts B., Olson S. *et al.* (1990). Correlates of hippocampus hypoplasia schizophrenia. *Proceedings of the American Psychiatric Association (Annual Meeting)* p. 304. New York: APA.

Nimgaonkar V., Wessely S., Murray R. M. (1988). Prevalence of familiality, obstetric complications and structural brain damage in schizophrenic patients. *British Journal of Psychiatry*; **153**: 191–7.

Nornes H. O., Das G. D. (1974). Temporal patterns of neuron genesis in spinal cord of rat: I. An autoradiographic study—time and sites of origin and migration and settling patterns of neuroblasts. *Brain Research*; **73**: 121–38.

Nowakowski R. S. (1987). Basic concepts of CNS development. *Child Development*; **58**: 568–95.

Nowakowski R. S., Rakic P. (1981). The site of origin and route and rate of migration of neurons to the hippocampal region of the Rhesus monkey. *Journal of Comparative Neurology*; **196**: 129–54.

O'Callaghan E., Gibson T., Colohon C. (1990a). Seasonality in schizophrenia: confinement of winter birth excess to patients without a family history.

O'Callaghan E., Larkin C., Kinsella A., Waddington J. L. (1990b). Obstetric complications, the putative familial-sporadic distinction, and tardive dyskinesia in schizophrenia. *British Journal of Psychiatry* (in press).

O'Callaghan E., Larkin C., Waddington J. C. (1988). Clinical correlates of obstetric complications in schizophrenia. *Schizophrenia Research*; **1**: 125.

O'Leary D. D., Stanfield B. B. (1985). Occipital cortical neurons with transient pyramidal tract axons extend and maintain collaterals to subcortical but not intracortical targets. *Brain Research*; **336**: 326–33.

Oppenheim R. W. (1981). Cell death of motor neurons in the chick embryo spinal cord V. Evidence on the role of cell death and neuromuscular function in the formation of specific connections. *Journal of Neuroscience*; **1**: 141–51.

Owen M. J., Lewis S. W., Murray R. M. (1988). Obstetric complications and schizophrenia. A computed tomographic study. *Psychological Medicine*; **18**: 331–9.

Owen M. J., Lewis S. W., Murray R. M. (1989). Family history and cerebral ventricular enlargement in schizophrenia: a case control study. *British Journal of Psychiatry*; **154**: 629–34.

Pinto-Lord M. C., Evrard P., Caviness V. S., Jr. (1982). Obstructed neuronal migration along radial glial fibres in the neocortex of the reeler mouse. A Golgi–E.M. analysis. *Developmental Brain Research*; **4**: 379–93.

Rakic P. (1971). Neuron–glia relationship during granule cell migration in developing cerebellar cortex: a golgi and electron microscopic study in *Macaca rhesus*. *Journal of Comparative Neurology*; **141**: 283–312.

Rakic P. (1988). Intrinsic and extrinsic determinants of neocortical parcellation: a radial unit model. In: *Neurobiology of Neocortex* (Rakic P., Singer J. W., eds.), pp. 5–27. Chichester: Wiley.

Rakic P., Bourgeois J. P., Eckenhoff M. F. *et al.* (1986). Concurrent overproduction of synapses in diverse regions of the primate cerebral cortex. *Science*; **232**: 232–5.

Randall P. L. (1983). Schizophrenia, abnormal connections and brain evolution. *Medical Hypotheses*; **10**: 247–80.

Raper J. A., Chang S., Kapthammer J. P., Rathigen F. G. (1988). Growth cone guidance and labelled axons. In: *The Making of the Nervous System* (Parnavelas J. G., Stern C. D., Stirling R. V., eds.), pp. 188–203. Oxford: Oxford University Press.

Reveley M. A. (1985). CT scans in schizophrenia. *British Journal of Psychiatry*; 146: 367–71.

Reveley A. M., Reveley M. A. (1983). Aqueduct stenosis and schizophrenia. *Journal of Neurology, Neurosurgery and Psychiatry*; 46: 18–22.

Reveley A. M., Reveley M. A., Clifford C. A., Murray R. M. (1982). Cerebral ventricular size in twins discordant for schizophrenia. *Lancet*; i: 540–1.

Reveley A. M., Reveley M. A., Murray R. M. (1984). Cerebral ventricular enlargement in non-genetic schizophrenia: a controlled twin study. *British Journal of Psychiatry*; 144: 89–93.

Risch N. (1990). Linkage strategies for genetically complex traits 1. multilocus models. *American Journal of Human Genetics*; 46: 222–8.

Sacchetti E., Vita A., Calzeroni A. *et al.* (1987). Neuromorphological correlates of schizophrenic disorders. In: *Etiopathogenetic Hypotheses of Schizophrenia* (Cazullo C. L. *et al.*, eds.). Lancaster: MTP Press.

Sacchetti E., Vita A., Giobbio G. M. *et al.* (1989). Risk factors in schizophrenia. *British Journal of Psychiatry*; 155: 266–7.

Schugart K., Utset M. F., Fienberg A. *et al.* (1989). Homeobox containing genes: implications for pattern formation during embryonic development in the mouse. In: *Genetics of Neuropsychiatric Diseases* (Wetterberg L., ed.). London: Macmillan.

Schulz S. C., Koller M. M., Kishore P. R. *et al.* (1983). Ventricular enlargement in teenage patients with schizophrenia spectrum disorder. *American Journal of Psychiatry*; 140: 1592–5.

Schwarzkopf S. B., Bogerts B., Olsen S. C. *et al.* (1990a). Ventriculomegy in sporadic schizophrenia. *Proceedings of the American Psychiatric Association (Annual Meeting)* p. 128. New York: APA.

Schwarzkopf S. B., Nasrallah H., Olsen S. C., Coffman J. A. (1990b). Low family history in schizophrenia winter births. *Proceedings of the American Psychiatric Association (Annual Meeting)* p. 128. New York: APA.

Shur E. (1982). Season of birth in high and low genetic risk schizophrenics. *British Journal of Psychiatry*; 140: 410–15.

Slater E., Beard A. W., Glithero E. (1963). The schizophrenia-like psychoses of epilepsy. *British Journal of Psychiatry*; 109: 95–150.

Smith D. W. (1976). *Recognizable Patterns of Human Malformation: Genetic, Embryologic and Clinical Aspects.* Philadelphia: W. B. Saunders.

Stirling R. V., Summerbel D. (1988). Motor axon guidance in the developing chick limb. In: *The Making of the Nervous System* (Parnavalas J. G., Stern C. D., Stirling R. V., eds.), pp. 228–47. Oxford: Oxford University Press.

Suddath R. L., Christison G., Torrey E. F. *et al.* (1989). Quantitative magnetic resonance imaging in twin pairs discordant for schizophrenia. *New England Journal of Medicine*; 322: 789–94.

Suddath R. L., Christison G. W., Torrey E. F. *et al.* (1990). Anatomical abnormalities in the brains of monozygotic twins discordant for schizophrenia. *New England Journal of Medicine*; 322: 789–94.

Sutcliffe J. G., Milner R. J., Gottesfield J. M., Reynolds W. (1984). Control of neuronal gene expression. *Science*; 225: 1308–15.

Taylor D. C. (1975). Factors influencing the occurrence of schizophrenia-like psychosis in patients with temporal lobe epilepsy. *Psychological Medicine*; 5: 249–54.

Temple S., Raff M. C. (1986). Clonal analysis of oligodendrocyte development in culture: evidence for a developmental clock that counts cell divisions. *Cell*; **44**: 773–9.

Turner S. W., Toone B. K., Brett-Jones J. R. (1986). Computerised tomographic scan changes in early schizophrenia. Preliminary findings. *Psychological Medicine*; **16**: 219–25.

Vita A., Sacchetti R., Valvassori G., Cazzullo C. L. (1988). Brain morphology in schizophrenia: a 2–5 year CT scan follow-up study. *Acta Psychiatrica Scandinavica*; **78**: 618–21.

Waddington J. L., O'Callaghan E., Larkin C. (1990). Physical anomalies and neurodevelopmental abnormality in schizophrenia: new clinical correlates. *Schizophrenia Research*; **3**: 90.

Weinberger D. R. (1987). Implications of normal brain development for the pathogenesis of schizophrenia. *Archives of General Psychiatry*; **44**: 660–9.

Wetts R., Herrup K. (1982). Cerebellar Purkinje cells are descended from a small number of progenitors committed during early development: quantitative analysis of Lurcher chimeric mice. *Journal of Neuroscience*; **2**: 1494–8.

Wiesel T. N. (1982). Postnatal development of the visual cortex and the influence of environment. *Nature*; **299**: 583–91.

Yakovlev P. I., Lecours A. R. (1967). The myetogenetic cycles of regional maturation of the brain. In: *Regional Development of the Brain in Early Life* (Minowski A., ed.), pp. 3–70. Oxford: Blackwell Scientific.

9 The familial aggregation of affective disorders: relation to symptom severity and social provocation

PAUL BEBBINGTON, RANDY KATZ AND PETER McGUFFIN

CASE DEFINITION AS A PREREQUISITE OF GENETIC EPIDEMIOLOGY

Depressed mood is an extremely common human experience, and one that does not usually require elaborate explanation. When people are sad, they and their friends and relatives usually know why. The cause is clear and almost always a social event like a bereavement or a disappointment. However, there are limits to interpretation: sometimes the supposed cause seems inadequate to explain the degree of distress and sometimes no cause can be convincingly identified. In such cases it is reasonable to regard the disturbance as an illness worthy of investigation and study (Bebbington, 1987). This is particularly so in the case of the conditions covered by the term manic-depressive illness, but the exact range of disorders to be included is still unclear.

It is worth dwelling on this problem of where to draw the line in the decision to include potential cases. Case definition is crucial for drawing up representative samples of particular disorders so they can be investigated scientifically. It is obviously important for different investigators to feel confident that they are discussing the same phenomena. If researchers choose a definition of disorder that includes much milder cases than those studied in other centres, their findings will be very hard to interpret.

The problem of case definition in affective disorders is particularly acute for genetic researchers. This is because the demonstration that particular disorders run in families must be based on comparisons between groups of subjects, certainly the probands and their relatives, and often unrelated members of the local population as well. In order for these comparisons to be valid, the same methods of case definition must be used in each group.

Case definition has been greatly improved in recent years by the development of standardized interviews such as the Present State Examination (PSE; Wing et al., 1974) and the Schedule for Affective Disorders and Schizophrenia (SADS; Endicott and Spitzer, 1978), coupled with clearly described or operationalized classificatory schedules such as the *International Classification of Diseases* (ICD; World Health Organization, 1978) or the revised third edition of the *Diagnostic and Statistical Manual of Mental Disorders* (DSM-IIIR; American Psychiatric Association, 1987). It is probably fair to say that, as a group, genetic researchers have been slow to take advantage of such instruments, although this is changing. In recent years, there has been a positive explosion of psychiatric population surveys, particularly using the Diagnostic Interview Schedule (DIS; Robins *et al.*, 1981) and the PSE (Wing *et al.*, 1974). These provide consistent values for the prevalence of affective disorder in the general population. For major depressive disorder, the values range from 1.3 to 3.4% for men and from 3 to 7.1% for women. Depression defined by the PSE-ID-CATEGO system has a somewhat higher prevalence, ranging from 2.5 to 5% for men and from 6 to 10% for women (Bebbington, 1990).

EPIDEMIOLOGICAL PITFALLS IN GENETIC RESEARCH

The establishment of consistent rates of prevalence in the general population seems to offer opportunities to genetic researchers, allowing them to make secure comparisons with the prevalence of affective illness in the relatives of probands. However, there are several reasons why this may be a snare.

First, the thresholds used to provide prevalences of this order are really quite low. This is illustrated by Bebbington *et al.* (1989): it appears that high period prevalences are reflected in extremely high morbid risks for depression. Geneticists are particularly concerned with morbid risk as it allows them to control for differing age structures in the groups they wish to compare. Based on data from the Camberwell Community Survey (Bebbington *et al.*, 1981), it was calculated that around half the male and over two-thirds of the female inhabitants of Camberwell would experience an episode of depression by the age of 65 years. Such values leave little room for the effects of familiality—if nearly everyone becomes depressed anyway, having a family history is unlikely to make much demonstrable difference. This is a good argument for geneticists to concentrate on more severe disorders. However, as these are much rarer in general populations, it is not feasible to mount community surveys of the size needed to establish reliable prevalences for them. The geneticist may then be thrown back on the use of referred patients to establish morbid risk (see, for example, Sturt *et al.*, 1984).

As if this reservation about the use of community survey findings as reference data for genetic studies was not enough, there are others. The calculation of morbid risk requires good information about the timing and nature of first episodes of disorder. This is rarely available—the methods used in the Epidemiological Catchment Area (ECA) studies were not impressive in this respect (Bromet *et al.*, 1986), and our own study (Bebbington *et al.*, 1989) would have been improved by the use of more structured techniques for obtaining such information, like the Past History Schedule (PHS; McGuffin *et al.*, 1986). In order to provide good estimates of morbid risk, population surveys need to be designed deliberately for the purpose. To date, no such survey exists.

The final worry about using community survey data is the possibility that the frequency of depression is increasing as the century proceeds. Klerman (1988) has recently reviewed the relevant evidence. He rehearses the distinction between age, period and cohort effects. Cohort effects imply variations in the morbid risk of depression according to date of birth. If there is no cohort effect, or there is an actual reduction in depressive experience with later birth date, cross-sectional surveys would be expected to show an increase in lifetime prevalence in older subjects, as they have had a longer life in which to get depressed. In fact, a consistent *decline* in lifetime prevalence with age is seen in a number of studies, including our own (Bebbington *et al.*, 1989). This suggests a cohort effect of increasing, and possibly earlier, incidence of depression in subjects with later birth dates (Klerman *et al.*, 1985; Gershon *et al.*, 1987; Lavori *et al.*, 1987). Overall it implies that people are perhaps becoming increasingly suscept-ible to depression, although we shall argue that there are other interpre-tations.

These illustrations are persuasive, but depend crucially on the subject's ability to remember past episodes. Such episodes are likely to be more remote and thus easier for older subjects to forget, and this may account for the findings described by Klerman (1988). Estimates of lifetime prevalence are of doubtful validity (Bromet *et al.*, 1986), and Hasin and Link (1988) have now also raised the possibility that older subjects are less able or less willing to recognize past disturbances in their functioning as psychological in nature. Despite this, the possibility of increasing proneness to depres-sion in sequential birth cohorts clearly merits very serious attention. If established, it must be taken into account in calculations of the familiality of affective disturbance.

STRATEGIC APPROACHES TO THE GENETICS OF AFFECTIVE DISORDERS

In the face of reservations like these, the genetic epidemiology of affective disorders must be approached with a degree of caution. Fortunately there are additional techniques that can be used to investigate the familiality of these conditions. One technique that might aid our understanding is the deliberate variation of the criteria for disorder. Farmer *et al.* (1987) examined the familiality of schizophrenia by varying the defining criteria and observing the effect on concordance among twins (see also Chapter 5).

The variation in their definitions of schizophrenia lay in the inclusiveness or otherwise of the criteria. This proved a useful approach and can be adapted to the study of other disorders.

An aspect of affective conditions well suited to analysis of this type is their severity. This can be defined in terms of the character or number of symptoms, or the degree of disability. Severity can be used to create categories for comparison, or treated as a continuous variable. In either case the relationship with familiality can be explored, and this is clearly an important strategy in the light of the difficulties in deciding thresholds for recognizing depression that we have expounded above.

Let us accept that mild depressions are commonplace responses to various adversities. Genetic influences should consequently be more important for the rarer, severe conditions and also in those conditions that do not seem to have been brought about by unfortunate circumstances. This ought to be reflected in greater familiality, although familiality might equally indicate cultural transmission.

There is limited evidence from the literature research concerning the relationship between the severity of affective conditions and their familial transmission. Most genetic studies have been of the more severe forms (McGuffin and Katz, 1989). The pattern is consistent with an average lifetime risk of affective illness of just under 10% in the first-degree relatives of unipolar probands, and about twice that in those of bipolar probands. Twin data provide strong support for a genetic basis (Gershon *et al.*, 1976; Bertelsen *et al.*, 1977). McGuffin and Katz (1986) have analysed twin data assuming a multifactorial threshold model, and concluded that genes rather than the family environment are responsible for most of the variation in liability. Adoption studies confirm that the genetic basis for bipolar disorder is strong, more so than in unipolar disorder.

How do these findings compare with those of genetic investigations in less severe depressive disorders? There are relatively few such studies. However, they suggest the relatives of 'neurotic' depressives have higher rates of affective disorder than members of the general population, although familiality is less than in the more severe forms (Stenstedt, 1966; Perris *et al.*, 1982). Moreover, twin studies of neurotic depression indicate that the major source of familial aggregation is not genetic but environmental. In particular, concordance does not differ greatly between monozygotic (MZ) and dizygotic (DZ) forms (Slater and Shields, 1969; Torgersen, 1986). Shapiro (1970) did find MZ/DZ differences, but his 'non-endogenous' disorders would still be regarded as quite severe, as all of his probands had received in-patient treatment.

Our brief review permits us to conclude tentatively that both severe and mild affective disorders run in families. However, familial aggregation is more prominent, and more likely to reflect shared genes than shared culture, in the severe disorder. We must also conclude that the strategy of researching familiality by observing its relationship with the severity of affective disturbance has not been adequately exploited.

Examining the severity of illness in probands with and without a family history of affective disorder allows tests of the predictions (1) that familial disorders are more severe, and (2) that the severity of the proband's disorder increases as the criterion of illness in relatives is made more stringent, that is, restricted to more severe disorders. The second prediction, if confirmed, suggests the possibility that, to an extent, severe disorders 'breed true'.

The picture can be amplified by examining the relationship between the type of illness in proband and relative. The subdivision of affective disorder into the traditional 'endogenous' and 'neurotic' symptom types is in part a reflection of severity—so, for instance, CATEGO classes R and D (retarded depression and depressive psychosis) have generally higher symptom scores than classes N and A (neurotic depression and anxiety states) (Wing and Morris, 1981).

We think it reasonable to consider three potential mechanisms underlying the severity/familiality relationship. The first is a multifactorial liability/threshold model with two thresholds representing a severe and mild form of disorder (Reich *et al.*, 1972). It is assumed that a variable termed 'liability to develop the disorder' is continuously distributed within the population, being determined by a large number of small factors. It is further postulated that the two forms of disorder occupy the same continuum of liability and differ quantitatively rather than qualitatively. Thus those individuals whose liability exceeds a certain threshold manifest the common or 'broad' form of illness, while those whose liability exceeds a second, more extreme threshold exhibit a less common, more severe, 'narrow' form of disorder. Relatives of affective probands will have an augmented mean liability compared with the general population, and this will be greater for the relatives of narrow-form probands than for the relatives of broad-form probands. Hence more relatives of narrow-form probands than broad-form probands will be affected (Fig. 9.1). In addition, the affected relatives of narrow-form probands will comprise a mixture of narrow- and broad-form cases, while the relatives of broad-form probands will predominantly have the broad form. Finally, the relations of narrow-form probands will have a greater risk of broad-form disorder than the relatives of broad-form probands.

In the second model, the two classes of disorder arise from relatively few factors, probably genes, and these are different for each condition. This means that relatives will tend to share the genes underlying the proband's particular form of disorder, and the conditions will therefore breed true and be independent of each other.

It is theoretically fairly simple to distinguish between these models. In the first case, relatives of narrow-form probands will be at higher risk for broad-form disorders, and at much higher risk for narrow-form disorders than relatives of broad-form probands. In the second model, relatives of narrow-form probands will be at high risk of narrow-form disorders, but their risk of broad-form disorders will be that of the general population.

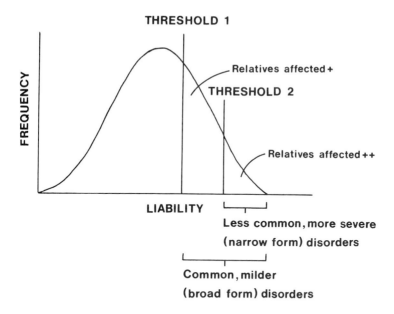

Fig. 9.1 *Threshold multifactorial (MF) model*

Relatives of broad-form probands will have a high risk of broad-form disorders, but the general population risk for narrow-form disorders.

This looks like a straightforward distinction, but it is made less clear by the possibility that intermediate models provide a better account of the data. In particular, it seems likely that a dual threshold model is underpinned by a few major factors (genes) and a range of minor factors (genes, social factors). This model is illustrated in Fig. 9.2 and gives intermediate predictions. One would expect the relatives of narrow-form probands to have a risk of broad-form conditions around that of relatives of broad-form probands—perhaps a little more or a little less, but greater than the general population risk.

The strategy of relating familiality to the severity of depressive illness is logically connected with that relating it to the degree of social provocation. This second approach ought in theory to be equally illuminating, but has again not been used to the full. The earliest hints about interactions between social and biological influences emerge from studies that were primarily genetic. Stenstedt (1952) suggested that those patients whose illnesses seemed related to obvious environmental factors had fewer family members affected than did those where there was no clear precipitant. An attempt to follow up this suggestion was reported by Pollitt (1972), who considered the roles of both familial diathesis and potential stresses together. He found that the morbid risk of depression among relatives of the depressed proband whose illness arose 'out of the blue' was higher, at about 21%, than when the proband's illness was 'justifiable', where the

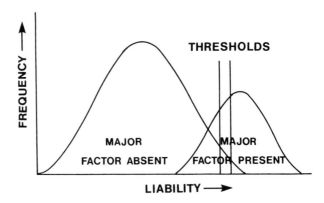

Fig. 9.2   *Interaction of major and minor factors accounting for illness*

morbid risk in relatives was between 6 and 12%. 'Justifiable' illnesses comprised those following either a severe physical stress or some psychological trauma.

THE CAMBERWELL DEPRESSION STUDY

Our own Camberwell Collaborative Depression Study was an attempt to examine the relationship between the form and severity of depressive conditions, their degree of social provocation, and the extent to which other family members were likely to suffer from similar conditions.

It comprised an investigation of 76 female and 54 male cases of recent onset depression, and of their first-degree relatives. The design and methods of the study are described in detail elsewhere (Bebbington *et al.*, 1988; McGuffin *et al.*, 1988a,b). The probands were sampled on the basis of an initial or renewed out-patient contact, although a substantial proportion had previous or subsequent in-patient treatment.

They were essentially cases of acute, uncomplicated, unipolar depression. Probands within the age range of 18 to 64 years were selected, who had no evidence of personality disorder or alcohol dependence but had experienced an acute onset of depression following a period free of disorder of at least six months. All patients from the Camberwell area of South London referred with a possible diagnosis of depression to the Bethlem and Maudsley Hospitals were screened, and those born of British or Irish parents were interviewed by one of two psychiatrists to establish their psychiatric status. Because of the somewhat stringent sampling criteria, it proved necessary to augment the male proband series with a small number of patients presenting at the Maudsley Hospital who were resident in areas adjacent to Camberwell.

The PSE (Wing *et al.*, 1974) was used to provide a cross-section of psychiatric symptoms during the past month. In addition, a natural history schedule covered longitudinal aspects, past episodes and dates of onset. Where preceding episodes of illness had occurred, ratings were carried out from hospital case notes using the Syndrome Checklist (SCL; Wing *et al.*, 1974). A hierarchical approach was adopted to combine CATEGO classes from multiple episodes (Wing and Sturt, 1978).

The Life Events and Difficulties Schedule (LEDS) of Brown and Harris (1978) was used by a separate interviewer to establish a history of adversity in the 6-month period before onset. Events and onset were carefully dated. Events were rated for threat, independence and focus, using the panel method of Brown and Harris (1978).

A proband's family was considered 'in scope' for the study once the second interview with the proband had been completed. An attempt was made to interview personally all available first-degree relatives, as well as their spouses where the couple had children aged 18 years or older.

The current mental state was again established through the PSE. However, the focus of interest in relatives is not just on their current state, but on their lifelong experience of illness. We therefore augmented the conventional PSE with a PHS (McGuffin *et al.*, 1986) designed to elicit previous episodes of depression and other psychiatric disorders, and to identify the most severe episode. The PHS effectively replaces the first question of the conventional PSE, and each subsequent obligatory PSE question is asked concerning 'lifetime ever' occurrence and the worst episode, as well as the past month in the conventional way. This approach has been shown to afford good inter-rater reliability, and good agreement between interview-derived CATEGO classification of past episodes and CATEGO classes derived from rating of hospital case records (McGuffin *et al.*, 1986). The current mental state was again established through the PSE.

The LEDS was again used to derive a 6-month history of life events, before onset in current cases, before interview for current non-cases, and before datable past episodes. A detailed family history of psychiatric and physical illnesses was taken from each informant, using a semi-structured format. Where inconsistencies arose between informants, an attempt was made to resolve these and to arrive at a consensus. Where there was a history of hospital treatment or treatment by a family practitioner for psychiatric symptoms, copies of summaries of the medical case notes were obtained. Such records were rated using the SCL by a rater blind to the interview information.

In addition to providing CATEGO classes equivalent to the ICD classification, PSE data can be represented by summary measures of severity. The first is the total PSE symptom score, the second is the Index of Definition (ID; Wing *et al.*, 1978). The latter is essentially a symptom score weighted in favour of certain symptoms of diagnostic significance.

We were thus able to draw on a number of indications of severity in the probands. First is the CATEGO class. The division between CATEGO classes R and D and CATEGO classes N and A corresponds to one concept of severity: the R and D classes are associated with the presence of symptoms that are more 'endogenous', and disorders of this type can be regarded as being further from the pattern of normal distress. However, it is possible to come across cases in CATEGO classes N and A that must be regarded as severe in the light of the large numbers of symptoms they display. It is therefore appropriate to employ the overall symptom score as a complementary measure of severity. While correlating with the CATEGO class, this is not completely predicted by it. The measure of severity afforded by the ID shares aspects of the categorical and the dimensional approaches, as symptoms used to define categories are given added weight in the establishment of ID levels. We did not use a measure of social disability, and were thus unable to determine severity in that particular manner. In this chapter, we describe results based only on the CATEGO class of the probands, although in future publications we will analyse our data in terms of the other measures of severity available to us.

The decision concerning measures of severity in the relatives was not self-evident. We would have preferred to use equivalent measures in probands and relatives, but there was particular doubt about the continuous measures in relatives. We felt we could place little reliance on symptom scores relating to episodes long past. We did use the conventional ID level of 5 or greater to indicate current illness in relatives. However, a simpler, but narrower and possibly more robust, measure of the severity of 'lifetime ever' disorder will be adopted in this report. Thus, relatives who have ever had an episode of illness falling into a CATEGO depression category (N, D or R) were classified as cases if the episode had resulted in psychiatric referral. They were placed in a 'severe' category if they had been treated as in-patients, and in a 'moderate' category if they had received only out-patient treatment.

The affective status of relatives will be presented below in a variety of different ways. We will consider both current illness and lifetime prevalence of illness (i.e. including any illness that has occurred up to and including the present). Frequency of illness among relatives will also be expressed as morbid risk to age 65. We will adopt an approach which is a modification of the method of Strömgren. The age of onset distribution of depression in the probands was transformed to normality by taking the natural logarithm. The log age for each relative was then converted to a 'standard score', and weights (the proportion of the period of risk lived through by unaffected relatives) were then obtained by direct reference to the standard normal integral.

Out of a total of 130 potential probands, 124 completed their second interview and their families were therefore deemed 'in scope' for a family interview study. Twenty-four probands refused permission for their families to be contacted, six had no known living biological relatives, and in nine families all relatives refused to be interviewed. This left a total of 83 families available for interview. However, as described elsewhere (McGuffin *et al.*, 1988a), cooperative probands with cooperating family members did not differ significantly in terms of age, sex, socioeconomic status or CATEGO class from non-cooperative probands.

A total of 244 out of 315 first-degree relatives (77%) were personally interviewed, and for the remaining 71 historical information was obtained from the proband and at least one other first-degree relative. In addition, we were able to obtain case notes, hospital summaries and/or letters from treating psychiatrists for 47 out of 49 relatives (96%) who had at some time received hospital treatment for psychiatric disorders.

Principal findings

In Table 9.1, we present familiality in relation to the form of the proband's illness. When familiality is defined as affective illness in the relative requiring hospital treatment, there is a clear difference between probands suffering from disorders in categories R and D and those with disorders in categories N and A. The morbid risk of such disorder in the relatives of probands in the first category is 15.2%, over twice that in the relatives of the remaining probands.

The picture changes when the definition of relatives' disorders is broadened to include those occasioning any hospital treatment. There is now no difference between the proband groups. This indicates that the relatives of probands in our 'endogenous' categories have a greater morbid risk for severe disorders but a smaller one for mild disorders than those of probands in 'neurotic' categories.

Our findings concerning adversity and familiality were also contrary to expectation. We were unable to show an inverse relationship between antecedent stress in the proband and familial diathesis in terms of frequency of depression in first-degree relatives. Indeed, the morbid risk in relatives for depression of moderate severity and above was slightly higher where the proband had experienced life events or chronic difficulties in the 3-month period before the onset of depression. The highest lifetime prevalence of depression was found in the relatives of probands who had experienced both life events and chronic difficulties preceding the onset of their disorder, but neither difference between the groups of relatives classified according to these proband characteristics proved to be significant (McGuffin *et al.*, 1988b). These findings cannot be regarded as completely contradictory to those of Pollitt (1972) because the majority of precipitants of disorder in Pollitt's 'justifiable' group of depressed probands consisted of infections or other physical stressors. In our series, none of the 83 probands appears to have important physical factors contributing to the onset of the depression. Nevertheless, our results do present a serious challenge to the division of depression into familial/non-reactive and non-familial/reactive categories. This corresponds to our inability to demonstrate a difference in the association of life events with onsets of

Table 9.1 Proband illness type and relatives' morbid risk

Proband's worst ever diagnosis	Definition of relative's illness	N of relatives affected	BZ	Morbid risk (%)	r (±SE)
A + N +	In-patient treatment only	5	73.7	6.8	0.21 ± 0.13
	Any hospital treatment	18	77.7	23.1	0.36 ± 0.10
R + D +	In-patient treatment only	17	111.5	15.2	0.43 ± 0.08
	Any hospital treatment	31	119.6	25.9	0.41 ± 0.07

BZ = age corrected denominator calculated by modified Strömgren method
r = correlation in liability
SE = standard error

'endogenous' or 'neurotic' patterns of depression (Bebbington *et al.*, 1988).

To examine the relationship between familiality of depression and life events in greater detail, we compared the personally interviewed, first-degree relatives with a representative sample from the community from whom data had been collected using virtually identical methods of assessment (Bebbington *et al.*, 1981). These findings are briefly summarized in Table 9.2. There are three main points to note. First, as we have already observed, current cases were significantly more frequent among first-degree relatives than in the community. Second, the association between recent life events and current disorder in the community sample is marked and striking, whereas in first-degree relatives the association is weak. Third, we have found that not only does current illness appear to aggregate in families, but so also do recent life events. The increased rate of life events among first-degree relatives compared with the community sample is highly significant and remains so even when all potentially confounding proband-related events are removed. Furthermore, when we plotted life events over time in the relative sample (McGuffin *et al.*, 1988b), we did not find a peak of life events in close proximity to the proband's onset of illness. It therefore seems unlikely that the high rate of events (all of which were judged to be 'independent' or 'possibly independent' by our panel of raters) was associated either with the turmoil created by the onset of the proband's disorder or by certain life events that impinged both upon the proband and other family members. A logistic regression analysis, taking current disorder as the response variable, showed that both the experience of life events and being a first-degree relative had significant effects, but there was also a highly significant interaction between the effects of life events and family loading. This was because, as we have already indicated, the effect of recent life events on current illness is large in the general population but small for those who are a first-degree relative of a depressed proband.

Table 9.2 Life events and current disorder in first-degree relatives and community control cases—proband-related events excluded

	% Community sample (N = 289)	% Relatives (N = 244)
With recent life events	7.3	28.7
Cases among subjects with recent life events	57.1	21.4
Cases among subjects without recent life events	7.5	14.8
Total cases	11.1	17.2

Interpretation of findings

Our findings show only a small and non-significant inverse relationship between presence of adversity before onset of depression and family loading. They thus run counter to the (meagre) findings in the existing record. Nevertheless, we feel that they must be accorded considerable credence in view of the sophisticated techniques on which they are based. They are particularly interesting in the light of our earlier discussion of threshold liability models, as they are exactly what would be expected under the model presented in Fig. 9.2. It will be remembered that this model illustrates a dual threshold deriving from the influence of a few major factors, probably genetic, and many minor factors that are likely to be both genetic and social. It leads to the prediction that the relatives of narrow-form probands will have much more in the way of narrow-form disorder than broad-form relatives but a roughly equivalent risk of broad-form disorders. This is borne out by the data in Table 9.1, which suggest that the risk of broad-form disorders (represented by treatment for depression not as an in-patient) is actually less in the relatives of narrow-form than of broad-form probands, although still quite high. If the model in Fig. 9.2 is indeed the appropriate one, it would predict the absence of a relationship between overall familiality and severity. We will explore this in later publications.

The findings concerning the relationship of adversity and familiality are also extremely complex and require careful interpretation. Our simple starting hypothesis was that both family loading and threatening life events have a causal relationship with depression and that there would be an inverse relationship between the two. However, we are obliged to reject this. We might, therefore, consider alternative and more radical hypotheses—for example, that a common familial factor predisposes both to depression and to a propensity to experience (or report) life events. Similar results are reported by Kendler and colleagues in Chapter 10. It could be tempting to speculate that the association between life events and depression, which has been repeatedly observed in community studies, is a spurious one induced by the fact that both affective illness and tendency to experience life events are caused by the same familial factor. However, this does not fit well with our finding based on the proband sample alone, where there is a clear temporal relationship between life events and subsequent onsets of depression.

We are left with the conclusion that the tendency to experience (or to report) life events and the tendency to experience depressive symptoms are both familial. These tendencies appear to be inextricably bound up with each other, so that given our present data, no simple model readily explains the relationship. One obvious, familial, explanatory variable might be social class. However, not only is there a lack of relationship between depression and social class in our data but there is a lack of relationship between frequency of adversity and social class. We are currently exploring the relationship between life events, depression and personality (including cognitive factors and attributional style). However, preliminary results (Katz and McGuffin, 1987) do not suggest a relationship between propensity to experience life events and conventional dimensions such as those measured on the Eysenck Personality Questionnaire (Eysenck and Eysenck, 1975).

REFERENCES

American Psychiatric Association (1987). *DSM-IIIR: Diagnostic and Statistical Manual of Mental Disorders* (revised). Washington DC: APA.

Bebbington P. E. (1987). Misery and beyond: the pursuit of disease theories of depression. *International Journal of Social Psychiatry*; **33**: 13–20.

Bebbington P. E. (1990). Population surveys of psychiatric disorder and the need for treatment. *Social Psychiatry and Psychiatric Epidemiology*; **25**: 33–40.

Bebbington P. E., Brugha T., MacCarthy B. *et al.* (1988). The Camberwell Collaborative Depression Study. I. Depressed probands: adversity and the form of depression. *British Journal of Psychiatry*; **152**: 754–65.

Bebbington P., Hurry J., Tennant C. *et al.* (1981). The epidemiology of mental disorders in Camberwell. *Psychological Medicine*; **11**: 561–80.

Bebbington P. E., Katz R., McGuffin P. *et al.* (1989). The risk of minor depression before age 65: results from a community survey. *Psychological Medicine*; **19**: 393–400.

Bertelsen A., Harvald B., Hauge M. (1977). A Danish twin study of manic-depressive disorders. *British Journal of Psychiatry*; **130**: 330–51.

Bromet E. J., Dunn L. O., Connell M. O. *et al.* (1986). Long-term reliability of diagnosing lifetime major depression in a community sample. *Archives of General Psychiatry*; **43**: 435–40.

Brown G. W., Harris T. O. (1978b). *Social Origins of Depression*. London: Tavistock.

Endicott J., Spitzer R. (1978). A diagnostic interview: the schedule for affective disorders and schizophrenia. *Archives of General Psychiatry*; **35**: 837–44.

Eysenck H. J., Eysenck S. B. G. (1975). *Manual of the Eysenck Personality Inventory*. London: Hodder and Stoughton.

Farmer A., Katz R., McGuffin P., Bebbington P. E. (1987). A comparison between the Present State Examination (PSE) and the Composite International Diagnostic Interview (CIDI). *Archives of General Psychiatry*; **44**: 1064–8.

Gershon E. S., Bunney W. E., Leckman J. F. *et al.* (1976). The inheritance of affective disorders: a review of data and hypotheses. *Behaviour Genetics*; **6**: 226–71.

Gershon E., Hamovit J. H., Guroff J. J., Nurnberger J. I. (1987). Birth cohort changes in manic and depressive disorders in relatives of bipolar and schizoaffective patients. *Archives of General Psychiatry*; **44**: 314–19.

Hasin D., Link B. (1988). Age and recognition of depression: implications for a cohort effect in major depression. *Psychological Medicine*; **18**: 683–8.

Katz R., McGuffin P. (1987). Neuroticism in familial depression. *Psychological Medicine*; **17**: 155–62.

Klerman G. L. (1988). The current age of youthful melancholia: evidence for increase in depression among adolescents and young adults. *British Journal of Psychiatry*; **152**: 4–14.

Klerman G. L., Lavori P. W., Rice J. *et al.* (1985). Birth-cohort trends in rates of major depressive disorder among relatives of patients with affective disorder. *Archives of General Psychiatry*; **421**: 689–93.

Lavori P. W., Klerman G. L., Keller M. B. *et al.* (1987). Age–period–cohort analysis of secular trends in onset of major depression: findings in siblings of patients with major affective disorder. *Journal of Psychiatric Research*; **21**: 23–35.

McGuffin P., Katz R. (1986). Nature, nurture and affective disorders. In: *Recent Advances in the Biology of Affective Disorders* (Deakin J. F. W., Freeman H., eds.). British Journal of Psychiatry Special Publication. Ashford: Headley Bros.

McGuffin P., Katz R. (1989). The genetics of depression and manic depressive disorder. *British Journal of Psychiatry*; **55**: 294–304.

McGuffin P., Katz R., Aldrich J. (1986). Past and Present State Examination: the assessment of 'lifetime ever' psychopathology. *Psychological Medicine*; **16**: 461–6.

McGuffin P., Katz R., Aldrich J., Bebbington P. E. (1988a). The Camberwell Collaborative Depression Study. II. The investigation of family members. *British Journal of Psychiatry*; **152**: 766–74.

McGuffin P., Katz R., Bebbington P. E. (1988b). The Camberwell Collaborative Depression Study. III. Depression and adversity in the relatives of depressed probands. *British Journal of Psychiatry*; **152**: 775–82.

Perris C., Perris M., Ericsson U., von Knorring L. (1982). The genetics of depression: a family study of unipolar and neurotic-reactive depressed patients. *Archiv für Psychiatrie und Nervenkrankheit*; **232**: 137–55.

Pollitt J. (1972). The relationship between genetic and precipitating factors in depressive illness. *British Journal of Psychiatry*; **121**: 67–70.

Reich T., James J. W., Morris C. A. (1972). The use of multiple thresholds in determining the mode of transmission of semicontinuous traits. *Annals of Human Genetics*; **36**: 163–84.

Robins L. N., Helzer J. E., Croughan J. L., Ratcliff K. (1981). The NIMH Diagnostic Interview Schedule: Its history, characteristics and validity. In: *What is Case? The Problem of Definition in Psychiatric Community Surveys* (Wing J. K., Bebbington P., Robins L. N., eds.). London: Grant McIntyre.

Shapiro R. W. (1970). A twin study of non-endogenous depression. *Acta Jutlandica XLII* (publication of the University of Aarhus).

Slater E., Shields J. (1969). Genetical aspects of anxiety. In: *Studies of Anxiety* (Lader M. H., ed.). *British Journal of Psychiatry* Special Publication No. 3. Ashford: Headley Bros.

Stenstedt A. (1952). A study in manic depressive psychosis: clinical, social and genetic investigations. *Acta Psychiatrica Scandinavia Supplementum*; **79**.

Stenstedt A. (1966). Genetics of neurotic depression. *Acta Psychiatrica Scandinavica*; **42**: 392–409.

Sturt E. S., Kumakura N., Der G. (1984). How depressing life is: lifelong risk of depression in the general population. *Journal of Affective Disorders*; **7**: 109–22.

Torgersen S. (1986). Genetic factors in moderately severe and mild affective disorders. *Archives of General Psychiatry*; **43**: 222–6.

Wing J. K., Morris B. (1981). *Handbook of Psychiatric Rehabilitation Practice.* Oxford : Oxford University Press.

Wing J. K., Sturt E. (1978). *The PSE-ID-CATEGO System: A Supplementary Manual.* London: Institute of Psychiatry.

Wing J. K., Cooper J. E., Sartorius N. (1974). *The Measurement and Classification of Psychiatric Symptoms.* Cambridge: Cambridge University Press.

Wing J. K., Mann S. A., Leff J. P., Nixon J. M. (1978). The concept of a case in psychiatric population surveys. *Psychological Medicine*; 8: 203–17.

World Health Organization (1978). *Mental Disorders: Glossary and Guide to their Classification in accordance with the Ninth Revision of the International Classification of Diseases.* Geneva: WHO.

10 Life events and depressive symptoms: a twin study perspective

KENNETH S. KENDLER, MICHAEL C. NEALE,
ANDREW C. HEATH, RONALD C. KESSLER AND
LINDON J. EAVES

INTRODUCTION

Traditionally, causal explanations for depression have tended to emphasize *either* sociogenic/environmental *or* biologic/genetic factors. In the last two decades, however, increasingly rigorous studies have shown that both of these sets of risk factors are important. A more complete understanding of the aetiology of this condition is unlikely to occur without the consideration of both sets and, in particular, an examination of how they interact in the causal 'pathway' leading to depression.

In 1985, we began a longitudinal study of over 1000 pairs of unselected female twins from the Virginia Twin Registry with the specific goal of clarifying the interrelationship of genetic and environmental risk factors in the aetiology of the common psychiatric disorders in females: depression, anxiety (including generalized anxiety disorder, panic disorder and phobias), eating disorders and alcoholism. In this chapter, we examine results from the first wave of contact with the twins by mailed questionnaire. We will explore, using twin data analysed by structural equation modelling, the interrelationship between reported life events and levels of depressive symptomatology. In particular, we will attempt to answer two specific questions as follows.

1. To what extent are reported life events influenced by familial/ environmental and/or genetic factors, and does this influence change as a function of the degree to which the life event may be dependent or independent of the respondent's own behaviour?

2. Will the proportion of variance in depressive symptoms explained by genetic and/or familial environmental factors change as a function of the exposure to life events? In particular, will we see that genetic and/or familial environmental factors become more important given high versus low levels of exposure to stressful life events?

METHODS

This report is based on completed, mailed questionnaires returned from 824, female, same-sex, twin pairs, born on or after 1 January 1935, ascertained from the population-based, Virginia Twin Registry. Zygosity was determined by an algorithm incorporating self-report information on (i) physical similarity in childhood, (ii) similarity of physical features, and (iii) the frequency with which the twins were mistaken for one another as children. Such methods, when validated against blood typing, have been found to be over 95% accurate (see, for example, Kasriel and Eaves, 1976). In a subset of these twins, this information was supplemented by the review of photographs taken during the second wave of contact, which consisted of an extensive face-to-face interview. By this algorithm, 461 pairs were considered to be monozygotic (MZ) and 363 pairs were dizygotic (DZ). The age distribution of the twins is shown in Table 10.1.

Depressive symptoms were measured by the 20-item, Center for Epidemiologic Studies Depression Scale (CES-D; Radloff, 1977). Instructions to this scale request that the respondent report the level of depressive symptomatology experienced over the last week. The distribution of CES-D scores was highly positively skewed. As our methods of analysis assume normality, we examined several possible transformations of the CES-D score. The square-root transformation produced the most normal distribution, as assessed by measures of skewness and kurtosis, and was thus used for all subsequent analyses.

Undesirable life events were assessed by a self-report check-list adapted from the PERI Life Event Scale (Dohrenwend *et al.*, 1978). Respondents were asked to report life events experienced in the last year. A life-event score was obtained by summing the number of life events that the respondent endorsed. This distribution was also skewed and was approximately normalized by a $\log(x+1)$ transformation. The life-event inven-

Table 10.1 Distribution of matched twin pairs by year of birth

Year of birth	All twin pairs		MZ twin pairs		DZ twin pairs	
	N	%	N	%	N	%
1936–1941	17	2.0	11	2.4	6	1.6
1942–1946	57	6.9	27	5.9	30	8.3
1947–1951	125	15.2	55	11.9	70	19.3
1952–1956	148	18.0	92	20.0	56	15.4
1957–1961	163	19.8	85	18.4	78	21.5
1962–1966	186	22.6	112	24.3	74	20.4
1967–1971	128	15.5	79	17.1	49	13.5
TOTAL	824		461		363	

tory was heterogeneous with regard to two critical dimensions for our analysis. First, the life events differed in the degree to which they would, *a priori*, be expected to be shared by members of a twin pair. The total inventory, which consisted of 59 items, contained 15 items in which respondents were asked about stressful life events occurring in their co-twins. Nine further items described stressful life events that would obviously be shared by members of a twin pair: death, serious illness or serious personal crisis in parents, siblings or other relatives. For this report, we therefore analysed the full, 59-item inventory (in which stressful life events in the co-twin are treated as 'network' events for the respondent), a 44-item inventory (which eliminates the questions about stressful life events in the co-twin), and a 34-item inventory (which, in addition, eliminates the nine items about family members that would also be expected to be shared by the twins, plus an item that describes problems 'getting along with your twin').

Second, we also, before data analysis, categorized specific events from the 44-item inventory by the degree to which they may depend on the behaviour of the respondent. All the events were categorized into dependent ($n = 14$) e.g. serious marital problems, serious difficulties at work), possibly independent ($n = 9$) (e.g. laid off or fired from job, living in a bad neighbourhood) and independent ($n = 19$) (e.g. burglarized or robbed, death or serious personal injury of spouse, child, etc.). Two items, which were not easily classified in this regard, were excluded from these analyses.

Quantitative genetic modelling was done with the computer program LISREL (Joreskog and Sorbom, 1986), fitted to variance-covariance matrices, one each for MZ and DZ twins. These models have six degrees of freedom, with two variances (for twin 1 and twin 2) and one covariance for each zygosity. For the individual phenotype in question, we sought to divide the total variance into three components: specific environment, e^2 (i.e. environmental exposure not shared by members of a twin pair), common environment, c^2 (i.e. environmental experiences shared by members of a twin pair, which is assumed to be equal in MZ and DZ twins), and heritability or additive genetic effects, h^2. We were interested in comparing the fit of the three models: the full (or E,H,C) model, which incorporates specific, common environment and additive genetic variance; the E,H model, which assumes that additive genetic variance is the only source of twin resemblance; and the E,C model, which assumes that familial environment is the only source of twin resemblance. These models all assume the absence of non-additive genetic variance and assortative mating. Individual models were fitted by the method of maximum likelihood. The goodness-of-fit of a full model was assessed by a χ^2 goodness-of-fit test. The fit of subsidiary models was assessed by a likelihood ratio χ^2 test in which the degree of freedom equals the difference between the number of parameters in the full and the subsidiary model.

In addition to these standard, additive, univariate twin models, we also tested for the presence of genotype $\times$ specific environment and/or common environment × specific environment interaction for CES-D scores, as outlined by Heath *et al.* (1989) (see Fig. 10.1). Twin pairs were divided into three categories: those concordant for exposure to high levels of stressful life events, those concordant for exposure to low levels of stressful life events, and those discordant for exposure to levels of stress (in which one twin was exposed to high levels and the other twin to low levels of stressful life events). For these analyses, high and low levels of stressful life events were defined by a median split. These analyses, also done with LISREL, require as input six variance-covariance matrices: concordant exposed, concordant unexposed and discordant pairs, separately for MZ and DZ twins.

We proceeded with the analysis of this model in two steps. First, we estimated values for r_g and r_c that measure the degree to which the genetic and/or common environmental factors that influence symptoms of depression are the same in high- versus low-stress environments (see Fig. 10.1). Second, we examined whether the variance in CES-D scores accounted for by genetic and/or common environmental factors differs in exposed (or high-stress environments) versus unexposed (or low-stress environments). *Per* Heath *et al.* (1989) and Fig. 10.1, for exposed twins, we use the same symbols as above (E, H, C and e^2, h^2 and c^2), while for unexposed twins a (′) is added to the symbols (e.g. E′, H′, C′ and e'^2, h'^2 and c'^2).

RESULTS

Life events

Analysis of 59-, 44- and 34-item, life-event inventories

The results of model fitting to our full, 59-item, life-event inventories are given in Table 10.2. We found very high correlations in both MZ (+ 0.507) and DZ twins (+ 0.465). The full E,H,C model fitted well ($\chi^2 = 1.32$, d.f. = 3) and produced estimates for c^2 (0.438) that were much higher than for h^2 (0.064). The E,H model could be strongly rejected (likelihood ratio test: d.f. = 1, $\chi^2 = 21.90$), indicating that twin resemblance for the reporting of life events could not be explained solely by genetic factors. By contrast, the E,C model provided a good fit, with an estimate of c^2 (+ 0.488), which was quite similar to that found with the full model.

Results with the 44-item scale, which eliminated 15 items covering events in the co-twin, are shown in Table 10.3. As might be expected, the correlations, although still high, were somewhat lower in both zygosity groups: MZ, + 0.409; DZ, + 0.323. The full E,H,C model produced a good fit ($\chi^2 = 1.26$, d.f. = 3) and gave estimates for c^2 (0.238) that were higher than for h^2 (0.170). The E,H model could be rejected (likelihood ratio test: d.f. = 1, $\chi^2 = 5.49$), indicating that twin resemblance for the reporting of life events could not be explained solely by genetic factors. By contrast, the E,C model provided a good fit, with an estimate of c^2 of 0.371.

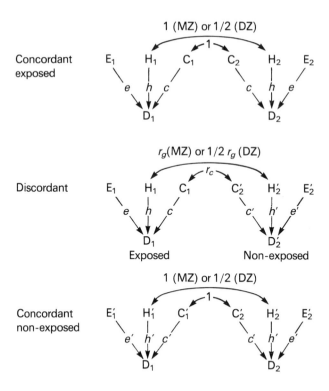

Fig. 10.1 *Path 'interaction' model in which pairs, separately for MZ and DZ twins, are divided into three groups: concordant for exposure (in this case defined as reporting above the median number of life events), discordant for exposure and concordant for non-exposure (defined as reporting the median number or less of life events). r_g and r_c refer, respectively, to the correlation in genetic and common environmental factors influencing depression scores (D) in exposed and unexposed individuals; e, h, c refer, respectively, to the paths from individual specific environment (E), additive genes (H) and common environment (C) to depression scores. Subscripts $_1$ and $_2$ refer to twin 1 and twin 2 in a pair. The prime symbol (') refers to the non-exposed condition, while the absence of a prime refers to the exposed condition*

Analysis of the 34-item, life-event scale, which eliminated death, serious illness or serious personal crises to family members common to both twins, produced results quite similar to those for the 44-item scale (Table 10.4). As might be expected, estimates for c^2 for the E,C model were slightly lower than with the 44-item scale (0.344).

Analysis of dependent, probably independent and independent life events

The results of the analysis of life events judged *a priori* as likely to be dependent on the respondent's own behaviour are given in Table 10.5. MZ and DZ twin correlations for the transformed life-event scores were $+0.315$ and $+0.220$, respectively. The E,H,C model fitted well ($\chi^2 = 0.79$,

Table 10.2 Total life events—59 variables—transformed by log $(x + 1)$

Model	Chi square	d.f.	p
(1) E,H,C	1.32	3	0.724
(2) E,H	23.22	4	0.000
(3) E,C	1.76	4	0.781

Model 1	Model 2	Model 3
$e^2 = 0.498$	$e^2 = 0.464$	$e^2 = 0.512$
$h^2 = 0.064$	$h^2 = 0.536$	$h^2 = 0.000$
$c^2 = 0.438$	$c^2 = 0.000$	$c^2 = 0.488$

MZ correlation matrix (n = 461)		· DZ correlation matrix (n = 363)	
1.000	0.507	1.000	0.465
0.507	1.000	0.465	1.000

e^2, proportion of variance due to individual specific environment.
h^2, proportion of variance due to additive genetic effects.
c^2, proportion of variance due to familial environment.

Table 10.3 Total life events—44 variables—transformed by log $(x + 1)$

Model	Chi square	d.f.	p
(1) E,H,C	1.26	3	0.739
(2) E,H	6.75	4	0.149
(3) E,C	3.47	4	0.482

Model 1	Model 2	Model 3
$e^2 = 0.592$	$e^2 = 0.566$	$e^2 = 0.629$
$h^2 = 0.170$	$h^2 = 0.434$	$h^2 = 0.000$
$c^2 = 0.238$	$c^2 = 0.000$	$c^2 = 0.371$

MZ correlation matrix (n = 461)		DZ correlation matrix (n = 363)	
1.000	0.409	1.000	0.323
0.409	1.000	0.323	1.000

e^2, proportion of variance due to individual specific environment.
h^2, proportion of variance due to additive genetic effects.
c^2, proportion of variance due to familial environment.

Table 10.4 Total life events—34 variables—transformed by log $(x+1)$

Model	Chi square	d.f.	p
(1) E,H,C	0.85	3	0.836
(2) E,H	5.48	4	0.242
(3) E,C	2.69	4	0.611

Model 1	Model 2	Model 3
$e^2 = 0.621$	$e^2 = 0.595$	$e^2 = 0.656$
$h^2 = 0.159$	$h^2 = 0.405$	$h^2 = 0.000$
$c^2 = 0.220$	$c^2 = 0.000$	$c^2 = 0.344$

MZ correlation matrix $(n=461)$		DZ correlation matrix $(n=363)$	
1.000	0.377	1.000	0.303
0.377	1.000	0.303	1.000

e^2, proportion of variance due to individual specific environment.
h^2, proportion of variance due to additive genetic effects.
c^2, proportion of variance due to familial environment.

Table 10.5 Dependent life events—transformed by log $(x+1)$

Model	Chi square	d.f.	p
(1) E,H,C	0.79	3	0.853
(2) E,H	1.96	4	0.743
(3) E,C	3.40	4	0.493

Model 1	Model 2	Model 3
$e^2 = 0.682$	$e^2 = 0.666$	$e^2 = 0.728$
$h^2 = 0.203$	$h^2 = 0.334$	$h^2 = 0.000$
$c^2 = 0.115$	$c^2 = 0.000$	$c^2 = 0.272$

MZ correlation matrix $(n=461)$		DZ correlation matrix $(n=363)$	
1.000	0.315	1.000	0.220
0.315	1.000	0.220	1.000

e^2, proportion of variance due to individual specific environment.
h^2, proportion of variance due to additive genetic effects.
c^2, proportion of variance due to familial environment.

d.f. = 3) and, in contrast to the results with the entire scale, produced estimates for h^2 (0.203) that exceeded the estimates for c^2 (0.115). Neither the E,H nor the E,C models could be rejected, indicating that we could not reject models in which the sole source of resemblance in reported dependent life events in twins were genetic or familial environmental factors.

The analysis of life events judged to be probably independent of the respondent's behaviour are shown in Table 10.6. The MZ and DZ twin correlations were +0.291 and +0.225, respectively. The major difference between these results and those for dependent life events is that, with the full model, the estimates for c^2 were slightly higher (0.137) and the estimates for h^2 were slightly lower (0.161). Otherwise, the general pattern of findings was the same.

By contrast, the results were quite different for the events judged highly likely to be independent of the respondent's behaviour (Table 10.7). The correlations in MZ and DZ twins were higher and more similar than those found with the previous categories: +0.387 and +0.347, respectively. The full (E,H,C) model fitted well ($\chi^2 = 3.72$, d.f. = 3) and produced estimates of c^2 (0.272) that now substantially exceeded those for h^2 (0.126). More significantly, the E,H model could now be rejected against the full model (likelihood ratio test: $\chi^2 = 7.61$, d.f. = 1), indicating that genes could not be the only source of twin resemblance for this category of life events. The E,C model could not, however, be rejected, and produced a substantial estimate for c^2 (0.368). Because death, illness and serious personal crisis in

Table 10.6 Probably independent life events—transformed by $\log (x + 1)$

Model	Chi square	d.f.	p
(1) E,H,C	4.67	3	0.198
(2) E,H	6.36	4	0.174
(3) E,C	6.30	4	0.178

Model 1	Model 2	Model 3
$e^2 = 0.702$	$e^2 = 0.681$	$e^2 = 0.740$
$h^2 = 0.161$	$h^2 = 0.319$	$h^2 = 0.000$
$c^2 = 0.137$	$c^2 = 0.000$	$c^2 = 0.260$

MZ correlation matrix ($n = 461$)		DZ correlation matrix ($n = 363$)	
1.000	0.291	1.000	0.225
0.291	1.000	0.225	1.000

e^2, proportion of variance due to individual specific environment.
h^2, proportion of variance due to additive genetic effects.
c^2, proportion of variance due to familial environment.

Table 10.7 Independent life events—transformed by log $(x+1)$

Model	Chi square	d.f.	p
(1) E,H,C	3.72	3	0.293
(2) E,H	11.33	4	0.023
(3) E,C	4.96	4	0.292

Model 1	Model 2	Model 3
$e^2 = 0.602$	$e^2 = 0.569$	$e^2 = 0.632$
$h^2 = 0.126$	$h^2 = 0.431$	$h^2 = 0.000$
$c^2 = 0.272$	$c^2 = 0.000$	$c^2 = 0.368$

MZ correlation matrix $(n=461)$		DZ correlation matrix $(n=363)$	
1.000	0.387	1.000	0.347
0.387	1.000	0.347	1.000

e^2, proportion of variance due to individual specific environment.
h^2, proportion of variance due to additive genetic effects.
c^2, proportion of variance due to familial environment.

parents and siblings were classified as independent events and would obviously be shared by both members of a twin pair, we also analysed a reduced list of independent life events, eliminating these events in first-degree relatives. The results (available on request) did not differ substantially for those found with the full list of independent events. For example, the MZ and DZ twin correlations were quite similar in value: $+0.359$ and $+0.352$, respectively.

The results of the full model for each of these analyses are summarized in Table 10.8. Two trends appear clearly. The more likely life events are to be dependent on the respondent's own behaviour, the greater the role for genetic effects. The more likely life events are to be independent of the respondent's own behaviour, the greater is the apparent role for familial/environmental effects.

Because the frequency of life events may change substantially over the life span, it was of interest to fit the above models while including age as a specific parameter (Heath *et al.*, 1989). As age is always the same for members of a twin pair, a strong age effect will inflate estimates of the familial environment. The results of these models indicated that the age effect on life events was quite modest; its inclusion produced only trivial decrements in the estimates of c^2.

CES-D

Table 10.9 shows the outcome of model fitting applied to the transformed

Table 10.8 Sources of variability in life events: estimates from best model

Life-event category	e^2	h^2	c^2
Dependent	0.682	0.203	0.115
Probably independent	0.702	0.161	0.137
Independent (Total)	0.632	0	0.368
Independent (Reduced)	0.645	0	0.355

e^2, proportion of variance due to individual specific environment.
h^2, proportion of variance due to additive genetic effects.
c^2, proportion of variance due to familial environment.

CES-D scores. The correlation in MZ twins ($+0.319$) only modestly exceeded that in DZ twins ($+0.247$). The full E,H,C model fitted very well ($\chi^2 = 0.72$, d.f. $= 3$) and produced estimates of $e^2 = 0.680$, $c^2 = 0.173$ and $h^2 = 0.147$. The deterioration in fit was not significant, by a likelihood ratio test, when either H or C was eliminated from the model.

Interaction models for levels of depressive symptoms

As outlined in Methods above, these models test for the presence of interactions between levels of reported life events and either genetic or common environmental factors (Fig. 10.1). We had defined 'exposed =

Table 10.9 Scaled depression score by CES-D—transformed by SQRT(x)

Model	Chi square	d.f.	p
(1) E,H,C	0.72	3	0.869
(2) E,H	3.35	4	0.502
(3) E,C	2.10	4	0.717

Model 1	Model 2	Model 3
$e^2 = 0.680$	$e^2 = 0.658$	$e^2 = 0.713$
$h^2 = 0.147$	$h^2 = 0.342$	$h^2 = 0.000$
$c^2 = 0.173$	$c^2 = 0.000$	$c^2 = 0.287$

MZ correlation matrix ($n = 457$)		DZ correlation matrix ($n = 360$)	
1.000	0.319	1.000	0.247
0.319	1.000	0.247	1.000

e^2, proportion of variance due to individual specific environment.
h^2, proportion of variance due to additive genetic effects.
c^2, proportion of variance due to familial environment.

high stress' as reporting more than the median number of life events, while 'unexposed = low stress' (noted by a [']) was defined as reporting the number of life events equal to or lower than the median value.

Do the same genes and common environment influence depression under low and high levels of stress?

Our first task in fitting these interaction models was to determine whether r_g and r_c differed significantly from unity. To test this, we fitted a series of models allowing one or both of these two correlations to take their maximum likelihood value versus fixing one or both to unity. We fitted these models to the twin data, subdivided by the 59-, 40- and 34-item, life-event inventories, as well as by life events classified as dependent, probably independent and independent. In none of these models was there a significant deterioration in fit when r_g and r_c were set to unity (results available on request). That is, we could not reject the hypothesis that the same genetic and common environmental factors influenced levels of reported depressive symptoms in individuals exposed versus non-exposed to high levels of environmental stress. All subsequent analyses fixed the values of r_g and r_c to one.

Does the magnitude of genetic and common environmental effects on depression differ in low- and high-stress environments?

Table 10.10 presents the results of model fitting using the 40-item, life-event inventory. In both MZ and DZ twins, the correlation in CES-D scores was highest in pairs concordant for exposure to high stress ($+0.389$ and $+0.252$, respectively), next highest for pairs discordant for such exposure ($+0.313$ and $+0.174$, respectively) and lowest for pairs concordant for non-exposure to high stress ($+0.162$ and $+0.149$, respectively). The full model, containing six parameters (E,H,C,E',H' and C'), fitted well ($\chi^2 = 4.93$, d.f. $= 12$). It produced estimates for h'^2 (0.266) that were substantially higher than for h^2 (0.118); c^2 also exceeded the estimates for c'^2, but the difference was less marked (0.129 versus 0.073, respectively). Models that constrained H=H' or C=C' could not be rejected as against the full model. However, the model that restricted both H'H' *and* C=C' could be rejected as against any of the other three models. These results indicate that there is significant interaction between exposure to high levels of stress and either genetic or common environmental factors, but we were unable to determine statistically whether the interaction occurs in one or the other or both.

The overall results were relatively similar using either the 59- or 34-item, life-event inventories (results available on request). The only noteworthy difference was that with the full model in these two analyses, the difference between c^2 and c'^2 was as large as or larger than the difference between h^2 and h'^2.

Table 10.10 Total life events—44 variables—median split transformed by SQRT(×)

Model	Chi square	d.f.	p
(1) E,H,C E',H',C'	4.93	12	0.960
(2) E,H,C E',C'	5.60	13	0.960
(3) E,H,C E',H'	5.09	13	0.973
(4) E,H,C E'	11.83	14	0.620

Model 1		Model 2	
Exposed	Non-exposed	Exposed	Non-exposed
$e^2 = 0.605$	$e'^2 = 0.809$	$e^2 = 0.633$	$e'^2 = 0.789$
$h^2 = 0.266$	$h'^2 = 0.118$	$h^2 = 0.120$	$h'^2 = 0.153$
$c^2 = 0.129$	$c'^2 = 0.073$	$c^2 = 0.247$	$c'^2 = 0.058$

Model 3		Model 4	
Exposed	Non-exposed	Exposed	Non-exposed
$e^2 = 0.596$	$e'^2 = 0.802$	$e^2 = 0.767$	$e'^2 = 0.720$
$h^2 = 0.334$	$h'^2 = 0.109$	$h^2 = 0.143$	$h'^2 = 0.174$
$c^2 = 0.070$	$c'^2 = 0.089$	$c^2 = 0.090$	$c'^2 = 0.109$

Correlation matrix			
	Concordant exposed	Discordant	Concordant non-exposed
MZ twins	0.389/98	0.313/162	0.162/197
DZ twins	0.252/91	0.174/128	0.149/141

For abbreviations, see text.

The results of the interaction model as applied to dependent life events are shown in Table 10.11. They differ substantially from those found with the full inventories. The full model estimates values of h^2 and c^2 that are slightly higher than the values of h'^2 and c'^2. However, the model that restricts H=H' *and* C=C' does not produce a significant deterioration in fit over the other models (e.g. versus the H=H' model—likelihood ratio test: $\chi^2 = 1.41$, d.f. = 1; not significant). A similar pattern is seen with probably independent life events, although the deterioration in fit with the constrained model (i.e. H=H', C=C') was greater but still not statistically significant.

The pattern is quite different when independent events are used to

Table 10.11 Dependent life events—median split transformed by SQRT(×)

Model	Chi square	d.f.	p
(1) E,H,C E′,H′,C′	10.44	12	0.578
(2) E,H,C E′,C′	10.54	13	0.649
(3) E,H,C E′,H′	10.92	13	0.618
(4) E,H,C E′	12.95	14	0.530

Model 1		*Model 2*	
Exposed	*Non-exposed*	*Exposed*	*Non-exposed*
$e^2 = 0.695$	$e'^2 = 0.800$	$e^2 = 0.705$	$e'^2 = 0.793$
$h^2 = 0.172$	$h'^2 = 0.146$	$h^2 = 0.125$	$h'^2 = 0.150$
$c^2 = 0.133$	$c'^2 = 0.054$	$c^2 = 0.170$	$c'^2 = 0.057$

Model 3		*Model 4*	
Exposed	*Non-exposed*	*Exposed*	*Non-exposed*
$e^2 = 0.688$	$e'^2 = 0.796$	$e^2 = 0.780$	$e'^2 = 0.744$
$h^2 = 0.267$	$h'^2 = 0.150$	$h^2 = 0.164$	$h'^2 = 0.191$
$c^2 = 0.045$	$c'^2 = 0.054$	$c^2 = 0.056$	$c'^2 = 0.065$

Correlation matrix			
	Concordant exposed	*Discordant*	*Concordant non-exposed*
MZ twins	0.269/95	0.284/167	0.191/195
DZ twins	0.219/74	0.238/136	0.029/150

For abbreviations, see text.

assign twins into exposed versus unexposed categories (Table 10.12). The full model estimates the value of h^2 (0.369) to be over six times greater than h'^2 (0.058), while c^2 is estimated to be slightly lower than c'^2. The constrained model (in which H = H′ and C = C′) can here be rejected against any of the other models (e.g. versus the H = H′ model—likelihood ratio test, $\chi^2 = 4.94$, d.f. = 1). Although the full model predicts a much greater change in H than in C on exposure to high levels of stress, the model in which H is constrained to equal H′ (while fitting worse than the model in which C = C′) cannot be rejected against the full model (likelihood ratio test, $\chi^2 = 1.22$, d.f. = 1).

Table 10.12 Independent life events—median split transformed by SQRT($\times$)

Model	Chi square	d.f.	p
(1) E,H,C E′,H′,C′	7.15	12	0.847
(2) E,H,C E′,C′	8.37	13	0.818
(3) E,H,C E′,H′	7.21	13	0.891
(4) E,H,C E′	13.31	14	0.502

Model 1		*Model 2*	
Exposed	*Non-exposed*	*Exposed*	*Non-exposed*
$e^2 = 0.504$	$e'^2 = 0.758$	$e^2 = 0.569$	$e'^2 = 0.737$
$h^2 = 0.369$	$h'^2 = 0.058$	$h^2 = 0.163$	$h'^2 = 0.187$
$c^2 = 0.127$	$c'^2 = 0.184 \cdot$	$c^2 = 0.268$	$c'^2 = 0.076$

Model 3		*Model 4*	
Exposed	*Non-exposed*	*Exposed*	*Non-exposed*
$e^2 = 0.510$	$e'^2 = 0.765$	$e^2 = 0.708$	$e'^2 = 0.686$
$h^2 = 0.334$	$h'^2 = 0.055$	$h^2 = 0.131$	$h'^2 = 0.141$
$c^2 = 0.156$	$c'^2 = 0.180$	$c^2 = 0.161$	$c'^2 = 0.173$

Correlation matrix n			
	Concordant exposed	*Discordant*	*Concordant non-exposed*
MZ twins	0.460/86	0.296/158	0.257/213
DZ twins	0.283/82	0.301/118	0.173/160

For abbreviations, see text.

DISCUSSION

We will discuss our major findings in turn. First, the reported number of life events correlated substantially in twins, with the correlation in MZ twins only slightly exceeding that in DZ twins. When reported events included those occurring to the co-twin, these correlations were in the range of +0.45–0.50. Excluding these events reduced the correlation to the +0.30–0.40 range. Model fitting could definitely reject a model in which resemblance in the number of reported life events in twins was due only to genetic factors. Models in which familial resemblance was due only to environmental factors could not be rejected. In general, the results were consistent with a substantial familial/environmental effect (as high as 0.40 if co-twin events were included, but only 0.20 to 0.25 if they were excluded), and a more modest genetic effect of around 0.15. These findings are consistent with those of McGuffin *et al.* (1988) who found, in a sample of depressed patients and community controls, that life events themselves were familial (see also Bebbington *et al.*, Chapter 9). Our findings also highlight the importance of examining the content of life events in assessing their degree of familial aggregation. That is, how much do life events aggregate in families because individual members are reporting the same event? This is a particular problem when 'network' events are included in life-event inventories. As family members are usually in each other's network, our finding that the inclusion of such events increases the apparent familial aggregation of life events is not unexpected.

Second, when life events were analysed via an *a priori* division into dependent, probably independent and independent of the respondent's behaviour, important differences emerge in the results of model fitting. For dependent life events, heritable influences could not be rejected and accounted for around 20% of the total variation, compared to around 10% for familial/environmental factors. By contrast, for independent life events, heritable influences, acting alone, could be clearly rejected; and the most parsimonious model included only individual specific and familial/environmental effects, with the latter accounting for around 35% of the total variation. These analyses are an example of the unique perspective twin studies can bring to longstanding problems in psychiatric epidemiology.

A major issue in the interpretation of the published life-event record is the degree to which life events may be products of, rather than causes of, psychopathology (Thoits, 1983). In response to this problem, many researchers have restricted their analysis to events that were judged either *a priori* or after an examination of the given situation to be independent of the respondent's behaviour. Our preliminary analysis supports the validity of this approach; genetic factors appear to play a significant role in the aetiology of dependent but not independent life events. It will be of particular interest in further analyses to determine whether the genes that influence the reporting of dependent life events also influence psychopathology.

An unexpected finding was that familial/environmental factors were *more* important in independent than in dependent life events. This finding could result from the fact that the preponderance of events in our inventory judged to be independent were death, serious illness or injury or serious personal crises occurring in people close to the twin. However, the estimates of familial environment for independent life events were not substantially reduced when parents, siblings or other relatives of the twin were eliminated from this list of people. It remains possible, however, that the high estimates of familial environment are an 'artifact' of measurement. Besides parents, siblings and other relatives, the other individuals on this list were spouse (brother-in-law of the co-twin), children (nieces/nephews of the co-twin) and 'someone else close to you' (likely to be a good friend of the co-twin). Information that might be helpful in further analyses aimed at characterizing the nature of familial influences on life events (and which is available in our data set) includes cohabitation status and frequency of contact with co-twin.

Third, depressive symptoms as measured by the CES-D scale were found to be modestly correlated in twins. Model fitting suggests that genetic and familial/environmental factors each account for about 15% of the variation, with the remaining 70% being accounted for by individual specific environment (which will include error of measurement). These findings differ from those of Jardine *et al.* (1984), who, using a shorter, 7-item scale in a large Australian twin series, could reject any role for familial/environmental factors in self-reported symptoms of depression in females, with estimates of heritability of around 35%. An item-by-item analysis of that depression scale did, however, reveal several items in which familial/environmental factors may be playing a significant aetiological role (Kendler *et al.*, 1986). There are several possible reasons for these differences, including sample error, differences in scales and differences in populations. Only further research can clarify this question. Our results here are consistent with those of a recently completed multivariate analysis of the CES-D in this sample (Silberg *et al.*, 1990).

Fourth, using a structural equation, 'interaction' model (Fig. 10.1), we found no evidence to reject the hypothesis that the genetic and familial environmental factors that influence depression in low-stress environments are the same as those which influence depression in high-stress environments. Although the power of these analyses may not be high, these findings are not consistent with the hypothesis that exposure to high levels of stress 'turns on' new genetic or familial environmental factors that are 'dormant' in low-stress environments.

Fifth, given that the same genetic and familial environmental factors influence depression in low- and high-stress environments, we then examined whether the importance of these factors in controlling the level of self-reported depression differed in the two environmental conditions. We found consistent evidence that genetic *and/or* familial environmental factors played a greater role in influencing depression in high-stress than in low-stress environments. Although we could clearly reject a model in which both genetic and familial environmental effects were the same in the low- and high-stress environments, we could not statistically determine whether it was just genetic effects that became more important (genotype × specific environment interaction), just familial environmental effects that became more important (familial × specific environment interaction) or both effects that became more important in high-stress environments. In fitting the full model, the evidence tended to favour genotype × environment interaction as the more important feature, but this finding was not stable across all analyses.

Finally, we examined whether the results of the interaction model would change as a function of the kind of life event considered. This was of potential importance because the 'interaction' model assumes that there is no genetic or familial environmental correlation between the exposure variable (life events) and the dependent variable (depressive symptoms). With dependent life events, no statistical evidence for interaction was found. By contrast, the evidence for interaction was quite strong when independent life events were considered. Given that we found no evidence for a genetic effect on independent life events, the observed interactive effect could not plausibly result from a genetic correlation between life events and depression. However, it remains possible that the results of the interaction model may be influenced by a familial environmental correlation between life events and depression. If this were the case, then pairs concordant for exposure to life events would also tend to have high levels of familial environmental factors that predispose to depression. It is difficult to see how this could cause the pattern of twin correlations found with our 'interaction' model; however, further theoretical and analytical work will be needed to clarify this difficult question.

As noted above, we were unable to determine whether the interaction involves genetic and/or familial environmental factors. Although not couched in this language, the outcome of earlier work is consistent with an interaction between current life-event exposure and familial environment. For example, Brown and Harris (1978) showed that risk for depression in individuals with exposure to a recent stressful life event was significantly greater in individuals who had than in those who had not experienced early maternal separation. Genotype × environment interaction, which has been widely found in animals and plants (Mather and Jinks, 1982) has also been reported, using adoption study designs, for both alcoholism (Cloninger *et al.*, 1981) and antisocial behaviour (Cadoret, 1982).

In summary, in earlier work (Kendler and Eaves, 1986) we have proposed that:

a complete understanding of the etiology of most psychiatric disorders will require an understanding of the relevant genetic risk factors, the relevant environmental risk factors, and the ways in which these two risk factors interact.

In particular, we focused on the potential importance of what we termed 'genetic control of exposure to the environment' (genotype–environment correlation) and 'genetic control of sensitivity to the environment' (genotype × environment interaction). Our ongoing twin study in Virginia was planned to elucidate precisely these mechanisms. In this preliminary report, based only on the first wave of contact using mailed questionnaires, we have presented evidence supporting our contention that the 'pathway' from genotype to psychiatric symptoms may be more complex than simply the addition of genetic and environmental vulnerabilities. Genes and familial environment appear to play a significant role in the reporting of the 'environmental' factor type of life events. Of particular interest, we found evidence that either genes or familial environmental factors influence the sensitivity of individuals to environmental stress.

In further work, we will hope to clarify the significance of these findings in two ways. First, these results should be confirmed with more sophisticated genetic models. For example, we will examine, in a single multivariate analysis, the genetic and common environmental variance and covariance of our three classes of life events: dependent, probably independent and independent. A more difficult problem is to develop an interaction model that relies on a continuous measure of the environment rather than the simple dichotomization used here. Second, we will attempt to replicate these preliminary findings both in a larger questionnaire sample including male twins and in our second wave of data collection, in which personal interviews were used to obtain a more detailed assessment of life events and a detailed psychiatric assessment, which will allow depression to be assessed both as a qualitative phenotype (i.e. a 'disorder') and as quantitative phenotype (i.e. a 'depression score').

ACKNOWLEDGEMENTS

This research was supported by grant MH-40828 from the United States National Institutes of Mental Health. Leroy Thacker MS assisted with the data analysis.

REFERENCES

Brown G. W., Harris T. (1978). *Social Origins of Depression: A Study of Psychiatric Disorder in Women*. New York: Free Press.

Cadoret R. J. (1982). Genotype–environment interaction in antisocial behavior. *Psychological Medicine*; **12**: 235–9.

Cloninger C. R., Bohman M., Sigvardsson S. (1981). Inheritance of alcohol abuse—cross fostering analysis of adopted men. *Archives of General Psychiatry*; **38**: 861–8.

Dohrenwend B. S., Krasnoff L., Askenasy A. R., Dohrewend B. P. (1978). Exemplification of a method for scaling life events: the PERI life events scale. *Journal of Health and Social Behavior*; **19**: 205–29.

Heath A. C., Neale M. C., Hewitt J. K. *et al.* (1989). Testing structural equation models for twin data using LISREL. *Behavior Genetics*; **19**: 9–35.

Jardine R., Martin N. G., Henderson A. S. (1984). Genetic covariation between neuroticism and symptoms of anxiety and depression. *Genetic Epidemiology*; **1**: 89–107.

Joreskog K. G., Sorbom D. (1986). LISREL VI. Mooresville, Ind: Scientific Software.

Kasriel J., Eaves L. J. (1976). A comparison of the accuracy of written questionnaires with blood-typing for diagnosing zygosity in twins. *Journal of Biosocial Science*; **8**: 263–6.

Kendler K. S., Eaves L. J. (1986). Models for the joint effect of genotype and environment on liability to psychiatric illness. *American Journal of Psychiatry*; **143**: 279–89.

Kendler K. S., Heath A., Martin N. G., Eaves L. J. (1986). Symptoms of anxiety and depression in a volunteer twin population: the etiologic role of genetic and environmental factors. *Archives of General Psychiatry*; **43**: 213–21.

Mather K., Jinks J. L. (1982). *Biometrical Genetics: The Study of Continuous Variation*. London: Chapman and Hall.

McGuffin P., Katz R., Bebbington P. (1988). The Camberwell collaborative depression study: III. Depression and adversity in the relatives of depressed probands. *British Journal of Psychiatry*; **152**: 775–82.

Radloff L. S. (1977). The CES-D scale: a self-report depression scale for research in the general population. *Applied Psychological Measurements*; **1**: 385–401.

Silberg J. L., Heath A. C., Kessler R. *et al.* (1990). Genetic and environmental effects on self-reported depressive symptoms in a general population twin sample. *Psychiatry Research* **24**: 197–212.

Thoits P. A. (1983). Dimensions of life events that influence psychological distress: an evaluation and synthesis of the literature. In: *Psychosocial Stress: Trends in Theory and Research* (Kaplan H. B., ed.), pp. 33–102. New York: Academic Press.

11 *Genetic markers and affective disorder*

PETER McGUFFIN AND MATTHEW P. SARGEANT

One of the problems faced by the geneticist in attempting to study affective illness is also shared by researchers in epidemiology. This is to answer the fundamental question, what do we mean by 'a case' of affective disorder? Understanding the root of this problem does not require a great deal of clinical experience or sophistication; most clinicians would readily agree that affective disturbance, usually depression or depression-mixed-with-anxiety, is one of the most widespread of symptoms. Furthermore, comparatively short-lived bouts of a depressive *syndrome*, i.e. depressed mood accompanied by typical associated symptoms of depression, have been shown to be surprisingly prevalent in the general population. Thus, using a broad definition of what constitutes 'a case' yields prevalences that are high, often in excess of 10%. This is true not just in modern urban communities (Bebbington *et al.*, 1981) but also in rural settings (Brown and Prudo, 1981) and in developing countries (Orley and Wing, 1979).

From the geneticist's viewpoint, prevalence estimates alone are of limited value because what is really required is the frequency of being affected by the disorder at some time in life. This is commonly expressed as *morbid risk* or *lifetime expectancy* (also called lifetime incidence) of developing a disorder. Calculating this is complicated by the fact that unaffected individuals included in the study broadly fall into two groups, those who are unaffected now and who will remain unaffected, and those who are unaffected now but will become affected at some point in the future.

One way of calculating morbid risk is based on the method of Strömgren, the Danish psychiatrist (and this in turn is an elaboration of a method proposed by Weinberg, a German physician-geneticist). Details of this are given in a paper by Bebbington *et al.* (1989), who used figures from an earlier population survey (Bebbington *et al.*, 1981) to estimate the risk up to the age of 65 years of becoming 'a case' of depression in an area of South London defined by the old Borough of Camberwell. Over 70% of women and just under a half of all men were likely to be affected by minor depression at some stage in their adult lives and, as a consequence of this, Bebbington *et al.* (1989) suggested that broad definitions of depression are probably of limited use in genetic studies. Indeed, for a disorder which is so common that at some stage most women are affected, it might be more profitable to focus genetic studies on the families of those who are apparently immune to depression!

As a result of their findings, Bebbington *et al.* therefore suggested that genetic studies of affective disorder might sensibly take as a starting point probands who have had hospital-treated depression and that this could provide a means of focusing on the more severe, and possibly therefore the more 'biological' types of disorder. This proposal is somewhat problematical in that other factors, which are not just concerned with severity or symptoms, may influence hospital referral, for example, sex, social class or proximity to hospital clinics. Nevertheless, in practice, it is the approach that most investigators have taken. We will, therefore, for the remainder of this chapter follow the same pragmatic path and assume that it is reasonable to take severe, hospital-treated depression as the starting point for genetic studies. We will first consider the evidence that there is a genetic contribution to severe affective disorder before going on to discuss possible modes of transmission, and then we will review the work accomplished so far in using genetic markers in studies of association and linkage. Finally, we will consider the future prospects and likely benefits of such studies.

THE EVIDENCE FOR GENETIC INFLUENCES

Family studies

As mentioned in Chapter 2, the first and necessary piece of evidence that a disorder is genetic is that it tends to run in families. There is no doubt that this is true of manic-depressive illness, and Kraepelin (1922) was among the first to remark on this, noting that hereditary factors were apparent in 80% of his patients. Subsequent studies, using a narrow Kraepelinian definition, consistently confirmed that the disorder was more common in relatives of index cases than in the general population (Slater and Cowie, 1971). However, over the past 20 years or so it has become the rule in family studies to follow the suggestion of Leonhard (1959), who divided the Kraepelinian entity, manic-depressive illness, into two parts, bipolar (BP) disorder, in which there are episodes of both mania and depression (or less commonly of mania alone), and unipolar (UP) disorder, where there are attacks only of depression. This distinction was first used in family studies by Angst (1966), a Swiss psychiatrist, and independently, in the same year, by Perris (1966) in Sweden. Although Perris found that there was a striking degree of homotypia, that is a tendency for relatives of UP and BP probands to 'breed true' and fall ill with the same type of disorder, the findings of Angst were more complex. Among the relatives of probands with UP disorder there was an increase only of UP illness but among the relatives of BP there was an excess of both UP and BP disorder.

Most subsequent studies fit with the pattern described by Angst. McGuffin and Katz (1986) reviewed 12 studies and calculated that the weighted, average, morbid risk of severe affective disorder was 19.2% in the first-degree relatives of BP probands and 9.7% in the first-degree relatives of UP probands. On average, 7.8% of the relatives of BP probands had BP disorder while 11.4% had UP disorder. By contrast, the first-degree relatives of UP probands showed a high rate, 9.1%, only of UP disorder while the average morbid risk of BP disorder was 0.6%. These morbid risks have to be compared with population figures. For UP and BP disorder combined, or for severe affective illness requiring in-patient treatment, this is about 3%; for BP disorder the population morbid risk is under 1% (Reich *et al.*, 1982; Sturt *et al.*, 1984). Thus, both BP and UP disorder appear to be strongly familial but combining morbid risk figures in this way smooths over some of the difficulties in family studies, including the fact that there is a very large range in the figures from different studies, which may reflect differing diagnostic practices in different centres. Most studies have shown that families ascertained via BP probands contain a higher number of affected members. However, two investigations (Tsuang *et al.*, 1980; Rice *et al.*, 1987) have now found no substantial differences in the rates of disorder among the relatives of BP and UP probands. It is not certain why this is so but the large sample size in the study of Rice *et al.* makes sampling error an unlikely explanation. Nevertheless, their method of relying on a lifetime interview and including subjects in the BP category who gave retrospective accounts of untreated mania, so-called 'bipolar-II' disorder, probably produces a broader definition than the one usually used outside of the United States.

Twin studies

As has been mentioned in Chapter 2, and elsewhere in this book, familial aggregation is necessary to infer that a disorder is genetically influenced but it is not, on its own, enough. Studies of monozygotic (MZ) and dizygotic (DZ) twins provide one of the classical methods of assessing the relative contributions of genes and shared environment. Another advantage of twin studies is that if we merely want to assess whether genetic influences are present, there is no necessary recourse to population figures, as a significantly higher concordance rate in MZ than in DZ twins is in itself persuasive. Four published sets of results are summarized in Table 11.1 and are reasonably consistent in showing MZ concordance rates two to five times as large as DZ concordance rates, strongly suggesting the importance of genetic factors. The data reported by Gershon *et al.* (1975) were derived from a compilation of older studies where the investigators mainly had not differentiated UP from BP disorder. Bertelsen *et al.* (1977) based their research on Danish twin and psychiatric registers and did distinguish between subtypes of affective illness. They found a tendency for homotypia to occur, with 15 out of 19 affected, identical co-twins of UP

Table 11.1 Twin concordance for major affective disorder

Reference	MZ		DZ	
	N	*Concordance (%)*	*N*	*Concordance (%)*
Gershon *et al.* (1975)*	91	69	226	13
Bertelsen *et al.* (1977)**	69	67	54	20
Torgersen (1986)**	37	51	65	20
McGuffin and Katz (preliminary results)**	62	53	79	28

MZ = monozygotic; DZ = dizygotic.
* Combined figures from six earlier studies reporting pair-wise concordance.
** Systematic register-based studies reporting proband-wise concordance.

probands having UP disorder and 21 out of 27 identical twins of BP probands having BP disorder. This would not, however, suggest that UP and BP disorder are completely distinct at a genetic level, because, even allowing for diagnostic error and some UP subjects subsequently developing manic episodes, we cannot overlook the fact that 10 out of 46 affected co-twins had a different form of affective illness from their genetically identical probands.

Like the majority of family studies, the Danish twin study suggests that genetic influences are stronger in BP than in UP disorder. Taking the MZ:DZ concordance ratio as a rough guide, the Danish study shows a ratio of 3.5:1 when the proband had BP disorder compared with 2:1 when the proband had UP disorder. The preliminary results reported by McGuffin *et al.* (1990), like those of Torgersen (1986), were again based on a systematic sample obtained via a register. Both of these studies concentrated on UP disorder. The study by Torgersen was focused on moderately severe depression while that of McGuffin *et al.* included a substantial number of probands who had received only out-patient treatment so that it is perhaps not surprising that the results are similar. They suggest a genetic contribution to UP, major depression, albeit one which is less marked than for BP disorder, and are therefore not greatly different from the findings of Bertelsen *et al.* concerning UP disorder.

Adoption studies

Adoption studies represent the other, major, 'natural experiment' that can be exploited by geneticists studying complex conditions such as the affective disorders. It is perhaps surprising that adoption studies have received less emphasis in affective disorder than in schizophrenia and it is tempting to propose that this is because a genetic basis for affective illness is a less controversial topic.

Among the more clearcut results have been those of Mendlewicz and Rainer (1977), who showed that 28% of the biological parents of BP adoptees had affective illness compared with 12% of their adopting parents. The rate of affective illness in the biological parents of adoptees did not differ significantly from that in the parents of BP non-adoptees, of whom 26% were affected. Again, there was a suggestion that the two subtypes of affective disorder are not distinct entities, as the majority of affectively ill, biological parents of BP probands had UP rather than BP disorder. A smaller and less detailed study dealt mainly with UP illness and this time concentrated on the offspring of patients with affective disorder (Cadoret, 1978). Adopted-away offspring of patients with affective illness had higher rates of affective illness than those adoptees whose natural parents were psychiatrically well. Based mainly on health insurance records, the Swedish adoption study carried out by Von Knorring *et al.* (1983) unexpectedly found little evidence of a genetic or family environmental component in affective illness. However, a more recent report of Scandinavian data from Denmark (Wender *et al.*, 1986) found quite marked evidence of a genetic contribution to affective illness. 'Blindfold' assessments were made of hospital records and showed an 8-fold increase in UP depression and a 15-fold increase in suicide among the biological relatives of adoptees with affective illness compared with the adoptive relatives and relatives of matched control adoptees.

In summary, despite certain methodological difficulties concerning the problems of definition, to which we have already alluded, the data from family, twin and adoption studies are mainly consistent. They provide a persuasive body of evidence that genetic influences are important. However, before going on to discuss the pin-pointing of the genetic abnormalities further by use of genetic markers, it is important to discuss the possible modes of transmission of severe affective disorder. This is because, as discussed in Chapter 3, it is desirable to have some knowledge about models of inheritance in order to design and effectively interpret studies with genetic markers. This may be more complicated than it appears at first sight as, although 'loaded' pedigrees are sometimes encountered that appear to have a dominant-like pattern of transmission, a broader perspective compels the conclusion that we are not dealing with a simple Mendelian disease. Indeed, as we have discussed in Chapter 2, it could be misleading to pick out such families and assume that they provide examples of an inherited disorder with a simple model of transmission which differs from all other forms of manic-depressive illness.

MODE OF INHERITANCE

Liability/threshold models provide us with the best concept of framework for understanding the transmission of affective disorders and other common forms of familial mental illness (see Chapter 2). Here it is assumed that a variable termed 'liability to develop the disorder' is continuously distributed in the population such that only those whose liability at some time exceeds a certain threshold manifest the disorder. In general, statistical analyses have one of two possible aims. The first is to quantify genetic and environmental effects, and the second is to detect evidence of major genes. From the examples of comparatively simple analyses, given in Chapter 2, there is a suggestion that in severe affective illness, particularly when this includes BP disorder, the overwhelming contribution to variance in liability is genetic. The estimated heritability from Bertelsen's twin study (see above) is in excess of 80%. Similarly, major affective disorder, mainly of the UP type, receives a substantial genetic contribution with a heritability of about 50%. By contrast, the twin study results of Torgersen (1986) suggest that neurotic depression aggregates in families largely because of shared environment. In all of these examples, it is assumed that liability is normally distributed (or nearly normally distributed), and results from the additive combination of multiple, genetic and environmental effects. However, particularly with a disorder of high heritability, it is reasonable to speculate that a substantial contribution to liability comes from a major gene, the effects of which may or may not be modified by multiple genes of smaller effect (polygenes), or family environment.

The broad principles of segregation analysis are discussed in Chapter 2. Most modern studies are based on the concept of mixed model analysis (Morton and McLean, 1974), where a full model of major gene plus multifactorial background is compared with reduced models in which either major gene effects or polygenic effects are excluded. Alternatively, a test is carried out for the probability of transmission of a major gene which conforms to Mendelian expectations (Elston and Stewart, 1971). Most sophisticated of all, the mixed model concepts and the notion of transmission probabilities are combined together in a 'unified' model (Lalouel *et al.*, 1983). Applying the Elston and Stewart approach, Bucher *et al.* (1981) claimed to have rejected major gene effects in families ascertained via BP probands. However, using a data set that partially overlapped with that of Bucher *et al.*, O'Rourke *et al.* (1983) found that a major gene with or without a multifactorial background provided a satisfactory explanation of the transmission of affective illness. Similarly, using a larger sample of families, Rice *et al.* (1987) applied a mixed-model approach and found evidence for the presence of a major locus when they controlled for other possible confounding variables such as birth cohort effects and age of onset. However, on applying a more stringent test, they found that the major gene model compared unfavourably with a more general, vertical transmission model. Thus, when probabilities of transmission of the major gene were not constrained to Mendelian values, a significant improvement was found when a likelihood ratio test (see Chapter 2) was applied.

In summary then, analyses based on large or moderately large samples give at best only partial support for the hypothesis of major gene effects in bipolar illness. However, most of these analyses have assumed that the disorder is mainly homogeneous and cannot be taken as effectively ruling out major genes in some forms. We can, therefore, proceed to consider genetic marker studies with somewhat mixed and only partially satisfactory conclusions. Affective illness, particularly of the BP type, has a large genetic component, but the main justification for searching for major genes is there is no compelling evidence against their existence in at least some families.

GENETIC MARKERS

The term 'genetic marker' has been used in two rather different ways in psychiatric research. In the first and stricter sense, a genetic marker is an inherited characteristic which: (a) has a simple mode of transmission, and (b) is polymorphic (i.e. there are two or more alleles of a gene frequency of at least 1%). It follows that genetic markers must be capable of being reliably detected and are stable over time (i.e. they are not state dependent). Examples include 'classical' markers, such as blood groups, histocompatibility (HLA) antigens, certain plasma proteins and traits such as colour blindness, as well as DNA markers, so-called restriction fragment length polymorphisms (RFLPs) (see Chapter 1). The second, and much broader sense, in which the term 'genetic marker' has been applied (some would say misapplied) has been to be include virtually any biological finding that may be inherited and can be potentially related to psychiatric illness. Some examples here would be platelet monoamine oxidase, tests of neuroendocrine status or abnormalities of smooth-pursuit eye movements. In the remainder of this chapter, consideration will be restricted to the first type of genetic marker.

The relationship between genetic polymorphisms and disease can be investigated in two ways. In the first, the population study, the frequency of a particular phenotype in ill individuals is compared with that in healthy individuals drawn from the same ethnic group. This can provide evidence of an *association* between a particular marker phenotype and the disease. In the second method, families segregating for both the marker and the disease are studied. This may provide evidence of *linkage* (i.e. close proximity on the same chromosome between the marker locus and the locus for a gene which manifests as the illness). The distinction between association and linkage is an important one. The terms are sometimes confused but it is only under exceptional circumstances, which we will discuss later, that association reflects linkage or vice versa (see also Chapter 4).

Association

In psychiatry, as in other areas of medicine, studies of association have principally been concerned with classical markers, in particular blood groups and the human leucocyte antigen (HLA system). In affective illness, there has been some agreement that the blood group O is increased in BP patients compared with controls (Parker *et al.*, 1961; Masters, 1967; Mendlewicz *et al.*, 1974), and in BPs compared with patients with UP illness (Shapiro *et al.*, 1977). However, in one study, group O was found to be associated with involutional melancholia (Irvine and Miyashita, 1965), a diagnostic subtype that seemed to contain only unipolar cases. In yet another study (Flemebaum and Larson, 1976), group A was increased in both BP patients and the total sample of manic-depressive patients. Thus the overall picture is confused and inconsistent, which suggests that no true important association is present.

Similarly, a confusing picture has emerged from studies of the HLA system in affective illness. Again, the rationale for carrying out such studies is a proposed analogy between affective illness and other common familial diseases where the pathogenesis is obscure. For example, studies of HLA associations have provided important clues to the aetiology of the juvenile diabetes, ankylosing spondylitis and a variety of other conditions, most of which are thought to involve disordered immune mechanisms. The first report of an association between manic-depressive illness and HLA concerned the B7 and BW16 antigens, where one group of workers reported early, promising results (Shapiro *et al.*, 1976) and found that these held when they extended to a larger study (Shapiro *et al.*, 1977). Unfortunately, the reported associations were not found elsewhere (Johnson, 1978) but instead associations with a variety of other antigens were found (Bennaheim *et al.*, 1976; Stember and Fieve, 1976; Govaerts *et al.*, 1977; Targum *et al.*, 1979; Wentzel *et al.*, 1982) and indeed one group reported that the frequency of B7 was actually significantly decreased in manic-depressive patients (Beckman *et al.*, 1978). We have to conclude that the balance of evidence is against manic-depressive illness being an HLA-associated condition.

Other marker systems have received relatively little attention but one study took various polymorphic enzymes and plasma proteins into account and suggested an association between group-specific protein 1 (Gc1) and depressive spectrum disease (Tanna *et al.*, 1977). No independent replication of this has been forthcoming.

As will be evident from the dates of the studies quoted above, there has been recent disenchantment with association studies in affective disorder and this is probably mainly engendered by the inconsistent and contradictory findings so far. Moreover, there are other more practical drawbacks to association studies. These include the problem of diagnosis, which has been touched on earlier in the chapter, and the question of comparability of patient populations from different centres. Applying strict operational definitions of illness can ensure that a patient sample is phenotypically homogeneous but does not avoid the possibility that there is more than one underlying genotype. The selection of controls provides a further pitfall for the unwary: thus there may be a section of the population in which a particular marker and a certain disorder are common without there being any causal relationship. This phenomenon, called stratification, can lead to spurious associations. For example, HLA BW16 is more common in Ashkenazi Jews than in other white people often loosely described as 'caucasian', so that an excess of Jewish patients in an affectively ill sample could lead to the false conclusion that an association exists between the disorder and the antigen (Targum *et al.*, 1979).

The remaining problem concerns the statistical handling of the results. It has long been suggested (e.g. Weiner, 1962) that the conventional 5% level of significance is inappropriate in disease association studies where the prior probability of an association is remote. Thus, in a large number of studies when a disease is selected at random, 1 in 20 will yield 'significant' associations by chance alone. Similarly, in a study of a highly polymorphic system, such as HLA, which consists of many antigens, many different tests will be carried out and, on average, 1 in 20 tests will result in a 'significant' association. This statistical problem, called the Bonferroni inequality, can be corrected for by multiplying the obtained p values by the number of tests performed. However, this is probably an over-strict correction and runs the risk of a type 2 (false-negative) error (Svejgaard *et al.*, 1975), so that it is preferable to check apparent associations against the results of a second, independent study.

Despite these difficulties, association studies still do have a theoretical appeal. This is particularly true if we are dealing with conditions where liability to become ill may be contributed by many susceptibility loci of comparatively small effect (Sturt and McGuffin, 1985). For example, the association between duodenal ulcer, blood group O and secretor status is well established and has been consistently replicated but, if a threshold model is assumed, the association accounts for little over 1% of the variance in liability to develop the disorder (Edwards, 1965). As explained in Chapters 3 and 4, linkage between loci does not usually result in allelic association in populations. Therefore, if we can rule out stratification and set aside the theoretical possibility that selection is acting jointly on two loci, detecting association means either that a marker is very tightly linked with a susceptibility locus producing *linkage disequilibrium*, or that the marker gene itself has a *pleiotropic* effect. (This is a phenomenon whereby the same gene is expressed in two or more quite different and apparently separate ways.) Setting out to detect linkage disequilibrium involving loci 1 centimorgan (cM) apart (i.e. loci between which recombination occurs only once in every hundred meioses) could theoretically be accomplished in affective illness by studying 1500 evenly spaced polymorphisms (the human gene is about 3000 cM long). This would obviously involve a huge but not impossible amount of work.

Linkage

It is convenient to describe linkage studies on affective disorder under three headings corresponding to the types of marker investigated. These are: classical autosomal markers, X-linked markers and DNA polymorphisms.

Classical markers

Linkage studies involving the HLA system have provoked even greater interest and just as much confusion as the association studies. The first published report was based on families with affective illness in at least two generations (Targum *et al.*, 1979). Only one family suggested the presence of linkage, while the combined lod score for all families suggested that the close linkage was unlikely. However, a later report, based mainly on the analysis of sibships where two or more members of the family had affective disorder, claimed to have found 'a gene on chromosome 6 that can affect behaviour' (Weitkamp *et al.*, 1981). This provoked a great deal of media excitement as well as interest in the medical and scientific world. Although one further study provided evidence for HLA linkage to a gene for BP-II disorder (Turner and King, 1983), others (Johnson *et al.*, 1981; Goldin *et al.*, 1982; Suarez and Reich, 1984) produced results which threw much doubt on the question of HLA linkage. A recent re-analysis (Price, 1989) of the original data of Weitkamp *et al.* (1981) and other published and unpublished data sets used a variety of models of transmission of affective illness in lod score analysis, in addition to completing an analysis of affected sibling pairs. Linkage between affective illness and HLA could be excluded to a distance of 20 to 25 cM and there was no evidence of linkage heterogeneity.

Two studies have concentrated on families where one or more members had BP disorder (but are categorized as 'affected' relatives who have either UP or BP disorder) and have reported the results of lod score analysis with multiple blood groups and other classical markers (Johnson *et al.*, 1981; Goldin *et al.*, 1984). A third study based on a Pennsylvania Old Order Amish family (see below) was reported in less detail, but taken together the results effectively exclude linkage at a distance of at least 10 cM with ABO, Rhesus, the Duffy blood group locus, haptoglobin, group-specific component (Gc) and glutamine-pyruvate-transaminase (GPT). Interestingly, all three studies produced mildly positive scores with the MNS blood-group locus, giving a combined lod of 1.9 at a combination fraction of 0.2. This is probably worthy of follow up.

X-linkage

The first tangible evidence that an X-linked gene might be involved in the transmission of affective disorder came in the study of Reich *et al.* (1969), who reported two large pedigrees where the disorder cosegregated with colour blindness, a character now known to be on the long arm of X. However, the existence of many instances of father-to-son transmission, together with the results of recent studies using complex segregation analysis (e.g. Bucher *et al.*, 1981), would indicate that X-linkage can at best account for a minority of cases. A subsequent study (Mendlewicz and Fliess, 1974) strongly suggested linkage between manic-depressive disorder and deutan and protan colour blindness at a recombination fraction of 0.1, as well as linkage with the Xg blood-group locus. The lod score in both cases was impressively high but two major problems then arose. The first was that the Xg locus and colour blindness are now thought to be at virtually the opposite ends of the X chromosome, making the probability of finding a third locus within mapping distance of both very remote indeed. The second problem was that other studies failed to confirm X-linkage using colour blindness as a marker, with the most extensive data coming from a collaborative study in one American and three European centres (Gershon *et al.*, 1980). The combined data did not suggest linkage but there was considerable heterogeneity in that one pedigree strongly suggested linkage, eight were indeterminate and seven suggested no linkage. The investigators suggested that this may reflect true heterogeneity in BP disorder but that an alternative explanation was of a systematic bias of diagnosis or ascertainment affecting one or more pedigrees. This seemed especially likely as the pedigrees contributed by the American centre were homogeneous for non-linkage whereas the earlier American study of Mendlewicz and Fliess (1974) was homogeneous for linkage. It was concluded that the discrepancies between these two American series seemed too great to be accounted for by random sampling errors.

Controversy continued and a further re-analysis of data (Risch and Baron, 1982) was said to support a 'true heterogeneity' hypothesis. Further provocation came from a report by Baron *et al.* (1987) of linkage between X-chromosome markers and manic-depression in Israeli families, closely followed by a report of linkage in Belgian families between manic-depression and a polymorphic DNA marker on the long arm of the X chromosome using a probe for the blood clotting factor IX (Mendlewicz *et al.*, 1987). Together these results began to make the X-linkage hypothesis, previously enfeebled by controversy, regain its strength. However, it now seems that these recent findings are much less mutually supportive than they appeared at first because factor IX is located some distance from the glucose-6-phosphate dehydrogenase (G6PD) and the colour blindness loci that were used as markers in the Israeli study. This distance is probably about 40 cM, again making it unlikely that a manic-depression gene could be linked to all three loci. Therefore, if the findings of Baron *et al.* (1987) and Mendlewicz *et al.* (1987) are true, we probably need to postulate the existence of two, separate, affective-disorder genes on the long arm of the X chromosome.

DNA markers

The area of greatest interest as far as autosomal DNA markers are concerned has been the short arm of chromosome 11, where apparently very strong evidence of linkage of a gene for manic-depression was reported by Egeland *et al.* (1987). These workers identified several large pedigrees in which multiple members had affective disorder from among the Old Order Amish, a religious sect in Pennsylvania, USA. The Amish were attractive from the point of view of genetic linkage research because they are a close-knit community with large sibships and often three or more generations available for study. Furthermore, the fact that they are comparatively genetically isolated (i.e. there is little marrying-in to the community) increases the chances that depression found among the Amish is genetically homogeneous. An added advantage is that the diagnosis of affective illness is unlikely to be contaminated by alcohol or drug abuse, as these are rare among the Amish. Initial linkage studies, as mentioned earlier, used classical markers including blood groups and various protein polymorphisms (Kidd *et al.*, 1984). Subsequent research, using more than 20 RLFPs and some classical markers, also gave predominantly negative results (Kidd *et al.*, 1987). However, in a study concentrating on one large pedigree, there was evidence of linkage between a putative gene for bipolar affective disorder, the Harvey-*ras*-1 (H-*ras*) oncogene locus and the insulin (INS) locus situated on the p15 region of chromosome 11. The lod score with H-*ras* alone exceeded 4 (odds on linkage of 10 000 to 1) and multipoint mapping using both H-*ras* and INS data provided even stronger evidence for linkage.

At the same time as the publication of the positive Amish pedigrees, two other studies reported absence of linkage between BP disorder and chromosome 11p15 markers in Icelandic families and in non-Amish North American families (Detera-Wadleigh *et al.*, 1987; Hodgkinson *et al.*, 1987). The most likely initial explanation of one set of strongly positive results and two negatives seemed to be heterogeneity. Statistical analysis of the published results supported this (McGuffin, 1988) and it seemed plausible that the Amish community, descended from only about 30 pioneer couples, could have a form of affective disorder that was genetically distinct from that in Iceland or in other parts of the United States. A fourth study on an Irish pedigree proved negative (Gill *et al.*, 1988) but again this did not disturb the heterogeneity hypothesis. It was only after two years of follow-up work that the original positive linkage results from the Amish study began to look less certain. A re-analysis of the original data supported the published conclusions (Kelsoe *et al.*, 1989), but the addition of updated diagnostic information markedly altered the picture. In particular, two individuals previously classed as unaffected became ill with severe affective disorder and in both cases this meant that there had to be recombination between the disease and the marker loci. These and other less significant changes in the core pedigree reduced the lod scores dramatically both with H-*ras* and INS. Further information came from extensions of the core pedigree. In one of these extensions, close linkage with either H-*ras* or INS could be excluded up to a distance of 15 cM, and when the extensions together with the updated core pedigree were analysed, linkage up to a distance of 15 cM could be excluded in the entire material. Although it is still possible to postulate that two or more forms of genetically distinct BP disorder exist among the Amish and that both are segregating within the same large pedigree, this strains credulity. A more likely explanation is simply that there is not a gene for affective illness on chromosome 11p15.

CONCLUSIONS AND FUTURE PROSPECTS

We have seen that carrying out genetic marker studies in complex phenotypes such as affective illness is a hazardous pursuit. In the absence of clear knowledge about the mode of transmission of affective illness we have to make three assumptions in carrying out linkage studies. First, we assume that there is homogeneity within, if not between, pedigrees. Secondly, we assume that there is a gene of major affect for at least some forms of the disorder and thirdly, we need to suppose that the mode of transmission at least in large multiplex (multiply affected) pedigrees can be inferred 'approximately'. Fortunately, as discussed in Chapter 3, making false assumptions about the mode of transmission of a disease is unlikely to lead to the spurious detection of linkage if linkage does not, in fact, exist. However, mis-specification of the mode of transmission biases against the detection of linkage and incomplete penetrance inevitably reduces the efficiency of likelihood methods of analysis (Sturt and McGuffin, 1985).

Studies so far in affective illness have mainly been of the 'random search' type where, opportunistically, researchers use whatever markers are available in the hope of being fortunate enough to detect linkage. Although this is clearly a gamble, it is one that has paid off in disorders with more straightforward patterns of inheritance such as Huntington's disease (Gusella *et al.*, 1983). An alternative is to concentrate on potential 'candidate genes'. This entails choosing marker genes where the gene products have some putative relationship with the pathogenesis of affective illness. For example, we might focus on neuroreceptor genes or the genes for enzymes involved in the metabolism of monoamines. A third strategy aims for comprehensive cover of the entire human genome so that there is a systematic search throughout all 22 pairs of autosomes and the sex chromosomes. This is, of course, potentially a time-consuming and costly exercise. It must involve the testing of multiple markers to obtain comprehensive covering of the genome (probably in the region of 300). The data will need to be analysed in a range of different genetic models and probably using alternative sets of diagnostic categories (for example, a particular problem being how to categorize individuals with mild to moderately severe UP disorder in families selected for BP disorder). This means that we will once again run into the problem of multiple testing. Although, as we have mentioned, mis-specification of the mode of transmission should not throw up false positives, multiple testing, for the reasons we have also discussed earlier in the section on association studies, almost certainly will. The only satisfactory way of overcoming this problem is to attempt to replicate any positive findings.

In summary, then, we need to aim to collect large samples of large multiplex pedigrees and to search systematically through the human genome using a large number of markers. We then need to ensure that we have enough material available to check that any positive findings have not arisen by chance. The implication of all of this is that collaborative studies are required involving multiple clinical centres and laboratories. At the time of writing, collaborative projects are being set up both in Europe under the auspices of the European Science Foundation and in the United States by the National Institute of Mental Health. Together these ambitious projects begin to take psychiatry into the era of 'big science'. Although the yield so far from genetic marker studies in affective illness has been confusing and disappointing, we can be confident that if major genes exist (and not just polygenes of small effect), they will be detected by collaborative, systematic mapping programmes.

REFERENCES

Angst J. (1966). Zur Atiologie und Nosologie endogener depressiver Psychoses. *Monographen aus der Neurologie und Psychiatrie No. 112.* Berlin: Springer-Verlag.

Baron M., Risch N., Hamburger R. *et al.* (1987). Genetic linkage between X-chromosome markers and bipolar affective illness. *Nature*; **326**: 289–90.

Bebbington P., Katz R., McGuffin P. *et al.* (1989). The risk of minor depression before age 65: results from a community survey. *Psychological Medicine*; **19**: 393–400.

Bebbington P., Tennant C., Hurry J. (1981). The epidemiology of mental disorders in Camberwell. *Psychological Medicine*; **11**: 561–80.

Beckman L., Perris C., Strandman E., Waniby L. (1978). HLA antigens and affective disorders. *Human Heredity*; **28**: 96–9.

Bennaheim D. A., Troup G. M., Rada R. T. *et al.* (1976). HLA antigens in schizophrenia and manic depressive disorders. In: *HLA and Disease, 11–14.* Paris: Editions Inserm.

Bertelsen A., Harvald B., Hauge M. (1977). A Danish twin study of manic depressive disorders. *British Journal of Psychiatry*; **130**: 330–51.

Brown G. W., Prudo R. (1981). Psychiatric disorder in a rural and an urban population. I. Aetiology of depression. *Psychological Medicine*; **11**: 581–99.

Bucher K. D., Elston R. C., Green R. *et al.* (1981). The transmission of manic depressive illness—II. Segregation analysis of three sets of family data. *Journal of Psychiatric Research*; **16**: 65–78.

Cadoret R. (1978). Evidence for genetic inheritance of primary affective disorder in adoptees. *American Journal of Psychiatry*; **135**: 463–6.

Detera-Wadleigh S. D., Berretini W. H., Goldin L. R. *et al.* (1987). Close linkage of C-Harvey *ras*-1 and the insulin gene to affective disorder is ruled out in three North American pedigrees. *Nature*; **325**: 806–7.

Edwards J. H. (1965). Association between blood groups and disease. *Annals of Human Genetics*; **29**: 77–83.

Egeland J. A., Gerhard D. S., Pauls D. L. *et al.* (1987). Bipolar affective disorder linked to DNA markers on chromosome 11. *Nature*; **325**: 783–7.

Elston R. L., Stewart J. (1971). A general model for genetic analysis of pedigree data. *Human Heredity*; **21**: 523–42.

Flemebaum A., Larson J. W. (1976). ABO-Rh blood groups and psychiatric diagnosis: a critical review. *Diseases of the Nervous System*; **37**: 581–3.

Gershon E. S., Mark A., Cohen N. *et al.* (1975). Transmitted factors in the morbid risk of affective disorders. *Journal of Psychiatric Research*; **12**: 283–99.

Gershon E. S., Mendlewicz J., Gastpar M. *et al.* (1980). A collaborative study of genetic linkage of bipolar manic depressive illness and red/green colour blindness. *Acta Psychiatrica Scandinavica*; **61**: 319–38.

Gill M., McKeon P., Humphries P. (1988). Linkage analysis of manic depression in an Irish family using H-*ras* 1 and INS DNA markers. *Journal of Medical Genetics*; **25**: 634–7.

Goldin L. R., Clerget-Darpoux F., Gershon E. S. (1982). Relationship of HLA to major affective disorder not supported. *Psychiatry Research*; **7**: 29–45.

Goldin L. R., Cox N. J., Pauls D. L. *et al.* (1984). The detection of major loci by segregation and linkage analysis: a simulation study. *Genetic Epidemiology*; **1**: 285–96.

Govaerts A., Mendlewicz J., Verbanck P. (1977). Manic depressive illness and HLA. *Tissue Antigens*; **10**: 60–2.

Gusella J. F., Wexler N. S., Conneally P. M. *et al.* (1983). A polymorphic DNA marker genetically linked to Huntington's disease. *Nature*; **306**: 234–8.

Hodgkinson S., Sherrington R., Gurling H. *et al.* (1987). Molecular genetic evidence for heterogeneity in manic depression. *Nature*; **325**: 805–6.

Irvine D. G., Miyashita H. (1965). Blood types in relation to depression and schizophrenia. *Canadian Medical Association Journal*; **92**: 611–14.

Johnson G. F. S. (1978). HLA antigens and manic depressive disorders. *Biological Psychiatry*; **13**: 409–12.

Johnson G. F. S., Hunt G. E., Robertson S., Doran T. J. (1981). A linkage study of manic-depressive disorders with HLA antigens, blood groups, serum proteins and red cell enzymes. *Journal of Affective Disorders*; **3**: 43–58.

Kelsoe J. R., Ginns E. I., Egeland J. A. *et al.* (1989). Re-evaluation of the linkage of relationship between chromosome 11p loci and the gene for bipolar affective disorder in the Old Order Amish. *Nature*; **342**: 238–43.

Kidd K. K., Gerhard D. S. *et al.* (1984). Recombinant DNA methods in genetic studies of affective disorders. *Clinical Neuropharmacology* vol. 7, suppl. 1. New York: Raven Press.

Kidd J. R., Egeland J. A., Pakstis A. J. (1987). Searching for a major genetic locus for affective disorder in the Old Order Amish. *Journal of Psychiatric Research*; **21**: 577–80.

Kraepelin E. (1922). *Manic Depressive Insanity and Paranoia* (Barclay R. M., trans.). Edinburgh: Livingstone.

Lalouel J. M., Rao D. C., Morton M. E., Elston R. C. (1983). A unified model for complex segregation analysis. *American Journal of Human Genetics*; **35**: 816–26.

Leonhard K. (1959). *Aufleilung der Endogen Psychosen*. Berlin: Akademia Verlag.

Masters A. B. (1967). The distribution of blood groups in psychiatric illness. *British Journal of Psychiatry*; **113**: 1309–15.

McGuffin P. (1988). Major genes for major affective disorder. *British Journal of Psychiatry*; **153**: 591–6.

McGuffin P., Katz R. (1986). Nature, nurture and affective disorder. In: *The Biology of Depression* (Deakin J. W. K., ed.). London: Gaskell Press.

McGuffin P., Katz R., Rutherford J. (1990). Nature, nurture and depression. A twin study. *Psychological Medicine*.

Mendlewicz J., Fliess J. L. (1974). Linkage studies with X chromosome markers in bipolar (manic depressive) and unipolar (depressive) illness. *Biological Psychiatry*; **9**: 261–94.

Mendlewicz J., Rainer J. D. (1977). Adoption study supporting genetic transmission in manic-depressive illness. *Nature*; **268**: 326–9.

Mendlewicz J., Massart-Guiot T., Wilmotte J., Fliess J. L. (1974). Blood groups in manic depressive illness and schizophrenia. *Diseases of the Nervous System*; **35**: 39–41.

Mendlewicz J., Simon P., Sevy S. *et al.* (1987). Polymorphic DNA marker and X chromosome and manic depression. *Lancet*; **ii**: 1230–2.

Morton N. E., McLean C. J. (1974). Analysis of familial resemblance. III. Complex segregation analysis of quantitative traits. *American Journal of Human Genetics*; **26**: 489–503.

Orley J. H., Wing J. K. (1979). Psychiatric disorders in two African villages. *Archives of General Psychiatry*; **36**: 513–20.

O'Rourke D. H., McGuffin P., Reich T. (1983). Genetic analysis of manic depressive illness. *American Journal of Physical Anthropology*; **62**: 51–9.

Parker J., Theille A., Spielberger C. (1961). Frequency of blood types in a homogeneous group of manic depressive patients. *Journal of Mental Sciences*; **107**: 936–42.

Perris C. (1966). A study of bipolar (manic depressive) and unipolar recurrent depressive psychoses. *Acta Psychiatrica et Neurologica Scandinavica*; supplementum 42.

Price R. A. (1989). Affective disorder not linked to HLA. *Genetic Epidemiology*; **6**: 299–304.

Reich T., Clayton P. J., Winokur G. (1969). Family history studies v. the genetics of mania. *American Journal of Psychiatry*; **125**: 1358–69.

Reich T., Cloninger C. R., Suarez B., Rice J. (1982). Genetics of the affective disorders. In: *Handbook of Psychiatry. Psychosis of unknown aetiology* (Wing J. R., Wing L., eds.), pp. 147–59. Cambridge: Cambridge University Press.

Rice J. P., Reich T., Andreasen N. C. *et al.* (1987). The familial transmission of bipolar illness. *Archives of General Psychiatry*; **44**: 441–7.

Risch N., Baron M. (1982). X-linkage and genetic heterogeneity in bipolar-related major affective illness. Re-analysis of linkage data. *Annals of Human Genetics*; **46**: 152–66.

Shapiro R. W., Bock E., Rafaelsen O. J. *et al.* (1976). Histocompatibility antigens and manic depressive disorders. *Archives of General Psychiatry*; **33**: 823–5.

Shapiro R. W., Ryder L. P., Svejgaard A., Rafaelson O. J. (1977). HLA antigens and manic depressive disorders: further evidence of association. *Psychological Medicine*; **7**: 387–96.

Slater E., Cowie V. (1971). *The Genetics of Mental Disorders*. Oxford: Oxford University Press.

Stember R. H., Fieve R. R. (1976). Histocompatibility complex in affective disorders. Proceedings of the 129th Annual Meeting of the American Psychiatric Association, pp. 123–4. New York: APA.

Sturt E., Kamakura N., Der G. (1984). How depressing life is—lifelong morbidity risk for depressive disorder in the general population. *Journal of Affective Disorders*; **7**: 109–22.

Sturt E., McGuffin P. (1985). Can linkage and marker association resolve the genetic aetiology of psychiatric disorder: Review and argument (editorial). *Psychological Medicine*; **15**: 455–62.

Suarez B. K., Reich T. (1984). HLA and major affective disorder. *Archives of General Psychiatry*; **41**: 22–7.

Svejgaard A., Platz P., Ryder L. P. *et al.* (1975). HLA and disease associations—a survey. *Transplant Review*; **22**: 3–39.

Tanna V. L., Winokur G., Elston R. C., Go R. C. P. (1977). Blood markers and depressive disorders: an association study. *Comprehensive Psychiatry*; **18**: 263–9.

Targum S. D., Gershon F. S., Van Ferdeweugh M., Rosentine N. (1979). Human leukocyte antigen system not closely linked or associated with bipolar manic depressive illness. *Biological Psychiatry*; **14**: 615.

Torgersen S. (1986). Genetic factors in moderately severe and mild affective disorders. *Archives of General Psychiatry*; **43**: 222–6.

Tsuang M., Winokur G., Crowe R. (1980). Morbidity risks of schizophrenia and affective disorders among first degree relatives of patients with schizophrenia, mania, depression and surgical conditions. *British Journal of Psychiatry*; **137**: 497–504.

Turner W. J., King S. (1983). An autosomal dominant form of bipolar affective disorder. *Biological Psychiatry*; **18**: 63–88.

Von Knorring A. L., Cloninger C. R., Bohman M., Sigvardsson S. (1983). An adoption study of depressive disorders and substance abuse. *Archives of General Psychiatry*; **40**: 943–50.

Weiner A. S. (1962). Blood groups and disease. *Lancet*; **i**: 813.

Weitkamp L. R., Stancer H. C., Persand E. *et al.* (1981). Depressive disorders and HLA: a gene on chromosome 6 that can affect behaviour. *New England Journal of Medicine*; **305**: 1301–41.

Wender P. H., Kety S. S., Rosenthal D. *et al.* (1986). Psychiatric disorders in the biological and adoptive individuals with affective disorders. *Archives of General Psychiatry*; **43**: 923–9.

12 *The genetics of vulnerability to alcoholism*

S. HODGKINSON, M. MULLAN AND R. M. MURRAY

In the 1960s and 1970s, one could have been forgiven for thinking that alcoholism was a phenomenon determined only by psychological and sociocultural factors. A popular paperback of the period stated 'there is no doubt it is a familial condition, but its transmission does not obey biological laws. It works by example' (Kessel and Walton, 1965). The resurgence of interest in genetic models has been kindled by recent genetic epidemiological work (Bohman *et al.*, 1981; Cloninger *et al.*, 1981), as well as by the suggestions that there are biophysical differences between individuals at high risk for alcoholism and the rest of the population (Schuckit and Gold, 1988). Animal models of alcoholism have also been developed, although it is fair to state that the relevance of these to our understanding of human alcohol addiction remains debatable (Keane and Leonard, 1989). The development of recombinant DNA techniques, however, is an important advance. They offer the most direct route for detecting possible variation in the structure of specific genes thought to be implicated in the aetiology of alcoholism.

In this chapter a critique of classical genetic studies of alcoholism will be presented, the question of what exactly is inherited will be addressed, and current research trends in this rapidly growing field will be reviewed.

CLASSICAL GENETIC STUDIES

Family studies

In retrospect, it is surprising that family studies have so consistently shown a higher morbid risk of alcoholism in the relatives of alcoholics than controls. Surprising, because definitions of alcoholism have varied, often being neither standardized nor operationally defined even within the same study, and diagnoses have rarely been made by direct interview. In fact, of over 40 published family studies of alcoholism, only four have interviewed the relatives of probands directly with standardized diagnostic schedules and have similarly assessed control groups (Cotton, 1979; Merikangas, 1989). These studies indicate up to a seven-fold increase in risk to first-degree relatives of alcoholic probands compared with the relatives of controls. Male relatives consistently show higher rates than female relatives but the sex of the proband does not influence the rates in relatives; it seems that the higher rates of alcoholism in men are attributable to greater environmental exposure to alcohol rather than to genetic differences (Reich *et al.*, 1975). Curiously, one study that examined risk to half-siblings found it to be in excess of the risk to full siblings (Schuckit *et al.*, 1972). As such a finding is incompatible with any wholly genetic model of transmission, it emphasizes the possible role of intrafamilial environmental factors.

Twin studies

The classical twin approach has been extensively reviewed elsewhere (Murray *et al.*, 1983; Marshall and Murray, 1989), so we will not discuss it in detail here. Essentially, two main types of study have been carried out. The first has contrasted concordance rates for alcoholism in monozygotic (MZ) and dizygotic (DZ) twins. However, the results have been inconclusive (Table 12.1), probably because, as shown below, the 'equal environment' assumptions of the twin method may be violated by the fact that the drinking habits of one twin can affect those of the second member of the pair.

The other, and possibly more valuable, type of study examines drinking patterns in normal twins. The larger size of the samples investigated has enabled more sophisticated analyses to be carried out. These not only estimate variance due to additive genetic effects (VA) but also distinguish between variance due to specific environmental effects (VSE) and that due to those intrafamilial effects (e.g. family attitudes, imitation) common to both twins (VCE), which have confounded the smaller twin studies of alcoholism.

In one such study, Clifford *et al.* (1981, 1984) examined alcohol use in 494 twin pairs who completed a weekly drinking diary. A biometrical analysis (Fulker *et al.*, 1980) revealed that in males, VA and VSE made up 40% and 32%, respectively, of the total variance in weekly alcohol consumption, with VCE accounting for the remaining 28%. The position was more complicated in women, where there was a negative correlation for alcohol consumption in DZ twins. The explanation seemed to be that the drinking habits of one member of a DZ twin pair influenced the other in the opposite direction (i.e. the co-twin of a heavy-drinking twin might be 'turned off' drinking by witnessing problems in his or her twin). It is, of course, well known that the families of alcoholics not only contain an excess of alcoholics but also of teetotallers!

Paradoxically, similarity in drinking habits depended on whether the twins were living together or not. Among MZ twins, the correlation in weekly alcohol consumption was 0.79 for those cohabiting and 0.50 for those living apart. The comparable correlations for DZ pairs were 0.60 and 0.33 respectively. As MZ pairs tend to live together until later into adult

Table 12.1 Twin studies of alcohol abuse

Reference	Sex	No. of pairs	MZ	DZ	Concordance MZ	Concordance DZ	Concordance ratio MZ/DZ
Kaij (1960)	M	174[a]	32	142	0.53	0.28	1.9:1
Hrubec and Omenn (1981)	M	712[b]	271	441	0.26	0.12	2.2:1
Gurling et al. (1981)	M + F	69[c]	29	40	0.29	0.33	0.9:1

[a] Diagnosis based on interview and official records. The vast majority of cases were alcohol abusers rather than alcoholics.
[b] No interviews carried out. Information from military service, Veterans' Hospitals and questionnaires. Quality unknown.
[c] Sample derived from hospital twin register and assessed using standardized interviews.

life than DZ pairs, this implies that MZ and DZ twins are subject to differential environmental effects.

The best way of avoiding the above biases is to study pairs of twins reared apart. Kaprio *et al.* (1984) therefore compared 30 MZ and 95 DZ pairs separated before the age of 11 years with matched pairs reared together. The intrapair correlation in alcohol consumption was greater for twins reared together than for those who spent their adolescence apart, thus confirming a common family effect. But among men, concordance rates for heavy alcohol use were higher in MZ than DZ pairs, both among those reared together and among the separated pairs. This obviously implies a genetic effect.

Adoption studies

Adoption studies provide the most convincing evidence for genetic factors in predisposition to alcoholism. Clearly, if an individual has had no contact with an alcoholic biological parent after birth, then we can discount the influence of those mechanisms operating within the family environment (e.g. social modelling or the intrafamilial development of a disincentive to drink) that have complicated twin studies. The timing of adoption is therefore crucial in ruling out early postnatal influences as is the exclusion of the offspring of alcoholic mothers in whom intrauterine effects might have been operating.

Again, adoption studies up until the late 1970s have been discussed in detail by Murray *et al.* (1983). In essence, three out of four studies provide evidence for a genetic effect while the fourth was an early study with many methodological defects (Table 12.2). Cloninger *et al.* (1981, 1988) have now carried out a number of further analyses to test the conclusions drawn from the Stockholm adoption study of Bohman *et al.* (1981). As this study has been widely quoted, it is of value to review it.

In brief, the method used was to study a cohort of illegitimate children separated from their parents in infancy. Data on the biological and adoptive parents were obtained from National Temperance Board registrations, the Criminal Register, and National Health Insurance records (medical and psychiatric diagnoses). The severity of alcohol abuse in the adoptees was estimated according to the degree of contact with the National Temperance Board. Among the 862 adopted men, 151 had some record of alcohol abuse, of whom 64 were categorized as mild abusers, 36 as moderate abusers and 51 as severe abusers.

There was a significant correlation between the presence of any alcohol abuse in biological parents and that in adoptees, but more detailed analysis showed that the most severely abusing biological fathers had only moderately abusing sons. Similarly, criminality in the biological fathers was more closely related to moderate abuse in sons than to either mild or severe abuse. Alcohol abuse in the adoptive parents did not increase the risk in adoptees but a number of other variables in the preplacement environment

Table 12.2 A summary of the first four adoption studies on 'alcoholism'

Study	No. of probands		Age of separation compared to controls	Age and sex compared to controls	p value for inter-group differences
	Male	*Female*			
Roe and Burks (1945)	21	15	4 vs. 1.3 yrs	Index adoptees younger and more females	n.s.
Goodwin et al. (1973)	55	49	Both <6 weeks	Almost same	n.s. for females; <0.001 for males
Cadoret and Gath (1978)	4	2	Both 'at birth'	Unknown	<0.03 for 'definite' alcoholism
Bohman (1978)	131	197	3 yrs: probands 3 months later than controls	Almost same	<0.05 for males; n.s. for females

n.s. = not significant.
See Murray *et al.* (1983) for reference.

did: age at placement, rearing by the biological mother beyond the age of 6 months, and the extent of hospitalization before placement. Again, the increased risk introduced by each of these variables was not directly associated with the degree of alcohol abuse in the adoptees. Only in those adoptees with the appropriate background (namely the severe and mild abusers) did postnatal provocation increase the risk for alcoholism. The moderate abusers, by contrast, appeared to have inherited a predisposition whose expression was not increased by postnatal environmental factors.

This study has, therefore, led to the suggestion that there are two main subtypes of alcohol abuse. Type I or 'milieu-limited' abuse is said to occur in both men and women, and to be characterized by milder, adult-onset abuse with no history of criminality in the biological parents. Both a genetic predisposition and adverse environmental influences are necessary for the development of this type; the risk was found to double in the presence of both these aetiological factors.

Type II or 'male-limited' abuse, on the other hand, is said to be characterized by teenage onset of severe abuse, and associated with serious criminality in the biological fathers. The risk to adopted-away sons of such fathers was found to be increased by a factor of nine, regardless of postnatal environmental influences.

Cloninger (1987) proposes that these subtypes are associated with particular, inherited, neuroadaptive mechanisms, which are reflected as behavioural characteristics in the phenotype. Thus, type I alcoholism is said to show low novelty seeking, high harm avoidance and high reward dependence, whereas type II alcoholism is characterized by the opposite, i.e. high novelty seeking, low harm avoidance and low reward dependence. These three dimensions of personality are said to interact to produce the two types of alcoholic. This elaborate theory has not yet been tested independently, but the possibility of particular personality profiles underlying the transmission of alcoholism is inconsistent with the widely held view that there is no such thing as an alcoholic personality.

The findings of this study must be viewed with caution, as the phenotype chosen was quantified arbitrarily along a dimension of severity of abuse. It is certainly curious that the postnatal environment was important for the development of both mild and severe alcohol abuse but not for adoptees who had become moderate abusers. Surely, severe abusers were moderate abusers at an earlier point! The study can also be criticized on the grounds that the identification of alcohol abusers from the National Temperance Board is biased away from the quietly inebriate and towards law-breaking individuals in whom the co-occurrence of antisocial traits and personality disorder is likely to be especially common.

Nevertheless, the classification derived from this study has provided the impetus for much subsequent work. Early results have not altogether supported the hypothesis (Schuckit and Irwin, 1989), but it does seem that individuals with a positive family history of alcoholism are more likely to show many of the features encapsulated in the concept of 'type II abuse'.

Thus 'familial' alcoholics have an earlier age of onset and faster development of a more severe form of dependence than do those with no family history (Goodwin, 1983; Branchey *et al.*, 1989). Furthermore, familial alcoholics are more likely to have antisocial personalities than those without affected relatives (Penick *et al.*, 1978; Hesselbrock *et al.*, 1982). However, such findings do not prove that the aetiological factors operating in familial and non-familial cases are different in kind. They could merely differ in degree, with familial cases having a greater genetic liability. Thus, differences between familial and non-familial cases are compatible with both a model implying distinct heterogeneity and with the multifactorial model of transmission.

HIGH RISK STUDIES

In the search for predisposing influences, some researchers have chosen to investigate that group known to be at high risk for alcoholism, namely children of alcoholics. The aim is to derive tests that will distinguish those at high risk from those whose risk is low (Schuckit, 1988). Certain difficulties are immediately obvious. First, children of alcoholic mothers may be influenced *in utero* by excess alcohol consumption, and it is conceivable that such exposure might predispose to later alcohol abuse. Secondly, only about one-quarter to one-third of the sons of alcoholics become alcoholic themselves. From a purely empirical viewpoint, therefore, we should not expect huge differences between 'high risk' and control subjects, as the former group is likely to be diluted by a substantial number of individuals not necessarily genetically predisposed.

In general, 'high risk' studies have not found the sons of alcoholics to differ from the sons of controls in personality characteristics. However, there has been argument about the possible inheritance of predisposing cognitive deficits. Knopp *et al.* (1988), who compared 134 sons of alcoholics with 70 controls at age 19 years, found that on the majority of tests results were similar but the 'high risk' individuals performed more poorly on the vocabulary subtest of the WAIS, and made more errors on the Halstead–Reitan Category Test and the Porteus Maze. In a much smaller study, Tarter *et al.* (1984) also reported cognitive deficits among delinquents with an alcoholic father compared with those with a non-alcoholic father. Schuckit and Gold (1988) were unable to confirm these results but their subjects were university students and therefore probably an inappropriate group to study because absence of cognitive impairment is presumably a prerequisite for university entrance! Another way of examining the same question is to study pairs of MZ twins who are discordant for alcoholism. Thus, Gurling and Murray (1987) reported significantly poorer performance on a series of cognitive measures by alcoholic MZ twins compared with their normal-drinking co-twins; the degree of decrement was related to the severity of the drinking history.

This study obviously implies that the cognitive deficits are secondary to the excessive drinking and do not cause it.

Event-related potentials (ERPs) have also been examined in high risk studies. ERPs measure computer-averaged brain waves in reaction to various stimuli. One such ERP, the P300, is flattened in alcoholics. Begleiter *et al.* (1984) reported similar findings in the adolescent sons of alcoholics, implying that this might be a marker of some neurophysiological vulnerability. However, these measurements are technically difficult to make and subject to artefact, and attempts at replication have produced mixed results.

A number of studies have compared the response to a dose of alcohol of controls and the non-alcoholic offspring of alcoholics. Two features of the design of such studies are critical. The controls must be adequately matched for previous substance exposure, for age, sex, race, and height-to-weight ratio. Second, the effects of the alcohol challenge should be measured in comparison to a placebo challenge. If the alcohol challenge were easily distinguished from placebo by the test subjects, then the effects of anticipation could differentially influence psychological, physiological, and conceivably biochemical measures.

Despite these difficulties, some results indicate that 'high risk', morbidity-free cases have a less intense reaction to alcohol; such individuals have decreased feelings of intoxication for a given blood alcohol level (Schuckit, 1988). Differing hormonal profiles in response to an alcohol challenge have also been detected; blood ACTH, cortisol and prolactin and urinary epinephrine levels were decreased in sons of alcoholics as compared to controls (Schuckit *et al.*, 1987a,b). Although these studies seem to be consistent, they mainly originate from one laboratory and, as a consequence, need to be replicated.

ALCOHOL CHALLENGE STUDIES IN TWINS

Normal twins have also been used to examine genetic influences on the response to alcohol. The heritability estimates for blood ethanol elimination that were derived from early studies ranged from 0.46 to an unlikely 0.98 (see review in Marshall and Murray, 1989). However, these studies were too small to estimate genetic variance accurately. Martin *et al.* (1985a), therefore, gave a dose of alcohol to 206 pairs of Australian twins; the heritabilities for peak blood alcohol concentration and rate of elimination of alcohol were 0.62 and 0.50, respectively. The results from 40 pairs who underwent repeat testing suggested that all the repeatable variation in the way that people metabolize alcohol is inherited. Only about 12% of the non-repeatable variation could be attributed to differences in drinking experience, and some of these effects were quite ephemeral: for example, consumption of alcohol on the previous evening was associated with higher blood alcohol concentrations during absorption and lower readings during elimination. In general, it seemed that although short-term environmental factors influenced alcohol metabolism, particularly in the absorption phase, the repeatable variance in peak blood alcohol concentration and rate of elimination was due mainly to genetic factors.

Martin *et al.* (1985b) also investigated psychomotor performance and physiological variables in their twins after alcohol. The measures, of course, showed differences between subjects in the sober state. But for many of the tests, extra variation was uncovered by alcohol ingestion. This was particularly true for motor coordination, body sway, and systolic blood pressure. An analysis of covariance showed that most of the additional variance exposed by alcohol was genetic in origin. Thus, there are genetic differences between individuals that determine how an individual will perform a given task under the influence of alcohol. The genes controlling these responses appear quite independent of those that determine the individual's general level of performance when alcohol free.

Significant correlations were found between performance and blood alcohol concentrations, but this accounted for little of the genetic variance exposed by alcohol. Martin *et al.* (1985a,b) concluded that, as blood alcohol concentration seemed to exert such a minor influence on variation in psychomotor deficits, future studies should focus on stages of metabolism subsequent to the initial breakdown of alcohol for the source of this genetic variation.

GENETIC MARKERS

The search for genetic markers of alcoholism is well under way but the results so far have been equivocal. Alcoholism has run the gauntlet of association studies with most of the traditional marker systems including ABO, MNS and HLA (Winokur *et al.*, 1976; Corsico *et al.*, 1988). Other phenotypic markers that have been examined and produced similar confusing results include taste sensitivity and colour blindness (Cruz-Coke and Varela, 1966).

The most interesting findings so far are those of Hill *et al.* (1988), who examined blood group markers using the affected sib-pair method of genetic analysis (Green and Woodrow, 1977). The advantages of this approach are that it is robust to the problems of unknown mode of transmission, incomplete penetrance, and age-related penetrance. It is, therefore, particularly suited to the study of alcoholism where these parameters are difficult to estimate. In Hill's study of 30 nuclear families there was suggestive evidence of linkage between alcoholism and the MNS locus on chromosome 4; to date these findings have not been replicated.

An alternative approach is to examine genetic systems that conceivably might be involved in the pathogenesis of alcoholism or its consequences. For instance, there is considerable evidence that immunological mechanisms are implicated in the development of cirrhosis. It was, therefore, natural to speculate that the HLA system, which is concerned in the control of immune responses, could be associated with some immune-related aspects of alcohol-induced liver damage. In fact, several studies of HLA association and alcoholic cirrhosis have implicated the HLA-B8, B40 and B13 alleles (Melendez *et al.*, 1979; Bell and Nordhagen, 1980; Saunders *et al.*, 1982). There is no association of these alleles with alcoholism without accompanying hepatic cirrhosis (Corsico *et al.*, 1988).

ALCOHOL-METABOLIZING ENZYMES

We have already noted that there is substantial interindividual variation in the effects of alcohol, and that this is, in part, under genetic control. Could this be consequent upon differences between individuals in the activity of the enzymes which metabolize alcohol, and might such differences contribute to susceptibility to alcoholism?

Ethanol is metabolized in the liver by class I alcohol dehydrogenase (ADH) and aldehyde dehydrogenase (ALDH). These enzymes process over 90% of the ethanol ingested, and because of this both have been investigated extensively. Class I ADH protein subunits are coded for by three non-allelic genes, ADH1, ADH2 and ADH3, the latter two being polymorphic (Smith *et al.*, 1973). Chromosome mapping studies have revealed that all three class I ADH genes are located on the long arm of chromosome 4, between q21 and q24. It is of interest that the MNS locus is also located on 4q. A variant enzyme at the ADH2 locus, known as 'atypical ADH', is particularly active, and differs in frequency in different ethnic groups. It has been suggested that this may account for some racial differences in the speed of alcohol metabolism, but the published studies have been equivocal (Agarwal and Goedde, 1987).

The acetaldehyde produced by the action of ADH is further oxidized to acetate in a reaction catalysed by ALDH. The genes for ALDH1 and ALDH2 have been localized and sequenced. Mitochondrial ALDH2, the gene for which is on chromosome 12 (Hsu *et al.*, 1986), accounts for most acetaldehyde oxidation in Caucasian populations but approximately half of all Japanese and Chinese have a point mutation on the ALDH2 gene, which results in a relatively inactive variant of the enzyme (Yoshida *et al.*, 1984; Shibuya and Yoshida, 1988a). As a consequence, acetaldehyde accumulates after alcohol ingestion, causing vasodilation, flushing, tachycardia and muscle weakness (Goedde and Agarwal, 1987). This reaction is similar to that produced by disulfiram, an inhibitor of ALDH.

Goedde *et al.* (1979) suggested that this unpleasant reaction to alcohol might partly account for the lower consumption of alcohol among Orientals. This lower consumption holds not just in Asia, but also among those of Oriental extraction living in the USA. The ALDH2 hypothesis was supported by the discovery that the *per capita* alcohol consumption in two Japanese cities was related to the differing proportions of their populations that had the deficient isoenzyme. Thus, the mean alcohol consumption in a city in which only 25% of the population had the deficiency was almost double that in a city in which 50% of the population had the deficient ALDH2 variant.

Further studies have demonstrated that Japanese alcoholics differ from their fellow countrymen in that less than 5% have the defective variant and more than 95% the active type so common in Europe (Shibuya and Yoshida, 1988b; Goedde *et al.*, 1989). Thus, it seems that among Japanese at least, the possession of the ALDH2 variant protects against the development of alcoholism, presumably by rendering heavy drinking much less rewarding.

Although no such dramatic findings have been reported among Caucasians, these studies are important not only because they demonstrate that alterations in a single enzyme can predispose against alcoholism but also because they show that what were thought to be culturally determined differences in alcohol consumption were, in fact, genetically determined.

MAPPING ALCOHOL-RELATED BEHAVIOURAL TRAITS IN MICE

It follows from the above that a strategy based on an understanding of the genetic control of alcohol metabolism may be more profitable than an attempt at 'random' linkage marker studies. One way of pursuing this strategy is to examine inbred strains of mice (Plomin *et al.*, 1980). In doing so, one can study a well-defined series of biochemical pathways in an animal of distinct genetic lineage, and examine behaviours such as alcohol preference, alcohol tolerance and withdrawal. As variation at the level of DNA sequence between mouse and human is relatively small, biochemical correlates of behavioural profiles in the mouse may be relevant to human alcoholism.

Recently, interesting work has shown that, in mice bred for either high or low propensity to seizures on alcohol withdrawal, differences exist in the degree of up-regulation of neuronal calcium channels induced by chronic alcohol ingestion. The number of dihydropyridine-sensitive calcium channels increases in both withdrawal seizure-resistant (WSR) and withdrawal seizure-prone (WSP) mice, but the increase in the WSP strain is much greater (J. Littleton, personal communication).

Thus, by breeding animals for characteristic behaviour patterns or neurochemical profiles that are paralleled in human alcoholism, it may be possible to locate genes of potential aetiological significance. Recombinant DNA techniques are particularly suited to identifying 'candidate genes' from mouse studies because of the extensive knowledge of the mouse genome map. A number of strategies are available to map genetic loci in the mouse, and by the use of linkage groups common to both mouse and human (synteny), then to establish their location on human chromosomes.

Perhaps the most powerful approach in behavioural and pharmacological studies is the use of recombinant inbred strains (Eleftheriou and Elias, 1975). Thus, through a series of intermatings, lines of mice are bred which represent a unique series of haplotypes; within each line, all offspring are almost genetically identical, i.e. the alleles are fixed to homozygosity. The phenotypic variation between inbred lines (in, for example, ion channel activity or ethanol-modified motor activity) may then be used to determine a genetic relationship between correlated phenotypes (Goldman *et al.*, 1985). In an excellent review, Harris and Allan (1989) show how evidence was derived for a role of GABA-stimulated chloride channels in ethanol and benzodiazepine intoxication. By using such genetic tools it should be possible to begin to dissect the pharmacological processes involved in chronic alcohol ingestion.

CONCLUSIONS

Even the most 'dyed in the wool' geneticist must accept that environmental factors are crucial to the development of alcoholism. Thus, the elucidation of the 'environmental' components in the aetiology of alcoholism is of great importance, not least because this will allow the genetic components to be viewed in the appropriate context. The underlying message from this cursory glance at genetic research is that alcoholism must be seen from a number of different points of view. There is strong evidence for a significant genetic component, but the traditional simple approaches to the investigation of Mendelian disorders are not directly applicable. Rather than conceive of the genetic predisposition to alcoholism as a single-gene effect, or even as several, single, major loci (to account for genetic heterogeneity), it is more appropriate to consider a model based on many interacting components, each contributing only a small percentage of the overall risk.

Already, genetic components have been identified that act as protective or susceptibility factors, for example in alcohol sensitivity and alcoholic liver disease. In addition, animal studies have identified specific genetic effects that govern some behavioural responses to alcohol ingestion. Whatever the phenotypic form predispositions take, they will ultimately be reduced to the molecular level of DNA. At present, however, alcoholism is recognized by a range of behavioural manifestations, and a 'quantum leap' is required to move from the level of DNA mutation to the 'catch all' concept of 'alcoholism'.

In attempting to bridge this gap, laboratory studies need to proceed in conjunction with careful clinical investigations. There are some hopeful precedents. For example, in coronary heart disease, which also has a complex, polygenic, multifactorial aetiology, the disease phenotype was first subdivided and the highly familial form due to monogenic hypercho-lesterolaemia identified. Then, molecular techniques were applied to relevant 'endophenotypes', e.g. the enzymes that regulate cholesterol synthesis and levels of fibrinogen. In a similar way, progress in the field of alcoholism is likely to come from painstakingly elucidating the genetic control of alcohol preference, metabolism and dependence, and the molecular mechanisms underlying susceptibility to end-organ disorders such as liver cirrhosis and Korsakoff's syndrome. In our view, this is a more logical approach than crudely asking 'is alcoholism genetic, and if so what is the responsible gene?'

REFERENCES

Agarwal D. P., Goedde H. W. (1987). Genetic variation in alcohol metabolising enzymes: implications in alcohol use and abuse. *Progress in Clinical Biological Research*; **241**: 121–39.

Begleiter H., Porjesz B., Bihari B., Kissin B. (1984). Event-related brain potentials in boys at risk for alcoholism. *Science*; **225**: 1493–6.

Bell H., Nordhagen R. (1980). HLA antigens in alcoholics with special reference to alcoholic cirrhosis. *Scandinavian Journal of Gastroenterology*; **15**: 453–6.

Bohman M., Sigvardsson S., Cloninger C. R. (1981). Maternal inheritance of alcohol abuse: cross-fostering analysis of adopted women. *Archives of General Psychiatry*; **38**: 965–9.

Buydens-Branchey L., Branchey M. H., Noumair D. (1989). Age of alcoholism onset: I. Relationship to psychopathology. *Archives of General Psychiatry*; **46**: 225–30.

Clifford C. A., Fulker D. W., Gurling H. M. D., Murray R. M. (1981). Preliminary findings from a twin study of alcohol use. In: *Twin Research 3, Part C. Epidemiological and Clinical Studies* (Gedda L., Parisi P., Nance W. E., eds.), pp. 47–52. New York: Alan R. Liss.

Clifford C. A., Fulker D. W., Murray R. M. (1984). Genetic and environmental influences on drinking patterns in normal twins. In: *Alcohol Related Problems* (Krasner N., Madden J. S., Walker R. J., eds.), pp. 115–26. New York: Wiley.

Cloninger C. R. (1987). Neurogenetic adaptive mechanisms in alcoholism. *Science*; **236**: 410–16.

Cloninger C. R., Bohman M., Sigvardsson S. (1981). Inheritance of alcohol abuse: cross-fostering analysis of adopted men. *Archives of General Psychiatry*; **38**: 861–8.

Cloninger C. R., Sigvardsson S., Bohman M. (1988). Childhood personality predicts alcohol abuse in young adults. *Alcoholism Clinical and Experimental Research*; **12**: 494–505.

Corsico R., Pessino O. L., Morales V., Jmelninsky A. (1988). Association of HLA antigens with alcoholic disease. *Journal of Studies in Alcoholism*; **49**: 546–50.

Cotton N. (1979). The familial incidence of alcoholism. *Journal of Studies in Alcoholism*; **40**: 89–116.

Cruz-Coke R., Varela A. (1966). Inheritance of alcoholism. Its association with color blindness. *Lancet*; **ii**: 1282–4.

Eleftheriou B. E., Elias P. K. (1975). Recombinant inbred strains: a novel approach for psychopharmacogenetics. In: *Psychopharmacogenetics* (Eleftheriou B. E., ed.). New York: Plenum Press.

Fulker D. W., Eysenck S. B. G., Zuckerman M. (1980). A genetic and environmental analysis of sensation seeking. *Journal of Research into Personality*; **14**: 261–81.

Goedde H. W., Agarwal D. P. (1987). Polymorphism of aldehyde dehydrogenase and alcohol sensitivity. *Enzyme*; **37**: 29–44.

Goedde H. W., Harada S., Agarwal D. P. (1979). Racial differences in alcohol sensitivity: a new hypothesis. *Human Genetics*; **51**: 331–4.

Goedde H. W., Singh S., Agarwal D. P. *et al.* (1989). Genotyping of mitochondrial aldehyde dehydrogenase in blood samples using allele-specific oligonucleotides: comparison with phenotyping in hair roots. *Human Genetics*; **81**: 305–7.

Goldman D., Nelson R., Deitrich R. A. *et al.* (1985). Genetic brain polypeptide variants in inbred mice and in mouse strains with high and low sensitivity to alcohol. *Brain Research*; **341**: 130–8.

Goodwin D. W. (1983). Familial alcoholism. *Substance and Alcohol Actions and Misuse*; **4**: 129–36.

Green J. R., Woodrow J. C. (1977). Sibling method for detecting HLA-linked genes in disease. *Tissue Antigens*; **9**: 31–5.

Gurling H. M. D., Murray R. M. (1987). Genetic influence, brain morphology and cognitive deficits in alcoholic twins. In: *Genetics and Alcoholism* (Goedde H. W., Agarwal D. P., eds.), pp. 71–82. New York: Alan R. Liss.

Gurling H. M. D., Murray R. M., Clifford C. A. (1981). Investigations into the genetics of alcohol dependence and into its effect on brain function. In: *Twin Research 3, Part C. Epidemiological and Clinical Studies* (Gedda L., Parisi P., Nance W. E., eds.), pp. 77–87. New York: Alan R. Liss.

Harris R. A., Allan A. M. (1989). Alcohol intoxication: ion channels and genetics. *FASEB Journal*; **3**: 1689–95.

Hesselbrock V. M., Stabenau J. R., Hesselbrock M. N. *et al.* (1982). The nature of alcoholism in patients with different family histories for alcoholism. *Neuropsychopharmacology and Biological Psychiatry*; **6**: 607–14.

Hill S. Y., Aston C., Rabin B. (1988). Suggestive evidence of genetic linkage between alcoholism and the MNS blood group. *Alcoholism Clinical and Experimental Research*; **12**: 811–14.

Hrubec Z., Omenn G. S. (1981). Evidence of genetic predisposition to alcoholic cirrhosis and psychosis. *Alcoholism Clinical and Experimental Research*; **5**: 207–15.

Hsu L. C., Yoshida A., Mohandas T. (1986). Chromosomal assignment of the genes for human ALDH1 and ALDH2. *American Journal of Human Genetics*; **38**: 641–8.

Kaij L. (1960). *Alcoholism in Twins*. Stockholm: Almqvist and Wiksell.

Kaprio J., Koskenvuo M., Langinvainio H. (1984). Finnish twins reared apart. IV: Smoking and drinking habits. A preliminary analysis of the effect of heredity and environment. *Acta Genetica Medica Gemellologica*; **33**: 425–33.

Keane B., Leonard B. E. (1989). Rodent models of alcoholism: a review. *Alcohol and Alcoholism*; **24**: 299–309.

Kessel N., Walton H. (1965). *Alcoholism*, p. 71. London: Penguin.

Knopp J., Teasdale T., Goodwin D. W. *et al.* (1988). Premorbid characteristics in high risk and low risk individuals of developing alcoholism. In: *Genetic Aspects of Alcoholism*, Proceedings of the Satellite Symposium on Alcohol and Genetics, Sapporo, Japan (Kiianmaa K., Tabakoff B., Saito T., eds.), **137**: 117–26. Helsinki: The Finnish Foundation for Alcohol Studies.

Marshall E. J., Murray R. M. (1989). The contribution of twin studies of alcoholism research. In: *Genetics and Alcoholism* (Goedde H. W., Agarwal D. P., eds.). New York: Alan R. Liss.

Martin N. G., Oakeshott J. G., Gibson J. B. *et al.* (1985b). A twin study of psychomotor and physiological responses to an acute dose of alcohol. *Behavioral Genetics*; **15**: 305–47.

Martin N. G., Perl J., Oakeshott J. G. *et al.* (1985a). A twin study of ethanol metabolism. *Behavioral Genetics*; **15**: 93–109.

Melendez M., Vargas-Tank L., Fuentes C. *et al.* (1979). Distribution of HLA histocompatability antigens, ABO blood groups and Rh antigens in alcoholic liver disease. *Gut*; **20**: 288–90.

Merikangas K. R. (1989). Genetics of alcoholism: a review of human studies. In: *Genetics of Neuropsychiatric Diseases* (Wetterberg I., ed.), pp. 269–71. London: Macmillan.

Murray R. M., Clifford C. A., Gurling H. M. D. (1983). Twin and adoption studies: how good is the evidence for a genetic role. In: *Recent Developments in Alcoholism* vol. 1 (Galanter M., ed.), pp. 25–48. New York: Plenum Press.

Penick E., Read M., Crowley P. *et al.* (1978). Differentiation of alcoholics by family history. *Journal of Studies in Alcohol*; **39**: 1944–8.

Plomin R., DeFries J. C., McClearn G. E. (1980). *Behavioural Genetics: A Primer*. San Francisco: Freeman.

Reich T., Winokur G., Mullaney J. (1975). The transmission of alcoholism. In: *Genetic Research in Psychiatry* (Fieve R. R., Rosenthal D., Brill H., eds.), pp. 259–71. Baltimore: Johns Hopkins University Press.

Saunders J. B., Wodak A. D., Haines A. *et al.* (1982). Accelerated development of alcoholic cirrhosis in patients with HLA-B8. *Lancet*; **i**: 1381–4.

Schuckit M. A. (1988). Multiple markers of the response to ethanol in sons of alcoholics and controls. In: *Genetic Aspects of Alcoholism*, Proceedings of the Sat. Symposium on Alcohol and Genetics, Sapporo, Japan (Kiianmaa K., Tabakoff B., Saito T., eds.), **137**: 107–16. Helsinki: The Finnish Foundation for Alcohol Studies.

Schuckit M. A., Gold E. (1988). A simultaneous evaluation of multiple markers of ethanol/placebo challenges in sons of alcoholics and controls. *Archives of General Psychiatry*; **45**: 211–16.

Schuckit M. A., Irwin M. (1989). An analysis of the clinical relevance of type 1 and type 2 alcoholics. *British Journal of Addiction*; **84**: 869–76.

Schuckit M. A., Gold E., Risch C. (1987a). Plasma cortisol levels following ethanol in sons of alcoholics and controls. *Archives of General Psychiatry*; **44**: 942–5.

Schuckit M. A., Gold E., Risch S. C. (1987b). Serum prolactin levels in sons of alcoholics and control subjects. *American Journal of Psychiatry*; **144**: 854–9.

Schuckit M., Goodwin D., Winokur G. (1972). A study of alcoholism in half-siblings. *American Journal of Psychiatry*; **128**: 122–5, 259–71.

Shibuya A., Yoshida A. (1988a). Frequency of the atypical aldehyde dehydrogenase-2 gene (ALDH 2/2) in Japanese and Caucasians. *American Journal of Human Genetics*; **43**: 741–3.

Shibuya A., Yoshida A. (1988b). Genotypes of alcohol-metabolising enzymes in Japanese with alcohol liver diseases: a strong association of the usual Caucasian-type aldehyde dehydrogenase gene (ALDH 1/2) with the disease. *American Journal of Human Genetics*; **43**: 744–8.

Smith M., Hopkinson D. A., Harris H. (1973). Studies on the properties of the human alcohol dehydrogenase isozymes determined by the different loci, ADH1, ADH2, ADH3. *Annals of Human Genetics*; **37**: 49–67.

Tarter R. E., Hegedus A. M., Goldstein G. *et al.* (1984). Adolescent sons of alcoholics. Neuropsychological and personality characteristics. *Alcoholism Clinical and Experimental Research*; **8**: 216–22.

Winokur G., Tanna V., Elston R., Go R. (1976). Lack of association of genetic traits with alcoholism: C3 Ss and ABO systems. *Journal of Studies in Alcoholism*; **37**: 1313–15.

Yoshida A., Huang I. Y., Ikawa M. (1984). Molecular abnormality of an inactive aldehyde dehydrogenase variant commonly found in Orientals. *Proceedings of the National Academy of Sciences (USA)*; **81**: 258–61.

13 Genes and the aetiology of eating disorders

J. L. TREASURE AND A. J. HOLLAND

The syndromes of anorexia nervosa and bulimia nervosa have a markedly different lineage. Anorexia nervosa can be traced back to the masterly clinical descriptions of Gull (1873) and Lasegue (1873) over a century ago, whereas it is just over a decade since bulimia nervosa was described (Russell, 1979). The two disorders share many features in common, for example, overvalued ideas about weight and shape, and extreme diets, but in bulimia nervosa bouts of massive overconsumption punctuate fasts. Strategies to avoid the metabolic consequences of binges include the induction of vomiting and the abuse of laxatives, diuretics and metabolic stimulants, and range from the ingenious to the frankly dangerous.

The aetiology of these disorders is unknown and it is unclear whether or not they have common origins. In the original series of Russell (1979), the symptoms of bulimia nervosa developed after an episode of anorexia nervosa, but neither the tenth revision of the *International Classification of Diseases* (ICD 10; World Health Organization, 1989) nor the revised third edition of the *Diagnostic and Statistical Manual for Mental Disorders* (DSM-IIIR; American Psychiatric Association, 1987) maintain this as a necessary criterion and the majority of cases now presenting to specialized clinics do not have such a history.

In the seminal descriptions of anorexia nervosa, familial factors were thought to be important in the development of the disorder. Gull (1873) reported that there was 'often something queer in the family history' and his treatment involved removing the patient from the family, into a nursing home where 'moral management' could be instigated. Greenhow (1873) concurred with this analysis, commenting that there was often a family history of insanity and that the illness flourished in certain 'moral surroundings'. More general aspects of Victorian society were also considered to be relevant: Playfair (1888) noted that the illness was 'of daily increasing frequency in this age of culture, overstrain and pressure'. Ryle (1936) returned, 50 years later, to the higher incidence of 'nervousness' in the immediate family and the relevance of an adverse family environment as he noted that some cases occurred in 'unhappy or ill-conducted homes', sometimes with 'spoiling by foolish parents'.

Cultural forces within the family (Minuchin *et al.*, 1975; Selvini-

Palazzoli *et al.*, 1978) or society (Orbach, 1978; Garner *et al.*, 1980; Brumberg, 1988; Patton, 1988) are still considered to be of primary aetiological importance in the development of eating disorders. Sociocultural mechanisms could explain the increasing incidence of anorexia nervosa (Szmukler *et al.*, 1985) and the increased prevalence in high risk groups such as ballet dancers and fashion models (Garner *et al.*, 1980). However, the study of Lucas *et al.* (1988) found that the incidence of the classic form of the disease, restricting anorexia nervosa, has not changed over the last 50 years. Also, sociocultural mechanisms fail to account for individual susceptibility.

Vulnerability may result from genetic or environmentally acquired, physiological or psychological traits. For example, there may be disturbance in hypothalamic function (Russell, 1970) or a tendency to obesity or a high growth rate (Crisp, 1967). Psychogenic formulations have evolved over the years and have included specific fears over impending sexuality and maturity (Waller *et al.*, 1940; Crisp, 1967), a disturbance in body image (Bruch, 1973; Slade, 1985) or low self-esteem (Grace *et al.*, 1985).

RECENT EVIDENCE FOR FAMILIAL FACTORS IN THE AETIOLOGY OF ANOREXIA NERVOSA

An initial approach to test the aetiological importance of the family is to identify cases amongst relatives. The next stage in the analysis is to identify what clinical features, if any, distinguish patients with affected relatives from patients with normal relatives: in other words, identify the clinical features that are most strongly familial or heritable. A further approach is then to identify familial clinical features, such as personality traits, that are not in themselves pathological but which are predictive of the extent of psychopathology in individuals and their relatives.

The familial incidence of eating disorders

A history of anorexia nervosa amongst the relatives is occasionally seen in clinical practice. Fig. 13.1 shows the pedigree of a patient presenting to our clinic. The diagnosis of anorexia nervosa in her great aunt and aunt had been made, perhaps because of ready access to medical care as two members of the family were medical practitioners. More often the diagnosis of anorexia nervosa was not made contemporaneously. Fig. 13.2 illustrates this: the clinical features and the objective evidence of severe weight loss at age 15 years are highly suggestive of anorexia nervosa in the grandmother. A history of bulimia nervosa amongst relatives is much harder to elicit: first, because the syndrome was not delineated until 1979, and, secondly, because the symptoms are covert and any weight loss is not striking.

The prevalence of anorexia nervosa in the first-degree relatives of

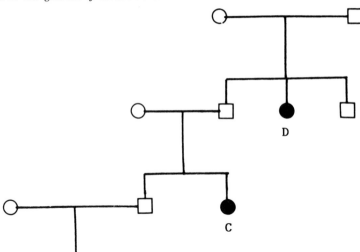

Fig. 13.1　*A family with anorexia nervosa in several generations: A presented to the eating disorders clinic aged 24 years with primary amenorrhoea (body wt. 39 kg; height 1.58 m), the onset of anorexia nervosa had been at 11 years. Her sister (B) developed anorexia nervosa at age 15 years with bulimic features but recovered three years later. The paternal aunt (C) developed anorexia nervosa when aged 15 years but recovered after five years and, although married, has no children. The paternal great-aunt (D) had anorexia nervosa when aged 17 years but never recovered from the illness: she never married, lived alone and remained thin with eccentric eating habits until her death. Many of the male members of the family were medical practitioners*

consecutive series of patients ranges from 5 to 10% (Theander, 1970; Morgan and Russell, 1975; Dally and Gomez, 1979; Crisp *et al.*, 1980). The lifetime risk of a relative having an eating disorder is 6% in comparison to the risk of 1% in the relatives of controls (Gershon *et al.*, 1983). Strober *et al.* (1985) found that 5% of female, first-degree relatives of a series of probands with eating disorder had a history of an eating disorder. The pooled risk of eating disorder was five times as great amongst female, first-degree relatives of patients with anorexia nervosa than in controls. Their findings also suggested that severe, restrictor-type anorexia nervosa and bulimia may segregate differentially in families.

The familial incidence of other psychiatric illnesses

It has been argued that 'there is no neurosis specific to anorexia nervosa, and no specific anorexia nervosa' (Kaye and Leigh, 1954), and that anorexia nervosa is merely a constellation of symptoms stemming from diverse psychopathology (Levy, 1938). Some justification for these views

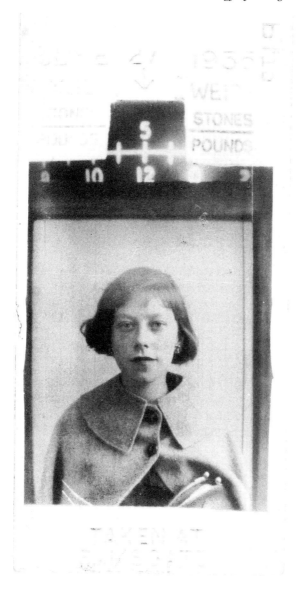

Fig. 13.2 *Photograph of the maternal grandmother of a current patient with anorexia nervosa. The photograph was taken when the grandmother was 15 years old in a seaside booth in which her weight was also recorded at 37 kg. The grandmother's weight loss led to admission to a nursing home for bed rest; the diagnosis of anorexia nervosa was not made at the time, although the family recognized the similarity with the granddaughter's illness*

arises from the observation of diverse psychiatric syndromes in the relatives. Sixty-six per cent of Kay and Leigh's 38 patients with severe chronic anorexia nervosa had psychotic or neurotic parents or neurotic siblings. This figure is much higher than that of Dally's (1969) series of 139 patients, where the incidence of psychological disturbance amongst the parents was 33%.

Unipolar depression has been shown to occur two to four times more frequently in the first-degree relatives of both anorexic and bulimic patients than in the general population (Winokur *et al.*, 1980; Gershon *et al.*, 1983; Hudson *et al.*, 1983; Rivinius, 1984). The only studies that failed to find such a pattern were those of Stern *et al.* (1984) and Theander (1970). Nevertheless, there is no evidence to support the hypothesis that anorexia nervosa and affective disorder are part of a common genetic spectrum, as the incidence of eating disorder amongst the relatives of patients with unipolar or bipolar depression was not increased. It was only amongst patients with eating disorders who had coexisting, persistent, depressive symptoms that an increased family history of affective disorder was found. This suggests that depression and eating disorder are transmitted independently, although the two disorders do coexist within a subgroup of patients (Strober *et al.*, 1986).

We have conducted a twin and family study of anorexia nervosa in which a sibling and parent were given a structured interview designed to elicit a history of abnormal eating behaviour, alcoholism and other psychiatric symptoms. The results are shown in Tables 13.1 and 13.2.

These findings suggest that the familial clustering of eating disorders in the families of bulimic probands is higher than in the families of restricting anorexia nervosa. There is also a higher prevalence of alcoholism in the families of twins with bulimia nervosa than in twins with anorexia nervosa but there are no significant differences for ratio of depression.

The prevalence of anorexia nervosa and bulimia nervosa differs markedly. In north-east Scotland the prevalence of anorexia nervosa is 1/1000 females and in Rochester, USA it is 2/1000 (Szmukler *et al.*, 1986; Lucas *et al.*, 1988). The prevalence of bulimia nervosa amongst schoolgirls in London (Johnson-Sabine *et al.*, 1988) or amongst female attenders at a general practitioner (King, 1986) is approximately 1%. Therefore, if the familial prevalence is compared with the population prevalence, restricting anorexia nervosa emerges as the more familial condition.

Which clinical features distinguish familial anorexia nervosa?

The clinical features of subjects with a positive family history of anorexia nervosa ($n = 22$) differ from those ($n = 45$) without such a history on only two features. Their weight falls to a significantly lower level (14.2 kg/m^2 vs. 15.6 kg/m^2; $p < 0.05$) and the illness develops at an earlier age (16.5 vs. 18.7 years).

Twin studies in eating disorders

Twins offer a unique opportunity to separate aetiological factors. First, an analysis of the concordance rate between monozygotic (MZ) and dizygotic

Table 13.1 The prevalence of eating disorders in the relatives of twins with eating disorders

First-degree female relatives	*29 cases of restricting anorexia nervosa* (N=77)			*38 cases of bulimia nervosa* (N=91)			
	Cases	(%)	70% CL*	Cases	(%)	70% CL	p (Fisher's 2-tailed)
History of anorexia nervosa	3	(3.9)	2–8%	4	(4.3)	2–8%	0.6
History of bulimia nervosa	2	(2.6)	1–6%	8	(8.8)	6–13%	0.17
Partial syndrome	4	(5.1)	3–9%	8	(8.8)	7–14%	0.55
Total eating disorder	9	(12)	8–17%	20	(22)	17–27%	0.12

* 70% confidence limit.

Table 13.2 The prevalence of depression and alcoholism in the relatives of twins with eating disorders

First-degree female relatives	*29 cases of restricting anorexia nervosa* (N=123)			*38 cases of bulimia nervosa* (N=160)			
	Cases	(%)	70% CL*	Cases	(%)	70% CL	p (Fisher's 2-tail)
Alcoholism	6	(4.8)	3–8%	19	(11.9)	9–15%	0.06
Depression	16	(13)	10–17%	29	(18.1)	15–22%	0.3

* 70% confidence limits.

(DZ) twins can establish whether genetic factors contribute to the aetiology. Moreover, any differences between MZ twins are usually taken to be non-genetic in origin and so a comparison of MZ discordant twins is a model to look at the environmental factors that predispose or protect against the development of a disorder. They thus provide a model of pathogenesis, the mechanisms by which defective gene products are linked to dysfunctional behaviour.

Reviews of twins with anorexia nervosa have consistently found an increased concordance rate for eating disorders in MZ than in DZ twins

(Askevold and Heiberg, 1979; Vandereycken and Pierloot, 1981; Garfinkel and Garner, 1982; Nowlin, 1983; Scott, 1986). It is difficult to draw conclusions from such reviews because of possible reporting bias and, in some cases, lack of definite information concerning the zygosity or whether the co-twins themselves had been interviewed. Some of these methodological difficulties were avoided in the earlier twin study by Holland *et al.* (1984). Thirty-four pairs of twins and a set of triplets were described. Of the 30 female-only pairs, 9 out of 16 (55%) MZ pairs were concordant for anorexia nervosa, whereas only 1 out of 14 (7%) DZ pairs was concordant. However, structured interviews to ascertain the form of the eating disorder were not used and these cases are a mixture of the restricting and bulimic forms of anorexia nervosa.

In a later study, we sought to overcome some of these methodological difficulties. Sixty-eight sets of female twins, of whom at least one had an eating disorder, were seen. Both twins, separately, were given structured interviews (the Eating Disorder Examination (EDE; Cooper and Fairburn, 1987) and the Diagnostic Interview Schedule (DIS; Robins *et al.*, 1981)) to determine the specific eating psychopathology and more general psychiatric symptoms. Zygosity was established by blood group analysis in all but two pairs, who were presumed to be dizygotic on the basis of differing eye colours. In order to obtain a large sample, twins were recruited from various sources and so there is a problem of ascertainment bias with the possibility that an excess of concordant MZ twins are in the sample. We also have only a small proportion of twins with bulimia nervosa without a history of anorexia nervosa.

Thirty of the twin pairs had restricting anorexia nervosa and 29 of the 38 (76%) cases with bulimia nervosa had a past history of anorexia nervosa. The pairwise and probandwise concordance rates are shown in Table 13.3. The findings on applying a simple path-analysis model using the HERIT computer program (McGuffin and Katz, 1986) are shown in Table 13.4. Genetic factors account for the greater part of the variation in liability to develop anorexia nervosa, whereas, for bulimia nervosa, cultural transmission is more important. Thus the increased prevalence of eating disorders amongst the co-twins with bulimia nervosa is probably accounted for by common exposure to detrimental, environmental (rearing) experiences. It should be noted that our sample is quite small and therefore the standard errors of our estimates are large. Nevertheless, our findings have received support from a larger study of eating attitudes in normal female twins where anorexia-like symptoms have a modest but significant heritability. By contrast, bulimia-like symptoms appear to have negligible heritability by significant family environmental effects (J. Rutherford, personal communication).

The clinical features of concordant and discordant monozygotic pairs

The clinical features of concordant, anorexic, MZ twins differed from

Table 13.3 Pairwise and probandwise concordance rates for restricting anorexia nervosa and bulimia nervosa in 68 twin pairs

	Concordance rate			
	Pairwise		Probandwise	
Diagnostic criteria	MZ (31)	DZ (29)	MZ (38)	DZ (30)
Eating disorder (anorexia nervosa or bulimia nervosa)	0.45	0.21	0.55	0.24
Restricting anorexia nervosa	0.51	0.08	0.59	0.08
Bulimia nervosa	0.25	0.33	0.36	0.38

Table 13.4 Estimates obtained using the HERIT and THRESH programs

Diagnostic criteria	Heritability	Common environment	Unique environment
Eating disorder (anorexia nervosa or bulimia nervosa)	0.35	0.49	0.16
Anorexia nervosa	0.76	0.19	0.05
Bulimia nervosa	0.03	0.81	0.16

those of the discordant MZ pairs in that their premorbid weight was lower (21.5 kg/m^2 vs. 23.4 kg/m^2), their weight fell to a significantly lower level (13.6 kg/m^2 vs. 15.2 kg/m^2), they had significantly fewer bulimic symptoms (5 vs. 1 on the bulimia subscale of the eating disorders' inventory), and there was a trend for the age of onset to be lower (17 vs. 18.7 years).

If, as has been argued (see above), anorexia nervosa is a non-specific type of neurosis, then it would follow that twins discordant for anorexia nervosa would tend to be concordant for other forms of neurotic illness. The lifetime prevalence of psychiatric disorders amongst MZ and DZ twins, discordant for eating disorder, is shown in Fig. 13.3. Subjects with an eating disorder had many other additional symptoms; over 70% had had a depressive illness. In contrast, the twins without an eating disorder had significantly fewer, additional psychiatric illnesses. These findings suggest that anorexia nervosa does not arise out of a general genetic predisposition to neurosis or from a cultural background which fosters neurosis.

Several conclusions can be tentatively drawn from these studies. First, there is a genetic contribution to the risk of developing restricting anorexia

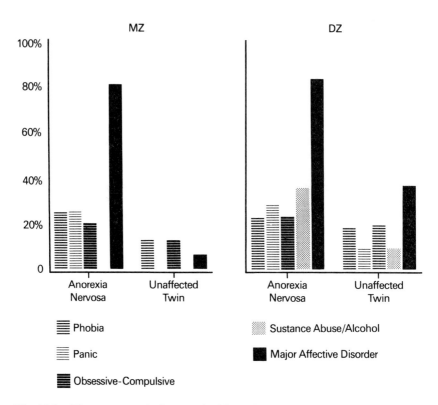

Fig. 13.3   *The percentage of subjects with additional psychopathology amongst probands and unaffected co-twins of twin pairs discordant for anorexia nervosa. Monozygotic (MZ) and dizygotic (DZ) twin pairs are shown separately*

nervosa at a young age. Secondly, eating disorders, especially bulimia nervosa, occurring in older women whose weight is above average, do not require a genetic predisposition and can develop in anyone exposed to the relevant, pathogenetic, environmental factors. These simple conclusions need to be considered in more detail. Models used to partition genetic and environmental, aetiological factors commonly assume that these effects are additive. We have argued (Holland *et al.*, 1988) that such models may be inappropriate for eating disorders and that an interactive model may be more valid. Additive models may overestimate the contribution of genetic factors because, if non-additive, gene–environment interactions exist, they will be included with purely genetic effects. Our clinical experience leads us to consider a model in which weight loss (caused by physical or psychological illness or by dieting) uncovers the genetic vulnerability in body weight/appetite control. We speculate that weight loss in genetically vulnerable individuals could result in the release of endogenous opiates. In turn, these could be reinforcing or addictive and result in the increased activity and alertness seen in patients with anorexia nervosa, which contrasts markedly to the apathy and retardation seen as a result of starvation in most people.

These aetiological considerations must be evaluated against the known epidemiological and clinical features of the disorder: the much greater female than male prevalence; the preponderance in social classes 1 and 2; the onset at the time of puberty. Anorexia nervosa has been recognized as a distinct illness for over a century (see above), and early descriptions of the disorder date from the seventeenth century (Morton, 1694), as would be consistent with an illness with a biological aetiology.

The female:male ratio is readily explained by a biological model. The control of weight and reproduction in females is intertwined, although the exact mechanisms are ill understood (Unvas-Moberg, 1989). The nutritional cost of pregnancy and lactation is large and it is probable that the physiological strategies to cover this involve changes in appetite and/or metabolism driven by hormonal signals. Such changes have also been observed during the menstrual cycle (Lissner *et al.*, 1988; Bisdee *et al.*, 1989).

Reciprocally, reproductive function is markedly affected in the female by changes in weight (Frisch, 1988). Dieting can rapidly interrupt the menstrual cycle (Pirke *et al.*, 1985). Central neurotransmitter function is altered during dieting (Goodwin *et al.*, 1987); serotoninergic function is more affected in women. It is possible that the hormonal fluxes at puberty disturb the weight set point or control of appetite in certain vulnerable individuals and this leads to a further disturbance in the hypothalamic function. This could explain the sex ratio and the time of onset of the disorder.

If weight loss does uncover the genetic vulnerability, this also could explain the onset in adolescence and the social class distribution, as these are associated with dieting behaviour (Nylander, 1971). In others, the emergence of sexual feelings, with the weight-related pubertal changes, may reawaken memories of earlier sexual abuse (Oppenheimer *et al.*, 1985) and lead to avoidance by weight loss.

It is unlikely that any major psychiatric disorder will be explained solely on the basis of a genetic vulnerability, although this may be a necessary condition. It is probable that the reaction of the family to their daughter's weight loss will alter the course of the illness. For example, conflict between the parents may render them impotent to change their daughter's behaviour, or disengagement within the family may result in the weight loss proceeding unheeded. In Western society, numerous secondary gains accrue from weight loss, which is deemed fashionable, attractive and an outward sign of self-discipline and control. Later, the consequences of starvation, such as depression, obsessionality, social withdrawal and sexual regression, serve to perpetuate the disorder.

Implications for management arise. The concept of an inherited predisposition should neither provoke, on the one hand, therapeutic nihilism nor, on the other, unrealistic expectations from genetic engineering! More usefully, parents can be absolved from the guilt of assuming that their behaviour 'caused' their daughter to develop anorexia nervosa and can be mobilized to combat a less shameful threat. Our interaction model would explain why weight restoration is needed to promote recovery. Nevertheless, skilled psychotherapeutic support is also required to minimize the cascade of secondary disabilities that arises once the illness becomes entrenched. Preventative measures should warn of the dangers of weight loss, especially for those who may be constitutionally vulnerable to develop anorexia nervosa.

In contrast, there is no genetically vulnerable group who are more at risk to develop bulimia nervosa. This behaviour is contagious (Chiodo and Latimer, 1983). Glamorized descriptions of eating disorders in the popular press, with revelations about the secret methods of weight loss, have probably contributed to its increasing prevalence. The symptoms of bulimia nervosa can be explained on the basis of homeostatic mechanisms used to restore weight to its set point (Editorial, 1988; Treasure, 1988). Although weight loss is probably the final common pathway in the aetiology of bulimia nervosa, the factors that lead to this behaviour becoming so highly valued are diverse.

In conclusion, the answer to the question frequently posed jokingly to those who treat patients with eating disorders: 'how can I catch anorexia nervosa for a few weeks?', is that probably, you cannot. But women can all too easily acquire the behaviours and become immersed in the hazardous habits of bulimia nervosa.

ACKNOWLEDGEMENTS

We are grateful to the Mental Health Foundation and the Society for Research into Anorexia Nervosa for their support of this project.

REFERENCES

American Psychiatric Association (1987). *DSM-IIIR: Diagnostic and Statistical Manual of Mental Disorders.* Washington DC: APA.

Askevold F., Heiberg A. (1979). Anorexia nervosa: two cases of discordant MZ twins. *Psychotherapy and Psychosomatics*; **32**: 223–8.

Bisdee J. T., James W. P. T., Shaw M. A. (1989). Changes in energy expenditure during the menstrual cycle. *British Journal of Nutrition*; **61**: 187–99.

Bruch H. (1973). *Eating Disorders, Obesity, Anorexia Nervosa and the Person Within.* New York: Basic Books.

Brumberg J. J. (1988). *Fasting Girls: The Emergence of Anorexia Nervosa as a Modern Disease.* Cambridge, Mass: Harvard University Press.

Chiodo J., Latimer P. R. (1983). Vomiting as a learned weight control technique in bulimia. *Journal of Behaviour Therapy and Experimental Psychiatry*; **14**: 131–5.

Cooper Z., Fairburn C. G. (1987). The Eating Disorder Examination: a semi-structured interview for the assessment of the specific psychopathology of eating disorders. *International Journal of Eating Disorders*; **6**: 1–8.

Crisp A. H. (1967). The possible significance of some behavioural correlates of weight and carbohydrate intake. *Journal of Psychosomatic Research*; **11**: 117–31.

Crisp A. H., Hsu L. K. G., Harding B., Hartshome J. (1980). Clinical features of anorexia nervosa: a study of consecutive series of 102 female patients. *Journal of Psychosomatic Research*; **24**: 179–91.

Dally P. (1969). *Anorexia Nervosa*. London: Heinemann.

Dally P., Gomez J. (1979). *Anorexia Nervosa*. London: Heinemann.

Editorial (1988). Slimming and serotonin. *Lancet*; **i**: 629.

Frisch R. E. (1988). Fatness and fertility. *Scientific American*; **258**: 70–7.

Garfinkel P. E., Garner D. M. (1982). *Anorexia Nervosa: A Multidimensional Perspective*. New York: Brunner Mazel.

Garner D. M., Garfinkel P. E., Schwartz D., Thompson M. (1980). Cultural expectations of thinness in women. *Psychological Reports*; **47**: 483–91.

Gershon E. S., Schreiber J. L., Hamont J. R. *et al.* (1983). Clinical findings in patients with anorexia nervosa and affective illness in relatives. *American Journal of Psychiatry*; **141**: 1419–22.

Goodwin G. M., Fairburn C. G., Cowen P. J. (1987). Dieting changes serotonergic function in women, not men: implications for the aetiology of anorexia nervosa? *Psychological Medicine*; **17**: 839–42.

Grace P. S., Jacobson R. S., Fullager C. J. (1985). A comparison of purging and non-purging bulimics. *Journal of Clinical Psychology*; **41**: 173–80.

Greenhow J. (1873). Proceedings of the Clinical Society of London. *British Medical Journal*; **1**: 527–9.

Gull W. (1873). Proceedings of the Clinical Society of London. *British Medical Journal*; **1**: 527–9.

Holland A. J., Hall A., Murray R. *et al.* (1984). Anorexia nervosa: a study of 34 pairs of twins and one set of triplets. *British Journal of Psychiatry*; **145**: 414–19.

Holland A. J., Sicotte N., Treasure J. (1988). Anorexia nervosa: evidence for a genetic basis. *Journal of Psychosomatic Research*; **32**: 561–71.

Hudson J. I., Pope H. G., Jonas J. M., Yorgelun Todd D. (1983). A family study of anorexia nervosa and bulimia. *British Journal of Psychiatry*; **142**: 133–8.

Johnson-Sabine E., Wood K., Patton G. *et al.* (1988). Abnormal eating attitudes in London schoolgirls—a prospective epidemiological study: factors associated with abnormal response on screening questionnaires. *Psychological Medicine*; **18**: 615–22.

Kay D. W. K., Leigh D. (1954). The natural history, treatment and prognosis of anorexia nervosa based on a study of 38 patients. *Journal of Mental Science*; **100**: 411–31.

King M. B. (1986). Eating disorders in general practice. *British Medical Journal*; **293**: 1412–14.

Lasegue E. C. (1873). On hysterical anorexia. *Medical Times Gazette*; **2**: 265–9.

Levy D. M. (1938). Maternal overprotection. *Psychiatry*; **1**: 561.

Lissner L., Stevens J., Levitsky D. A. *et al.* (1988). Variation in energy intake during the menstrual cycle: implications for food intake research. *American Journal of Clinical Nutrition*; **48**: 956–62.

Lucas A. R., Beard C. M., O'Fallon W. M., Kurland L. T. (1988). Anorexia nervosa in Rochester, Minnesota: a 45-year study. *Mayo Clinic Proceedings*; **63**: 433–42.

McGuffin P., Katz R. (1986). Nature, nurture and affective disorder. In: *The Biology of Depression* (Deakin J. F. W., ed.). London: Gaskell Press.

Minuchin S., Rosman B. L., Baker L. (1975). *Psychosomatic Families, Anorexia Nervosa in Context*. London: Harvard University Press.

Morgan H. G., Russell G. F. M. (1975). Value of family background and clinical features as predictors of long-term outcome in anorexia nervosa: four year follow-up study of 41 patients. *Psychological Medicine*; **5**: 355–71.

Morton R. (1694). *Phthisiologia: or, a Treatise of Consumptions*. London: Smith and Walford.

Nowlin N. S. (1983). Anorexia nervosa in twins: case report and review. *Journal of Clinical Psychiatry*; **44**: 101–5.

Nylander I. (1971). The feeling of being fat and dieting in a school population: epidemiologic interview investigation. *Acta Sociomedica Scandinavica*; **3**: 579–84.

Oppenheimer R., Howells K., Palmer R. L., Cahloner D. A. (1985). Adverse sexual experience in childhood and clinical eating disorders: a preliminary description. *Journal of Psychiatric Research*; **19**: 357–63.

Orbach S. (1978). *Fat is a Feminist Issue*. London: Paddington Press.

Patton G. C. (1988). The spectrum of eating disorder in adolescence. *Journal of Psychosomatic Research*; **32**: 579–84.

Pirke K. M., Schweiger U., Lemmel W. (1985). The influence of dieting on the menstrual cycle of healthy young women. *Journal of Clinical Endocrinology and Metabolism*; **60**: 1174–9.

Playfair W. C. (1888). Note on the so-called 'anorexia nervosa'. *Lancet*; i: 817–18.

Rivinius T. M. (1984). Anorexia nervosa and affective disorders: a controlled family history study. *American Journal of Psychiatry*; **14**: 1414–18.

Robins L. N., Helzer J., Cronghan J. *et al.* (1981). NIMH Diagnostic Interview Schedule. Washington University School of Medicine.

Russell G. F. M. (1970). Anorexia nervosa: its identity as an illness and treatment. In: *Modern Trends in Psychological Medicine* (Price J., ed.). London: Butterworth.

Russell G. F. M. (1979). Bulimia nervosa: an ominous variant of anorexia nervosa. *Psychological Medicine*; **9**: 429–48.

Ryle J. A. (1936). Anorexia nervosa. *Lancet*; ii: 893–9.

Scott D. W. (1986). Anorexia nervosa: a review of possible genetic factors. *International Journal of Eating Disorders*; **5**: 1–20.

Selvini-Palazzoli M., Boscolo L., Cecchin G., Prata G. (1978). *Paradox and Counterparadox*. New York: Jason Aronson.

Slade P. (1985). A review of body image studies in anorexia nervosa and bulimia nervosa. *Journal of Psychiatric Research*; **19**: 255–66.

Stern S. L., Dixon K. N., Hemzer E. (1984). Affective disorder in the families of women with normal weight bulimia. *American Journal of Psychiatry*; **141**: 1224–7.

Strober M., Morrell W., Burroughs J. *et al.* (1985). A controlled family study of anorexia nervosa. *Journal of Psychiatric Research*; **19**: 239–46.

Strober M., Salkin B., Borroughs J. *et al.* (1986). A family study of anorexia nervosa and depression. Paper presented at the annual meeting of the American Psychiatry Association, Washington, DC.

Szmukler G. I., Eisler I., Gillies C., Hayward M. E. (1985). The implications of anorexia nervosa in a ballet school. *Journal of Psychiatric Research*; 19: 117–82.

Szmukler G. I., McCance C., McCrone L., Hunter D. (1986). Anorexia nervosa: a psychiatric case register study from Aberdeen. *Psychological Medicine*; 16: 49–58.

Theander S. (1970). Anorexia nervosa: a psychiatric investigation of 44 female cases. *Acta Psychiatrica Scandinavica* (supplementum); 214: 1–194.

Treasure J. (1988). Psychopharmacological approaches to anorexia nervosa. In: *Anorexia and Bulimia Nervosa, Practical Approaches* (Scott D., ed.). London: Croom Helm.

Unvas-Moberg K. (1989). Neuroendocrine regulation of hunger and satiety. In: *Europe 1988*, Proceedings of the 1st European Congress on Obesity (Bjomtorp P., Rossner S., eds.). London/Paris: John Libby.

Vandereycken W., Pierloot R. (1981). Anorexia nervosa in twins. *Psychotherapy and Psychosomatics*; 35: 55–63.

Waller U. V., Kaufman M. R., Deutsch F. (1940). Anorexia nervosa: a psychosomatic entity. *Psychosomatic Medicine*; 2: 3–16.

Winokur A., March V., Mendels J. (1980). Primary affective disorder in relatives of patients with anorexia nervosa. *American Journal of Psychiatry*; 137: 695–8.

World Health Organization (1989). *International Classification of Diseases* 10th edn. Geneva: WHO.

14 *Growing together and growing apart: the non-genetic forces on children in the same family*

ROBERT GOODMAN

Over the last decade or so, some of the most striking conclusions reached by behavioural geneticists have concerned the environmental rather than the genetic determinants of human behaviour. I shall challenge some of these conclusions later in the chapter, but before doing so I shall summarize the relevant conclusions and the chain of reasoning that led to them. The views of behavioural geneticists have been expounded by Plomin and Daniels (1987), and I shall refer repeatedly to points raised in their initial article, in the accompanying, open peer reviews, and in their response to those reviews.

The methods of quantitative behavioural genetics were primarily devised to generate estimates on the heritability of a specific behavioural trait or constellation in a particular population. 'Heritability', in this context, refers to the proportion of the variance for that specific trait that can be attributed to genetic factors in that particular population. A heritability of 1.0 implies that the population's variability for that trait is entirely due to genes. If, as is usually the case, the heritability is less than 1.0, what accounts for the rest of the variance? The methods of quantitative behavioural genetics allow the remainder of the variance to be partitioned between two environmental factors, namely shared and non-shared environment. Shared environment refers to the environmental influences that are shared by relatives living together—poverty, for example, or exposure to atmospheric pollution. Non-shared environment refers to those environmental influences that are not shared by relatives living together—having a best friend who is a drug addict, being knocked down by a bus, and so on. Behavioural geneticists assess the effect of shared environment from the degree to which individuals reared together are more similar to one another than would be predicted on genetic grounds alone. The effect of non-shared environment is most straightforwardly estimated from the extent to which monozygotic (MZ) twins differ from one another despite growing up together and sharing all their genes—after allowing for differences that are simply due to unreliability of measurement.

It is worth noting at this stage that the division of environmental influences into shared and non-shared components is not as straightforward as it initially seems. Few, if any, of the environmental influences that act on two family members are either completely shared or stochastically independent. Many important influences are partly but not entirely shared. For example, twins are likely to experience similar but not identical parenting and schooling. From the standpoint of the behavioural geneticist, these partly shared influences contribute both to shared and non-shared environment. In effect, an imperfectly correlated environment has been resolved into two orthogonal components: a completely shared environment and an independent environment. The same environmental factor may result in a different mixture of shared and non-shared effects at different stages of the life cycle, or in different pairs of relatives. For example, if a pair of twins typically experiences more similar schooling than a pair of non-twin siblings, schooling will appear to contribute more to the shared environmental effect (and less to the non-shared environmental effect) when assessed by twin studies than when assessed by non-twin studies.

Plomin and Daniels review a large number of studies that have brought the methods of quantitative genetics to bear on measures of temperament and personality. The conclusions of these studies are certainly thought provoking. Genetic factors typically account for about half of the observed variance. After allowing for error variance, the contribution of environmental factors still seems substantial. The most surprising conclusion is that most of the environmental variance reflects non-shared environment, with shared environment making only a small contribution. This startling conclusion even emerges from studies of young twins who are still living together—a group who are particularly likely to share many aspects of their present and past environment. To provide just one numerical example, Loehlin's (1985) twin and adoption data suggest that non-shared environment accounts for about 25% of personality test variance, while shared environment only accounts for about 5%. The conclusion of Loehlin and Nichols' (1976) pioneering study of this phenomenon is worth repeating: 'Environment carries substantial weight in determining personality . . . but that environment is one for which twin pairs are correlated close to zero' (p. 92). Plomin and Daniels extend the argument for the supremacy of the non-shared over the shared environment beyond the domains of temperament and personality. They suggest that the environmental influences that affect the intelligence quotient (IQ) are also largely of the non-shared variety after adolescence. They also suggest that psychopathology is much more influenced by non-shared than by shared environment. In the case of schizophrenia, for example, they argue that a concordance rate of less than 50% in MZ twins demonstrates a major role for non-shared environment, whereas adoption studies fail to demonstrate any significant role for shared environment.

DOES SHARED ENVIRONMENT MATTER?

Plomin and Daniels (1987; p. 15) underline the potential importance of these conclusions by calling attention to some very radical implications.

Our new knowledge concerning the importance of nonshared environment may have its deepest implications for intervention. It is critical for interventionists to know that what parents do that is experienced similarly by their children does not have an impact on their behavioural development. If the effects of parents on their children lie in the unique environments they provide for each child, childrearing books need to be rewritten, and early childhood education and interventions aimed at the prevention of psychopathology need to be rethought.

I hope that these revolutionary thoughts stimulate all of us to re-examine previously unquestioned assumptions. Increasing attention to the factors that make children in the same family so different from one another is certainly a welcome change. At the same time, there are several reasons why we should pause before throwing away our child-rearing books, altering our modes of education and therapy, and abandoning our search for substantial effects attributable to shared environment.

The first reason for caution is the danger of extrapolating from one population to another. Studies of temperament and personality have relied primarily on affluent, well-functioning families who have volunteered to participate in research. Conclusions drawn from such studies may not apply to the deprived, deviant or abusing families who are over-represented in psychiatric practice. McCartney (1987; p. 33) summarizes this point well:

The shared environment is only unimportant when one considers good, middle-class environments that are functionally equivalent in some way. These environments, and not deprived environments, are the kinds that developmentalists tend to study. Thus, the implications of Plomin and Daniels' argument for intervention may not be as radical as is implied.

Plomin and Daniels overstate their case to make a point that needed making. It is worth noting, however, that the methods of quantitative behavioural genetics do *not* suggest that shared environment is unimportant for all psychological traits or behavioural disorders. As subsequently noted by Plomin *et al.* (1990), aggressive and antisocial behaviours in childhood and adolescence are important exceptions. Thus, in Stevenson and Graham's (1988) study of a population sample of adolescent twins, the intraclass correlation for aggressive and antisocial behaviours (as assessed by parent questionnaire) was 0.44 for MZ twins and 0.46 for same-sex, dizygotic (DZ) twins—persuasive evidence for a major effect of shared environment. Similarly, in their summary of existing twin studies of juvenile delinquency, McGuffin and Gottesman (1985) report that the average concordances for MZ and DZ twins were 87 and 72%, respectively, again suggesting that shared environment has a major impact. It is interesting, in passing, to note that twin studies suggest that antisocial behaviour in adult life owes more to genes and much less to shared environment (McGuffin and Gottesman, 1985). The decline of the shared environmental effect in adulthood may well be due, at least in part, to the fact that adult twins, who will mostly be living apart, do not share their environment to the same extent as adolescent twins, who will mostly be living together. To put this another way, a decline in the shared environmental effect in adulthood is inevitable unless aggressive and antisocial behaviours are entirely determined by early environment, irrespective of the individual's circumstances in adult life.

Whereas aggressive and antisocial behaviours have attracted a great deal of research, prosocial behaviours, such as helpfulness, kindness and generosity, have attracted rather less (see Radke-Yarrow *et al.*, 1983). Though prized by parents, teachers, friends, and society as a whole, remarkably little is known of the origins of prosocial behaviour. Although modern evolutionary theory suggests that a capacity for helpfulness and cooperation could be heritable, behavioural geneticists have not yet systematically examined the relative contributions of genetic and environmental factors to children's prosocial behaviours. Prosocial and antisocial behaviours in childhood are negatively correlated (Weir and Duveen, 1981), and may represent the opposite ends of a single behavioural dimension. If so, prosocial behaviours are likely to resemble antisocial behaviours in being particularly influenced by shared environment, at least in childhood. If shared environment does have a major impact on the development of both antisocial and prosocial behaviours, then most parents will conclude that shared environment is enormously important, even if it has little influence on other aspects of personality or psychopathology.

Quantitative behavioural genetics provides a unique perspective on the extent and nature of environmental influences on normal and abnormal psychological development. It is important to remember, however, that this perspective may be seriously distorting. There are several reasons for supposing that the assumptions and methods of quantitative behavioural genetics can inflate the apparent importance of non-shared environmental factors, and minimize the importance of shared environmental factors. Three possible sources of distortion seem particularly noteworthy: a lack of regard for the possible role of random factors in epigenesis; overestimation of measurement reliability; and failure to distinguish between independent and polarizing environments.

THE ROLE OF CHANCE IN BRAIN DEVELOPMENT

Plomin and Daniels (1987) repeatedly emphasize that MZ twins who have grown up together provide the most direct evidence for the importance of non-shared environment. When the behaviour of MZ twins differs reliably—that is, when the behavioural differences exceed what can be attributed to misclassification or measurement error alone—it is generally held to be self-evident that these differences must be the result of non-shared environmental factors. Thus Plomin and Daniels are echoing Gottesman and Shields (1982) and many others when they state that: 'Most schizophrenic identical twins do not have an affected cotwin. Because these are genetically identical pairs of individuals, nonshared environment must be the reason for these striking differences within pairs of identical twins' (p. 6). This is not necessarily so. Another possible cause for behavioural differences between identical twins must also be considered: the operation of chance in brain development.

In order to appreciate the possible role of random factors in brain development, it is worth reflecting on the manner in which genetic instructions are translated into neuronal organization (see Purves and Lichtman, 1985). An individual's genotype cannot directly determine the precise arrangement of every single neurone and synapse—there are no mechanisms for this to occur; in any case, the information content of the entire genome would be insufficient to permit billions of direct specifications. Instead, genetic instructions programme developing neurones to be self-assembling by specifying a remarkably economical two-stage process. In the first, 'additive' (or 'progressive') phase, developing neurones connect themselves together into a very rough approximation of the mature brain. In the rat, for example, the additive phase generates a corticospinal tract that contains axons from most cortical areas, including the visual cortex (Stanfield *et al.*, 1982). It appears, then, that the genetic programmes governing the initial formation of the corticospinal tract are not very specific, in the sense that they cannot stipulate which cortical areas do not need to contribute to the tract. There seem to be major constraints on how tightly specified these additive, self-assembling processes can be. Consequently, the fine tuning of neuronal organization depends principally on a subsequent wave of 'subtractive' (or 'regressive') processes (Cowan *et al.*, 1984), such as the elimination of corticospinal projections from the visual cortex (Stanfield *et al.*, 1982). This sort of two-stage, additive-then-subtractive sequence is but one instance of a common biological strategy, namely using partly random processes to generate a large number of variants on some particular theme, and then using selective processes to eliminate unwanted variants and/or reduplicate wanted variants. Other instances of such strategies include evolution by natural selection, trial-and-error learning, and the acquisition of a mature complement of B-lymphocyte clones.

If the mechanisms that translate genetic instructions into neuronal organization reflect chance as well as necessity, there is no reason to suppose that genetically identical individuals will develop identical nervous systems, even if they experience environments that are, to all intents and purposes, identical. This is a difficult assertion to prove, but two lines of evidence lend some support. First, there are precedents for assigning chance a role in human development. Thus chance is believed to affect the occurrence of left-handedness (Annett, 1985), the Lyonization of X chromosomes in females (Lyon, 1961; Vandenberg *et al.*, 1962), the specification of antibody idiotypes (Alt *et al.*, 1987), and the occurrence of situs inversus in individuals with Kartagener's syndrome (Afzelius, 1976). In each of these instances, chance rather than non-shared environment could account for discordance between MZ twins (see, for example, Revesz *et al.*, 1972; Burn *et al.*, 1986).

A second line of evidence suggesting that chance may play some role in neuronal development comes from experimental studies of homologous neurones in genetically identical animals (Levinthal *et al.*, 1975). In the water flea, *Daphnia magna*, for example, the number of neurones is small and the arrangement of neurones is predictable, with the result that it is possible to study the equivalent neurones in different animals. As water fleas reproduce by parthenogenesis, it is easy to study genetically identical individuals. As shown in Fig. 14.1, Levinthal *et al.* demonstrated marked differences in the pattern of dendritic branching between the homologous neurones of isogenic water fleas. Similar variations in dendritic branching have also been found in similar studies of homologous neurones in isogenic vertebrates (Levinthal *et al.*, 1975). Of course, these differences in dendritic development could reflect non-shared, external influences that have yet to be specified, but it is just as plausible that the exact pattern of dendritic branching is affected by random factors such as the Brownian movement of intracellular particles. If neuronal development is affected by external factors, these could justly be classified as environmental influences. On the other hand, it would surely be stretching the meaning of the term 'environment' too far to include the effects of random events at a subcellular level.

This issue of definition is far from trivial because the connotation of a word can influence our thinking. 'Environment' normally refers to those aspects of the physical and social world that surround and impinge on an individual. The term does not usually include those processes within an individual that are not driven by external factors. Consequently, if we label all non-genetic influences as 'environmental', we are likely to forget those non-genetic processes, such as the operation of chance in brain development, that are not environmental in the everyday sense of the word. Perhaps the current duo of genes and environment needs to be expanded into a trio of genes, environment, and epigenetic randomness. This is not to say that the role of chance in development is restricted to epigenetic randomness. On the contrary, randomness plays a part in the reshuffling of genes between generations, as well as in freak accidents, fortuitous meetings, and many other environmental contingencies. It seems likely, however, that this genetic and environmental randomness is compounded by an additional level of randomness that is inherent in the developmental process itself—a phenomenon that could be termed 'aleatory epigenesis'

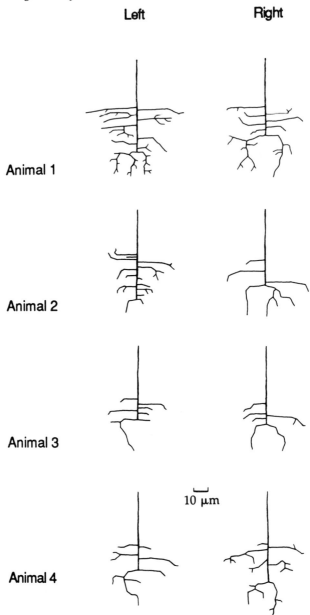

Left

Right

Animal 1

Animal 2

Animal 3

10 μm

Animal 4

Fig. 14.1   *Schematic representation of the branching patterns of dendrites from the homologous neurones on the left and right sides of the optic ganglion neurophil in four genetically identical water fleas. The order, position and relative lengths of all the branches have been maintained, but angular distortions were introduced in order to avoid overlapping. The differences between the four individuals demonstrate that dendritic branching is not completely genetically determined (adapted, with permission, from Levinthal et al., 1976)* (from aleatory: dependent on the throw of a die; hence, dependent on uncertain contingencies).

There is not yet any empirical evidence that aleatory epigenesis contributes to the psychological differences between MZ twins—but while the possibility exists, it is surely wrong to assume that reliable differences between MZ twins *prove* the existence of non-shared, environmental effects. In Kartagener's syndrome, a genetic defect in ciliary motility puts embryos at equal risk of developing normal or reversed visceral asymmetry; which path they follow appears to depend on chance (Afzelius, 1976). In schizophrenia, a genetic defect may also present the embryo with two distinct developmental paths, one leading to a normal brain, and the other to a preschizophrenic brain. Whether MZ twins follow the same or different paths may depend on external influences that have yet to be characterized. Alternatively, chance alone may determine whether or not the twins follow the same developmental path. At critical points in brain development, randomly generated differences on a microscopic scale may be responsible for marked differences in subsequent developmental trajectories. Given our current ignorance about the factors influencing brain development, it is premature to dismiss the possibility that chance plays a role in both brain and behavioural development.

MEASUREMENT ERROR

If neglecting the role of chance is one possible reason for overestimating the impact of non-shared environment, failing to make sufficient allowance for measurement unreliability is another. Plomin and Daniels (1987) argue that test–retest reliability is an adequate measure of how much of the difference between identical twins should be attributed to measurement error, with the rest of the difference being attributed to non-shared environment. Others argue that retest reliability can seriously underestimate the extent to which measurement error contributes to twin differences. Costa and McCrae (1987; p. 23) put this argument persuasively:

Many forms of error . . . exist, and retest reliability systematically underestimates some of these. Of two equally extraverted twins, the one who tends to use more extreme response categories will score higher on measures of extraversion; because styles of responding may be very stable, this source of error will not appear as retest unreliability. Similarly, two subjects may consistently understand a word or question differently.

This sort of unrecognized measurement error will inflate the apparent importance of the non-shared environment.

POLARIZING AND EQUALIZING EFFECTS

My final point about the distorting perspective of behavioural genetics concerns the potential inadequacy of distinguishing between just two sorts of environmental effects, namely shared and non-shared environmental effects. It seems helpful to recognize at least three sorts of environmental effects, accepting that many environmental influences will act in more than one way. 'Equalizing effects' represent instances when shared experiences influence family members in the same way. 'Independent effects' reflect the impact of experiences that impinge on just one family member. 'Polarizing effects' represent instances when the experience of living together causes family members to differentiate in opposite directions. Plomin and Daniels (1987) subsume both independent and polarizing effects under the rubric of 'non-shared environment'. This combination hides an important difference: the effective environments of family members are uncorrelated for independent effects but negatively correlated for polarizing effects (which are sometimes called 'contrast effects').

George Eliot (1876) wrote over a century ago that: 'some minds naturally rebel against whatever they were brought up in, and like the opposite: they see the faults in what is nearest to them'. I suspect that these and other polarizing effects do occur, both across and within generations. It seems plausible, for example, that siblings sometimes assert their sense of individuality by differentiating in opposite directions. Everyday experience inclines us to agree with George Eliot, but the scientific evidence for such effects is limited. The twin–twin transfusion syndrome is a striking example of a physical polarizing effect in which the *in utero* transfer of blood from one twin to the other results in one twin being small and anaemic, while the other twin is large and plethoric (Oski and Naiman, 1982). Three lines of evidence for psychological polarizing effects can be mentioned briefly. First, on various measures of temperament, the correlation between MZ twins is high, the correlation between parents and children is modest, and the correlation between DZ twins is low, absent, or even negative (Buss and Plomin, 1984). The difference between MZ and DZ twins is more marked than would be predicted from additive genetic effects alone, but could be explained by polarizing environmental effects or by non-additive genetic effects (cf. Lykken, 1982; Tellegen *et al.*, 1988). As non-additive genetic effects cannot explain why DZ correlations are lower than parent–child correlations, the overall pattern of correlations can most easily be explained by polarizing effects. Shields' (1962) finding that MZ twins were more alike on personality measures if they had been reared apart than if they had been reared together provides a second line of evidence for polarizing effects, though more recent studies of twins reared apart have not replicated these findings (Plomin *et al.*, 1988; Tellegen *et al.*, 1988). Finally, discrepancies between direct and indirect estimates of IQ heritability could also be due to polarizing environmental effects (Plomin and Loehlin, 1989).

Given the preliminary evidence for polarizing effects, it is important to consider what would happen if equalizing and polarizing effects operated simultaneously on the same trait. The consequences can be illustrated by an instructive though highly contrived example. Imagine a trait X that is affected just by the genes at time 1 (T1), by both genes and equalizing effects at time 2 (T2), and by genes, equalizing and polarizing effects at time 3 (T3). Figure 14.2 portrays changes in trait X in two siblings (A and B) who grow up together. At T1, siblings A and B differ because their genotypes differ. Moving from T1 to T2, both siblings experience an equalizing effect that boosts their level of trait X. Had they both grown up in another home, they might have experienced an equalizing effect that diminished their level of trait X. If the two siblings had been exposed to different equalizing effects by being adopted into separate homes, their resemblance at T2 would be less pronounced than if they grew up together. To put this another way, the correlation of reared-together siblings at T2 is higher than the correlation of reared-apart siblings at T2, that is, equalizing effects increase correlations. Moving from T2 to T3, siblings A and B assert their sense of individuality by polarizing in opposite directions on trait X. As a result of this sort of polarizing effect, the correlation of reared-together siblings at T3 is lower than at T2. Indeed, if the equalizing and polarizing effects are of comparable magnitudes, the correlations of reared-together and reared-apart siblings will be approxim-

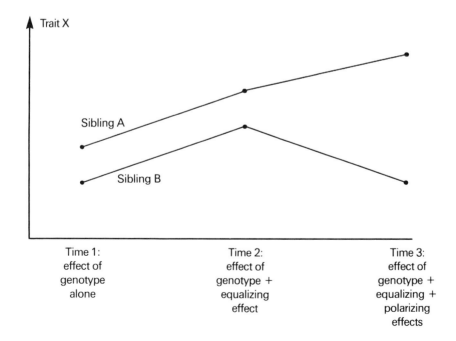

Fig. 14.2 *Equalizing and polarizing effects do not cancel out*

ately equal at T3. The equalizing and polarizing effects have cancelled one another out as far as correlations are concerned. In the real world, however, the effects have not cancelled out: moving in opposite directions from a shifted baseline is not the same as no change at all.

What will the quantitative behavioural geneticist make of all this? If the combination of equalizing and polarizing forces has no net effect on observed correlations, the behavioural geneticist will conclude that shared environment is irrelevant. At the same time, however, the non-genetic variance due to the equalizing and polarizing effects will not disappear, and the behavioural geneticist will end up attributing it all to non-shared environment. To return to our imaginary trait X, the behavioural geneticist will assume that the situation at T3 reflects a combination of genes and independent effects. The behavioural geneticist does not acknowledge the possibility that a combination of equalizing and polarizing effects can mimic an independent effect. Consequently, to the extent that equalizing and polarizing effects coexist, the variance due to this mixture will be attributed to non-shared environment. This methodological quirk is so surprising that it is worth reflecting somewhat further on its origins. Equalizing effects represent instances when the effective environments of two family members are positively correlated. Polarizing effects represent instances when the effective environments of two family members are negatively correlated. When equalizing and polarizing effects are balanced, the positive and negative correlations will cancel out and the effective environments of two family members will seem uncorrelated, leading to the erroneous conclusion that all the environmental variance is due to independent effects, i.e. non-shared environment.

If equalizing plus polarizing effects can be misinterpreted as independent effects, this is yet another reason for questioning behavioural geneticists' assertions that equalizing effects (shared environmental effects) explain very little, while independent effects (non-shared environmental effects) explain a lot. A behavioural geneticist might reply that the empirical findings are more parsimoniously, and therefore more scientifically, explained by independent effects than by a balanced mixture of equalizing and polarizing effects. This is a reasonable objection, but there are two counter-arguments. First, as described above, there is compelling evidence that growing up together results in a net equalizing effect for some traits, e.g. antisocial behaviour, and suggestive evidence that growing up together results in a net polarizing effect for other traits, e.g. activity level. It is both parsimonious and intuitively plausible to suppose that growing up together results in a mixture of equalizing and polarizing effects, with either the one or the other predominating for most traits. It is arguably less parsimonious to invoke some unknown force that allows equalizing and polarizing effects to act singly but prevents them ever acting together. Putting aside these considerations of parsimony, there is a second line of evidence that equalizing and polarizing effects may coexist. Twin and adoption studies provide persuasive evidence for equalizing effects on

IQ, at least in childhood (see Plomin and Daniels, 1987). At the same time, discrepancies between direct and indirect methods for estimating heritability suggest that polarizing effects also operate on IQ (Plomin and Loehlin, 1989). Although the evidence that equalizing and polarizing effects coexist is far from conclusive, behavioural geneticists should qualify their claim that equalizing effects are of little importance with the proviso that substantial equalizing effects might be masked by substantial polarizing effects.

In conclusion, independent and polarizing environmental influences may well account for some of the striking differences that exist between children in the same family. So too may random factors in brain development. At the same time, it is important to remember that equalizing environmental factors can account for some of the important psychological characteristics shared by children in the same family. The obituary for the shared environmental effect has been written too soon.

REFERENCES

Afzelius B. A. (1976). A human syndrome caused by immotile cilia. *Science*; **193**: 317–19.

Alt F. W., Blackwell K., Yancopoulos G. D. (1987). Development of the primary antibody repertoire. *Science*; **238**: 1079–87.

Annett M. (1985). *Left, Right, Hand and Brain: The Right Shift Theory*. London: Lawrence Erlbaum Associates.

Burn J., Povey S., Boyd Y. *et al.* (1986). Duchenne muscular dystrophy in one of monozygotic twin girls. *Journal of Medical Genetics*; **23**: 494–500.

Buss A. H., Plomin R. (1984). *Temperament: Early Developing Personality Traits*. Hillsdale, NJ: Lawrence Erlbaum.

Costa P. T., McCrae R. R. (1987). On the need for longitudinal evidence and multiple measures in behavioral-genetic studies of adult personality. *Behavioral and Brain Sciences*; **10**: 22–3.

Cowan W. M., Fawcett J. W., O'Leary D. D. M., Stanfield B. B. (1984). Regressive events in neurogenesis. *Science*; **225**: 1258–65.

Eliot G. (1876). *Daniel Deronda*, 1988 edn., p. 317. Oxford: Oxford University Press.

Gottesman I. I., Shields J. (1982). *Schizophrenia: The Epigenetic Puzzle*. Cambridge: Cambridge University Press.

Levinthal F., Macagno E., Levinthal C. (1975). Anatomy and development of identified cells in isogenic organisms. *Cold Spring Harbor Symposia on Quantitative Biology*; **40**: 321–33.

Loehlin J. C. (1985). Fitting heredity-environmental models jointly to twin and adoption data from the California Psychological Inventory. *Behavior Genetics*; **15**: 199–221.

Loehlin J. C., Nichols R. C. (1976). *Heredity, Environment, and Personality: A Study of 850 Sets of Twins*. Austin: University of Texas Press.

Lykken D. T. (1982). Research with twins: the concept of emergenesis. *Psychophysiology*; **19**: 361–73.

Lyon M. (1961). Gene action in the X-chromosome of the mouse (*Mus musculus* L.). *Nature*; **190**: 372–3.

McCartney K. (1987). The problem of documenting systematic nonshared environmental effects directly. *Behavioral and Brain Sciences*; **10**: 32–3.

McGuffin P., Gottesman I. I. (1985). Genetic differences in normal and abnormal development. In: *Child and Adolescent Psychiatry: Modern Approaches* 2nd edn. (Rutter M., Hersov L., eds.), pp. 17–33. Oxford: Blackwell.

Oski F. A., Naiman J. L. (1982). *Hematologic Problems in the Newborn* 3rd edn. Philadelphia: Saunders.

Plomin R., Daniels D. (1987). Why are children in the same family so different from one another? *Behavioral and Brain Sciences*; **10**: 1–60.

Plomin R., Loehlin J. C. (1989). Direct and indirect IQ heritability estimates: a puzzle. *Behavior Genetics*; **19**: 331–42.

Plomin R., Nitz K., Rowe D. C. (1990). Behavioral genetics and aggressive behavior in childhood. In: *Handbook of Developmental Psychopathology* (Lewis M., Miller S. M., eds.). New York: Plenum Press.

Plomin R., Pederson N. L., McClearn G. E. *et al.* (1988). EAS temperaments during the last half of the life span: twins reared apart and twins reared together. *Psychology and Aging*; **3**: 43–50.

Purves D., Lichtman J. W. (1985). *Principles of Neural Development*. Sunderland, Mass: Sinauer Associates.

Radke-Yarrow M., Zahn-Waxler C., Chapman M. (1983). Children's prosocial dispositions and behavior. In: *Mussen's Handbook of Child Psychology, vol. IV, Socialization, Personality, and Social Development* 4th edn. (Hetherington E. M., ed.), pp. 469–545. New York: John Wiley.

Revesz T., Schuler D., Goldschmidt B., Elodi S. (1972). Christmas disease in one of a pair of monozygotic twin girls, possibly the effect of Lyonization. *Journal of Medical Genetics*; **9**: 396–400.

Shields J. (1962). *Monozygotic Twins Brought Up Apart and Brought Up Together*. London: Oxford University Press.

Stanfield B. B., O'Leary D. D. M., Fricks C. (1982). Selective collateral elimination in early postnatal development restricts cortical distribution of rat pyramidal tract neurones. *Nature*; **298**: 371–3.

Stevenson J., Graham P. (1988). Behavioral deviance in 13-year-old twins: an item analysis. *Journal of the American Academy of Child and Adolescent Psychiatry*; **27**: 791–7.

Tellegen A., Lykken D. T., Bouchard T. J. *et al.* (1988). Personality similarity in twins reared apart and together. *Journal of Personality and Social Psychology*; **54**: 1031–9.

Vandenberg S. G., McKusick V. A., McKusick A. B. (1962). Twin data in support of the Lyon hypothesis. *Nature*; **194**: 505–6.

Weir K., Duveen G. (1981). Further development and validation of the prosocial behaviour questionnaire for use by teachers. *Journal of Child Psychology and Psychiatry*; **22**: 357–74.

15 *Autism as a genetic disorder*

MICHAEL RUTTER

In the first paper on the syndrome of autism, Kanner (1943) described it as innate and inborn. He drew attention to the abnormalities in infancy without evidence of prior normal development and to the intellectual, non-emotional qualities shown by many of the parents and grandparents. Subsequently, the supposed lack of parental warmth led many clinicians to abandon the notions of a constitutional deficit in the child and instead to postulate a psychogenic origin for autism. During the 1960s and 1970s, three sets of research findings caused a reappraisal and a growing appreciation that the syndrome probably usually had an organic basis of some type. First, empirical evidence failed to support early claims of abnormalities in autistic children's upbringing (Cantwell *et al.*, 1978). Secondly, it became clear that autism was usually associated with marked and persistent cognitive deficits (Hermelin and O'Connor, 1970; Rutter, 1979). Thirdly, follow-up (Rutter, 1970) and epidemiological studies (Deykin and MacMahon, 1979) showed that about a fifth to a quarter of autistic children developed epileptic fits, with the peak age of onset in adolescence.

Nevertheless, reviews during the 1960s (Rutter, 1967) and 1970s (Hanson and Gottesman, 1976) concluded that, although an organic aetiology was likely, genetic factors probably did not play a major role. Attention was drawn to the low rate of autism in sibs (non-systematic early data suggested a rate of not more than 2%), the lack of chromosome anomalies, and the similarities with syndromes associated with known brain trauma. It is now apparent that, even given the shaky data base, the logic in these early reviews was faulty in that it focused on the wrong features. Although the rate of autism in siblings was indeed low, it was much higher than the general population rate of 2–4 per 10 000, providing a strong pointer to genetic factors. The recognition that this was so, associated with the parallel finding of an apparently high familial loading for language delay (Bartak *et al.*, 1975), stimulated the first, systematic, twin study of autism (Folstein and Rutter, 1977), which suggested a strong genetic component. Subsequent research has produced findings in the same direction, although many questions remain unanswered. This chapter seeks to summarize the evidence that has accumulated on genetic influences during the last dozen years or so, and to discuss the dilemmas that remain, making a few suggestions on the way ahead.

TWIN STUDIES

In spite of advances brought about by molecular genetics, twin designs continue to provide some of the best tests for genetic influences (Rutter *et al.*, 1990a; Plomin *et al.*, 1991). Over the years there have been many case reports of autistic twins (reviewed by Smalley *et al.*, 1988; Silliman *et al.*, 1989), but these are not a satisfactory source for genetic data because of the tendency to over-report concordant monozygotic (MZ) pairs. Instead we need to focus on the larger-scale, population-based samples of twin pairs that include an autistic proband. The first was carried out by Folstein and Rutter (1977), who undertook a nation-wide search for such pairs in the UK, obtaining 11 MZ and 10 same-sex dizygotic (DZ) pairs. Both the absolute number and the MZ:DZ ratio was in keeping with the expectation based on the population incidence of autism and twinning. Zygosity was determined by blood groups except when it was obvious from genetically determined physical features. Three main findings emerged. First, there was a 36% pairwise concordance for autism in the MZ pairs compared with a 0% concordance in the DZ pairs—a difference significant at the 5.5% level. Second, there was an 82% concordance for serious cognitive abnormalities in the MZ pairs, compared with a 10% concordance in DZ pairs. This meant that five of the seven non-autistic co-twins in MZ pairs had cognitive abnormalities compared with only one of the ten non-autistic co-twins in DZ pairs—a statistically significant difference at the 2% level. This second finding suggested that what was inherited was a pattern of cognitive deficits that included, but was not restricted to, autism. Thirdly, biological hazards in the neonatal period accounted for about two-thirds of the cases of discordance for autism as traditionally diagnosed, but *not* for discordance on cognitive abnormalities or concordance for autism. The implication was that non-genetic factors such as brain trauma might play a contributory role in aetiology.

The finding that four of the eleven MZ pairs were concordant for autism but that a further five pairs were concordant for cognitive abnormalities raised two opposite queries. First, it is well known that language delay is more common in twins than in singletons (Rutter *et al.*, 1990b); could this be the explanation in spite of the marked MZ-DZ difference? A recent follow-up of the twin sample by Le Couteur *et al.* (1989a) indicated that this was unlikely because all the MZ co-twins without autism, but with a cognitive abnormality, showed substantial, continuing social difficulties that persisted into adult life. Second, could these instances of non-autistic cognitive impairment be viewed as mild cases of autism? A systematic, standardized, diagnostic interview (Le Couteur *et al.*, 1989b) was used at follow-up and the findings showed that none of the five co-twins met the *International Classification of Diseases* (ICD-10; World Health Organization, 1989) criteria for autism, although one was categorized as suffering from Asperger's syndrome. Two had attended normal schools and gone on to college or university. These cognitive/social impairments may prove to be part of the autism phenotype but, if so, the diagnostic criteria will have to be widened substantially.

Subsequently it was discovered that some cases of autism were associated with the fragile X anomaly (Folstein and Rutter, 1988; Smalley *et al.*, 1988). Accordingly, it was necessary to check whether the twin concordance findings were a consequence of this chromosomal abnormality. Cytogenetic analyses showed that one female MZ pair, discordant for autism but concordant for cognitive/social abnormalities, had the anomaly (Le Couteur *et al.*, 1988). There was also one other MZ pair, concordant for autism, that showed a non-replicated, low rate of fragile X expression, which was of uncertain significance.

The findings from this first twin study were striking but they were based on a small number of pairs, so that replication was necessary. Moreover, although diagnoses were made blind to pair and zygosity, standardized instruments were not used. Le Couteur *et al.* (1989a; and unpublished data) have recently undertaken a further, epidemiologically based, twin study using a sample obtained from a nation-wide survey of clinics, schools and parent organizations. For all twin pairs, zygosity was determined using blood groups and the diagnosis of autism was made according to operationalized ICD-10 criteria using the Autism Diagnostic Interview (ADI), a standardized investigator-based measure (Le Couteur *et al.*, 1989a). Fourteen MZ and 11 same-sex DZ pairs were found. One pair of MZ twins resulted from a triplet birth in which one child died in the neonatal period. In addition, there was one set of MZ triplets. As in the earlier study, the sample size and MZ:DZ ratio were very close to the expectations based on the population figures for autism and twinning. It should be noted that the proportion of DZ twin births has fallen markedly over the last 20 years (McGillivray *et al.*, 1988), so that same-sex DZ pairs are now less common than MZ twin births. There were no cases of fragile X in this new twin and triplet sample, and none of consanguinity. In this new sample, the MZ pairwise concordance rate (excluding the set of surviving triplets) for autism was 57%, with a 0% DZ pairwise concordance. The concordance rate for cognitive abnormalities was just under 90% in MZ pairs and about 10% in DZ pairs. It is evident that the results were very closely similar to those in the earlier twin study—replicating the findings for both autism and for cognitive/social abnormalities, although the field work was undertaken by different investigators and a different diagnostic instrument was used.

Before concluding that these findings indicate genetic influences, it was necessary to examine two possible confounding factors. First, concordance might be explicable on the basis of pre- and perinatal hazards, but the findings showed that this was unlikely. In the 11 concordant pairs, there were three instances of hazards only in the autistic proband and none where they affected both twins; in the 33 discordant pairs, hazards affected both twins in four pairs. Second, congenital anomalies are more common in twins than in singletons and somewhat more common in MZ than DZ twins (Rutter *et al.*, 1990a). Could this account for the concordance pattern? Anomalies were scored according to the Waldrop and Halverson (1971) system and it was found that the anomaly score did not differ between MZ and DZ pairs, between concordant and discordant pairs, or between autistic and non-autistic pairs. This possibility, too, could be rejected.

The pooled twin sample was also used to determine whether serious biological hazards (such as neonatal convulsions or a delay in breathing of five minutes or more) or major biological differences (such as a birth weight difference exceeding one pound) could account for the patterns of discordance. Serious hazards were less common in the second twin sample (as might be expected on the basis of improved obstetric and neonatal care). However, altogether, in the 33 discordant pairs there were 10 instances in which the hazards affected one twin only; in every instance this applied to the autistic and not to the non-autistic twin. The findings for biological differences went in the same direction but were less clearcut; in 8 out of 11 cases the autistic twin was disadvantaged. The results suggest that obstetric/neonatal hazards may serve to make the difference between a non-autistic cognitive/social deficit and overt autism in genetically predisposed individuals. However, two caveats need to be expressed. First, it is possible that at least some of the obstetric/neonatal complications may be a consequence of a genetically determined disorder, rather than a cause of the condition. Second, these findings cannot necessarily be generalized to singletons. Although twins and singletons with autism have been shown to be closely comparable in features such as sex ratio, intelligence quotient (IQ) distribution and so forth (Folstein and Rutter, 1977; Le Couteur *et al.*, 1989a), they do differ (as do non-autistic twins and singletons) in rates of severe pre- and perinatal complications. Such complications are only weakly associated with autism in singletons (Tsai, 1987).

Twin data on their own do not provide a satisfactory means for determining the mode of inheritance. However, the very high MZ:DZ concordance ratio makes straightforward, single, major gene models unlikely as the major explanation (Vogel and Motulsky, 1986). Mixed models or polygenic models of some type seem more likely.

The 64% probandwise MZ concordance rate for autism translates into a correlation of liability of 0.965 on the multifactorial model, using a population base rate for autism of 2 per 10 000. Obviously, this cannot be calculated for DZ pairs on the basis of a 0% concordance rate. However, the zero is probably an artefact of small numbers and a better estimate is provided by taking the rate in all siblings (including DZ co-twins). When the twin study sibships were pooled with the sibships from a parallel, family genetics study (Macdonald *et al.*, 1989), it was found that there were seven cases of autism in 229 sibs—a rate of 3% (see below). This produces a correlation of liability of 0.479. Broad heritability calculated from the MZ-DZ difference was 96.5%. When the calculation was repeated after exclusion of the two MZ pairs with possible or definite fragile X and the one MZ pair with familial retinoblastoma, the heritability was virtually identical (96.8%). There is no straightforward way of making the same calculations on the basis of the concordance figures for cognitive/social disabilities because their population base rate is not known. Nevertheless, it is obvious that they imply a similarly high level of heritability.

The only other population-based twin study has been that undertaken in Nordic countries by Steffenburg *et al.* (1989). In a sample of nine MZ and ten same-sex DZ pairs (excluding two MZ pairs with a definite or possible fragile X anomaly), the concordance rate for autism was 89% in MZ pairs and 0% in DZ pairs. As in the other twin studies, severe peri- or neonatal risk differentiated the autistic and non-autistic twins in discordant pairs (in all eight cases where the risk affected just one twin, the autistic twin was disadvantaged). The main differences from the findings of Folstein and Rutter (1977) and Le Couteur *et al.* (1989a) were the higher concordance rate for autism in MZ pairs and the absence of non-autism cognitive/social abnormalities in MZ co-twins. It is possible that this just reflects a very much broader concept of autism in Steffenburg's study. However, it may be relevant that the Nordic sample of twins was markedly atypical in its near-equal sex ratio (17 male and 14 female) and in its unusually high proportion with mental retardation (82%, with 50% severe retardation).

The only other twin series is that of Ritvo *et al.* (1985), who reported a 96% concordance in MZ pairs compared with 24% in DZ pairs. Their study is seriously flawed in terms of biased ascertainment (a major excess of MZ pairs), inappropriate analysis (the inclusion of opposite-sex DZ pairs), non-blind diagnosis, and lack of blood group testing of zygosity in many of the MZ pairs (Folstein and Rutter, 1988; Smalley *et al.*, 1988). The most striking aspect of their results is the very much higher concordance in DZ pairs (24%) than the rate in sibs (3%). If true, the difference suggests a powerful effect of shared environmental factors that have a greater effect on twins than singletons. However, because of the methodological shortcomings, there is every reason to view their findings with very considerable caution.

FAMILY STUDIES

For all their obvious strengths, twin designs have limitations (Rutter *et al.*, 1990a) and it is necessary to complement them with other designs, of which family genetic studies constitute a key variety. The first such study was undertaken by August *et al.* (1981), who found a 15% rate of cognitive abnormalities among the 71 siblings of autistic probands compared with 3% among the 38 siblings of Down's syndrome controls. Each sibling had individual psychological testing and of the eleven affected siblings of autistic probands, three had severe retardation (including one with autism), three had mild retardation (including one with autism), three had a learning disability, and two others had an IQ of less than 80. A further study by Baird and August (1985), using anamnestic data and records (rather than individual testing), found a rate of 20% cognitive disabilities among 51 siblings of 29 autistic probands; no control group was used. They noted that the familial loading was largely confined to autistic children with severe mental retardation. By contrast, Bartak *et al.* (1975) reported a family history of reading or language disabilities in a quarter of the families with an autistic boy whose IQ was 70 or greater (no normal control group was studied but the familial loading was similar to that found with a matched group of boys with a developmental disorder of receptive language). Piven *et al.* (1990), in a study of Kanner's cases (most of whom were *not* severely retarded), similarly found a familial loading for cognitive abnormalities, most of which did not involve mental handicap (there was no control group). Minton *et al.* (1982) undertook psychological testing with 50 siblings of 30 autistic subjects: some 7 to 10% (according to criteria) were mentally retarded, and there was a significant tendency for verbal IQ to be at least 15 points below performance IQs (10 out of 36 sibs compared with 2 out of 36 with comparable deficits in the opposite direction). Again, there was no control group but the findings were shown to differ from those expected on the basis of the standardized samples used in the test construction.

Findings on social characteristics of the parents of autistic children are sparse and somewhat contradictory. The parents have been found to be unremarkable with respect to neuroticism, introversion and obsessionality (Kolvin *et al.*, 1971; Cox *et al.*, 1975; Cantwell *et al.*, 1978), and findings have differed on whether or not they show an increase in thought disorder (Schopler and Loftin, 1969; Netley *et al.*, 1975; Lennox *et al.*, 1977). Cantwell *et al.* (1978) found that, compared with the parents of boys with developmental language disorders, parents of autistic boys were possibly more likely to show oddities of personality. Wolff *et al.* (1988) compared the parents of 21 autistic children with useful language with an individually matched group of parents of children with other forms of handicap. The parents in the two groups did not differ on empathy, sociability, or obsessionality (confirming earlier findings) but the parents of autistic children were much more likely to be definitely socially gauche (16/35 versus 0/39).

The most extensive, standardized data with appropriate controls are provided by the family genetic study undertaken by Macdonald *et al.* (1989). Direct assessments are now being made of first-degree relatives but the present findings are restricted to pedigree data. The coding of pedigrees was undertaken blind using case vignettes, good inter-rater reliability having been demonstrated. Preliminary findings, based on a sample of 78 autistic and 22 Down's syndrome probands, showed that 15% of the sibs of autistic individuals compared with 4.5% of the sibs of Down's syndrome individuals showed cognitive disabilities. Most of these involved specific disorders of speech and language rather than global mental handicap. Among the 21 affected sibs, there were ten with marked language delay, five with reading retardation alone (many of the language-delayed children also had reading difficulties), three with mental handicap (two of whom also had autism) and three with a severe disorder of articulation. A comparable difference between the groups was found for autistic-like social abnormalities (12% versus 0% for the sibs aged 16 years or older). The between-group differences for both cognitive and social abnormalities were statistically significant when analysed using a random effects model specifying familial clustering as a variable. This statistical method is necessary in order to take account of the fact that there may be several affected siblings in the same family. There was a 50% overlap between the cognitive and social abnormalities and both tended to be markedly less prevalent in the families of autistic subjects of normal intelligence. Thus, social abnormalities were found in about 20% of the sibs of mentally retarded probands (the rates being approximately equal in those with severe and those with mild retardation), but in less than 5% of those with a non-verbal IQ above 70. Similarly, cognitive deficits were found in about 20% of the sibs of mentally retarded probands compared with about 7% of the sibs of probands of normal intelligence. The familial loading was somewhat higher among the sibs of female probands than sibs of male probands but this difference fell well short of statistical significance. The familial loading was markedly less when the autistic proband had epileptic fits (4% versus 18%) but, because of small numbers, this difference fell short of statistical significance. There was no increased familial loading for epilepsy in the families of autistic subjects and none of the parental marriages was consanguineous.

The rates of both cognitive and social abnormalities were very much lower in parents than in sibs but the differences between the autism and Down's group were in the same direction. In the autism group, 5.2% of the parents were affected by some other type of abnormality compared with 2.1% in the Down's group.

The standardized Autism Diagnostic Interview (Le Couteur *et al.*, 1989b) and the standardized Autism Diagnostic Observation Schedule (Lord *et al.*, 1989) were used for all siblings with language delay and social abnormalities. Four sibs out of 140 met the ICD-10 criteria for autism (Macdonald *et al.*, 1989). The same methods were used in the twin study of Le Couteur *et al.* (1989a), producing three cases of autism among 89 sibs. The overall figure of 7 cases out of 229 gave an overall rate of 3% autism in siblings. This is some 100 times the rate found in most general-population epidemiological studies (Smalley *et al.*, 1988) and more than 10 times the population incidence that is found taking a very broad definition of autistic-like syndromes (Wing and Gould, 1979; Steffenburg and Gillberg, 1986). In their review, Hanson and Gottesman (1976) rightly pointed to the problems of older, unsystematic data. However, these new data using standardized diagnostic measures confirm the markedly raised rate of autism in the siblings of autistic probands.

Autism and schizophrenia

Over the years, there has been speculation that autism might be genetically related to schizophrenia. However, the evidence has been consistent in negating this suggestion. There are no reported cases of autism in the MZ co-twins of schizophrenic probands and no cases of schizophrenia in the MZ co-twins of autistic individuals. Moreover, family studies have shown no increase in the rate of schizophrenia in the parents or siblings of autistic individuals. Hanson and Gottesman (1976) estimated rates of 0.5% and 1.8%, respectively, pooling data across studies—figures that do not differ from those in the general population. These data must be treated with caution as they are based on rather unsystematic methods of assessment. Nevertheless, our own data (so far based on an incomplete sample) have produced comparable figures. Out of 175 parents assessed there has been only one doubtful case of schizophrenia and out of 100 adult siblings again only one case (this time definite)—rates of 0.6% and 1.0%, respectively.

Ritvo et al. (1989a) undertook an epidemiological study of autism in Utah, using a mixture of case records, solicited referrals and advertising in the media to elicit cases; a prevalence rate of 2.2 to 3.6 per 10 000 was found within the age range of 3 to 22 years. Twenty (9.7%) of the 207 families had more than one autistic child (Ritvo et al., 1989b). The overall sample of 241 autistic subjects included 13 with associated medical conditions (such as fragile X [see below] and Rett's syndrome) that could be aetiologically relevant. Unfortunately, these were not excluded from the study of autism in siblings (moreover, there was no systematic testing for fragile X), so that it is not known how these affected the findings. A recurrence risk for autism of 7% if the first autistic child was male was claimed, and one of 14.5% if the first autistic child was female; however, the difference between these two rates was not statistically significant. It is striking that these rates are well above the 2 to 3% found in all other investigations (Smalley et al., 1988; Macdonald et al., 1989). Ritvo et al. (1988) have also claimed to have identified seven parents with autism in the same study; however, adequate data on the childhood characteristics of the parents are lacking and the finding is out of keeping with all other studies (none of which has reported any cases of autism in parents). Freeman et al. (1989) undertook psychological testing of parents and, using a cut-off of one standard deviation, reported that the rate of cognitive impairment did not differ from that expected on the basis of standardization data; no control group was used and the tests chosen (Shipley Hartford and Wide Range Achievement tests), as well as the criteria for cognitive impairment, were rather different from those used by other investigators.

An earlier study by the same research group, based on a volunteer sample of 46 multiplex families, was used for segregation analysis (Ritvo et al., 1985). This produced results that were consistent with autosomal-recessive inheritance but not with multifactorial models. They made adjustments for the bias of sample ascertainment through multiplex families but necessarily this is a dubious procedure when using a volunteer sample involving other unknown biases, and many uncertainties remain regarding their findings. Autosomal-recessive inheritance is inconsistent with the observed marked excess of males among autistic individuals, unless some additional powerful modifying factor is postulated; the analyses undertaken assumed genetic homogeneity (which is not the case, as shown by the data for fragile X and single-gene disorders, as discussed in a later section of this chapter); they failed to adjust for family limitation after the birth of an autistic child (Jones and Szatmari, 1988); they failed to take account of the non-autistic, cognitive/social deficits that seem to be genetically associated with autism; and they assumed non-biased sampling of multiplex families. Spence *et al.* (1985) also carried out a linkage analysis using blood group polymorphisms and HLA; no evidence of linkage was obtained.

As already noted, the twin findings, as well as the family data, reported by the Ritvo group are markedly discrepant from those stemming from other research groups. Part of the explanation probably lies in various methodological limitations (as described above), but it may well be that, in addition, they have used different diagnostic criteria. Either way, the fact that their findings are not replicated by others indicates that caution is needed in their interpretation.

In summary, family studies show that autism is associated with a markedly increased familial loading for the same condition (although the absolute rate is quite low at around 3%) and an increased familial loading for cognitive and social deficits (perhaps especially for a combination of the two). Several studies have shown that most of these deficits occur in the absence of mental handicap. However, the studies of both August *et al.* (1981) and Baird and August (1985) differed in finding that the loading largely applied to mental retardation in siblings. It may be significant that their sample differed from others in being heavily weighted towards profound mental handicap; perhaps the type of familial loading differs for that subgroup.

Autism and mental retardation

With both types of familial loading, the question arises as to whether or not it is at all different from what might be expected in the case of probands with mental retardation *un*associated with autism (Reed and Reed, 1965). Thus, it might be suggested that the familial loading is just a function of the fact that autism is so often accompanied by mental handicap and not anything to do with autism as such. However, the evidence runs consistently against that hypothesis. The key point is that the familial loading for mental handicap (in the absence of autism) applied to mild, and not to severe, retardation (Nichols, 1984), whereas that in autism applies to both (Baird and August, 1985; Macdonald *et al.*, 1989). Moreover, Macdonald *et al.* (1989) found that the main loading was for specific language disorders and autistic-type social deficits in individuals of normal intelligence, rather than for mental retardation *per se*. Also, it is noteworthy that the familial loading in mild mental retardation applies to a group that is heavily skewed towards the socially disadvantaged, and the available data on autism suggest that the familial loading applies to middle-class, as much as to disadvantaged, families. It seems most unlikely that the familial loading for cognitive/social deficits associated with autism is a consequence of associated mental retardation.

The family findings, taken in conjunction with the twin data, point to a strong genetic component in autism. If genetic factors are important, it is necessary to go on to consider possible modes of inheritance. There are many reasons (including difficulties in defining the phenotype, the likelihood of genetic heterogeneity, and the problems created by arbitrary assumptions on penetrance—see Rutter *et al.*, 1990a) why it is difficult to use family data to test competing genetic models. As discussed already, the very high MZ:DZ concordance ratio found in twin studies argues against single, major gene effects as the explanation for most cases of autism. Smalley *et al.* (1988) have pointed out that the reported frequency of multiplex families is much too low for simple, autosomal-recessive inheritance, which in any case could not account for the marked male preponderance. However, because there is evidence that parents tend to limit their families after the birth of an autistic child if the child is not a first born (Jones and Szatmari, 1988), there is likely to be a lower than expected rate of affected siblings. This will complicate detection of mode of inheritance, as it does with some other seriously handicapping disorders (Brookfield *et al.*, 1988). A straightforward X-linked recessive inheritance can also be ruled out on the grounds that the observed prevalence of autism in females is too high.

An alternative is provided by multifactorial models in which a large number of additive, genetic and environmental effects create a normally distributed liability in the population that gives rise to overt disorder only above a particular threshold (Falconer, 1965). Emery (1986) has produced a useful list of guides to the possible operation of a multifactorial mode of inheritance. These include a weaker familial loading when probands have a milder disorder. The finding of Macdonald *et al.* (1989) that the loading was substantially less for probands whose autism was accompanied by a normal non-verbal IQ is consistent with this criterion, provided one can assume that the IQ level reflects the severity of the condition. A variant of the same criterion is the expectation that the familial loading should be greater in the case of the less frequently affected sex. Tsai and his colleagues (August *et al.*, 1981; Tsai *et al.*, 1981; Tsai and Beisler, 1983) reported findings that were weakly in line with the expectation, but were not able to control for IQ levels in comparing males and females. That control was possible in the analysis by Macdonald *et al.* (1989), with results again only weakly supportive. Thus, the available evidence is inconsistent with a straightforward operation of either single-gene or multifactorial models, and it seems that some type of mixed model involving the combination of two or more genes is more likely. However, the strong probability of genetic heterogeneity must be borne in mind. In that connection, it is necessary to consider the evidence that occasional cases of autism are associated with known medical conditions due to single, major genes.

ASSOCIATED SINGLE-GENE CONDITIONS AND CHROMOSOME ANOMALIES

The evidence on this topic has been reviewed by Reiss *et al.* (1986) and by Folstein and Rutter (1988). Both point out that occasional cases of autism have been associated with a wide range of medical conditions, but, until recently, the main interest has focused on phenylketonuria (PKU), and tuberose sclerosis. In both cases, the strength and specificity of the association are in doubt, although the evidence on tuberose sclerosis (Riikonen and Amnell, 1981; Hunt and Dennis, 1987) is much better than that on PKU. Reiss *et al.* (1986) suggested that autism is produced by damage to a developing, functional neuroanatomical system in the brain. As many different pathological processes can produce such damage, autism may be expected to be associated with a wide range of genetic (and non-genetic) disorders. However, in order to keep the findings in perspective, it is necessary to note that these single-gene and chromosome disorders account for only a small proportion of cases of autism as found in general-population, epidemiological studies. Thus, in Lotter's (1967; 1974) series of 32 definitely autistic and 22 possibly autistic children, there was just one case of tuberose sclerosis (and no other known genetic conditions). Wing and Gould's (1979) series of 74 'socially impaired' children, of whom 17 showed autism, included one case of tuberose sclerosis (not in the autistic subgroup), one case of PKU (again not in the autistic subgroup), and three cases of Down's syndrome (one in the autistic subgroup). Gillberg and Steffenburg's (1987) series of 46 cases of autism included just one case of tuberose sclerosis.

The one possible exception to this general pattern of only isolated cases associated with specific genetic conditions seemed to be provided by the fragile X anomaly, a fragile site on the X chromosome at q27.3, which is made manifest by culture in low folate media. It is now well established that the fragile X anomaly is found in some 5 to 10% of mentally retarded individuals (Turner *et al.*, 1986; Webb *et al.*, 1986; Kähkönen *et al.*, 1987), it being rare to detect the anomaly in normal individuals. This makes it second only to Down's syndrome as a known cause of mental handicap. It seemed obvious that it might also account for some cases of autism. An early paper reported a 5 to 20% incidence of fra(X) in autistic males (Blomquist *et al.*, 1985); this was accompanied by a rather overenthusiastic claim that some 20 to 25% of autistic individuals showed the fra(X)

(Gillberg and Wahlstrom, 1985); however, a pooling of samples produced the lower figure of 8% for the fra(X) (Brown *et al.*, 1986); and several recent studies of sizeable samples have produced figures of below 5% (Bolton *et al.*, 1989; Payton *et al.*, 1989). In the epidemiological sample of 41 autistic twin pairs of Le Couteur *et al.* (1989a), only one definitely showed the fra(X) and a further one showed inconsistent low levels of expression with less than 4% of cells positive—giving a rate of fra(X) between 2% and 5% calculated on the basis of fertilized ova, i.e. counting MZ pairs as one case (Bolton *et al.*, 1989). Similarly, Wahlstrom *et al.* (1989), in a population-based study of twins, found one case of fra(X) in 20 pairs, producing a rate of 5% (or 9% if a set of triplets is included). It may be concluded that there is a significant association between autism and the fragile X anomaly but that, probably, it does not account for more than 5% of cases.

The role of laboratory variations is brought out by the Gillberg and Wahlström's (1985) report, in which half of the 'positive' designations were based on just 1 to 2% of X chromosomes, whereas the prevailing view elsewhere is that one should require at least 3 to 4% with the fragile site at Xq27. The question arises, therefore, as to the meaning of low rates of fragile X expression. Bolton *et al.* (1989) have examined the issue in a study of families with more than one affected member but no member with a definite fragile X anomaly. Fourteen per cent of clinically non-affected individuals had 1 to 3% of cells with the fragile site on the X chromosome compared with 31% of clinically affected individuals—a statistically significant difference. The difference suggests that low fra(X) expression may have some clinical meaning. However, the relatively high rate in normals indicates that it is associated with a very high false-positive indication of clinical abnormality (and hence that it is of little diagnostic value at the individual level). Also, the fact that the low rates of fra(X) expression were evident in families *without* any member showing a definite fragile X anomaly indicates that it is most uncertain whether (or how) the two are connected. In addition, low levels of fra(X) expression proved to have rather low retest reliability, with the usual picture being a pairing of normal and low expression rather than low with high expression.

Apart from variations in cytogenetic criteria, it is evident that there has been substantial disagreement on the frequency with which fra(X) individuals show the autistic syndrome. Some have reported that as many as half do so (Levitas *et al.*, 1983; Hagerman *et al.*, 1986), others have put the figure at about 17% (Brown *et al.*, 1986), and yet others have found little difference between fra(X) and non-fra(X) retarded males in their rates of autistic symptomatology (Dykens *et al.*, 1988). More detailed behavioural assessments confirm the high frequency of social abnormalities (anxiety being more common than indifference) but indicate that it is less common for the clinical picture to take the form of autism, as usually diagnosed (Rutter *et al.*, 1990b).

In so far as autism is associated with the fragile X (albeit more weakly than once thought), the question arises as to whether the association is mediated by cognitive impairment or whether it represents some type of specific risk—perhaps because a gene for autism is located near the fragile X site (Gurling, 1986). Such specific risk no longer seems as likely now that it is clear that the proportion of autistic individuals with fra(X) is no higher (and may even be lower) than the proportion of mentally retarded individuals with fra(X). It is of interest that cerebellar abnormalities have been found to be associated with fra(X) (Reiss *et al.*, 1988b), as they have also with autism (Courchesne, 1989). Furthermore, it appears that the psychopathology associated with fra(X) may not be just a reflection of cognitive impairment: there are a few reports of the fra(X) in autistic individuals of normal intelligence (Blomquist *et al.*, 1985), and there are reports of a supposedly increased risk for psychopathology in fra(X) carriers (Fryns, 1986; Reiss *et al.*, 1988a). Carriers have a substantially raised rate of cognitive impairment (Fryns, 1986; Kemper *et al.*, 1986; Turner *et al.*, 1986; Webb *et al.*, 1986) but, although this accounts for some of the psychopathological risk, it does not account for all. The matter warrants further study.

At one time it was thought that the association between the fragile X anomaly and autism might shed light on the genetic mediation of autism more generally; that now seems less likely. It should be added that the further hope that identification of the fragile X anomaly would simplify genetic counselling because it would follow a straightforward, sex-linked, recessive pattern has also not been borne out (Pembrey, 1991).

DILEMMAS AND PROSPECTS

Two contrasting views of autism pervade the literature. First, there is the concept of autism as a broad, behaviourally varied, clinical grouping characterized by some form of organically determined, social impairment, but with very fuzzy boundaries and with many diverse aetiologies, both genetic and non-genetic (see, for example, Reiss *et al.*, 1986; Waterhouse *et al.*, 1989). According to this concept there is little point in searching for one or more genetic factors that are specific to autism. Rather, it is to be expected that the large, currently 'idiopathic' core will be gradually chipped away as more and more diverse causes are identified—just as is happening with mental retardation. Secondly, there is the concept of autism as a distinctive syndrome that, at its core, is likely to have a degree of aetiological specificity, even though it is probable that there will be more than one genetic variety (see, for example, Folstein and Rutter, 1988). Of course, as the evidence on associated conditions shows, it is apparent that *some* cases of autism arise in diverse ways; the question is whether ultimately this will prove to be the case with all or whether, instead, there will be a relatively cohesive central core with just a few autism-specific aetiologies.

At one time it was supposed that a wide range of environmental hazards, such as obstetric and neonatal complications, played a major role in the aetiology. That now seems much less likely. In the first place, the high MZ concordance (together with the low DZ concordance) suggests that it is likely to be unusual for genetic factors not to be involved. In the second place, the evidence on obstetric and neonatal complications shows that the association with autism is weak and that the main association is with minor, rather than major, complications (Tsai, 1987). Thus, there is no particular correlation with very low birth-weight or extremely premature gestation— unlike the situation with mental handicap. The same applies with other physical hazards. They may be important in occasional, individual instances but they seem to account for only a small proportion of cases of autism.

There are several reasons why the available evidence favours the second view, namely that autism-specific aetiologies are likely to be found. Perhaps the most crucial is the mass of evidence that differentiates autism from the general run of mental handicap, in spite of the fact that most autistic individuals are also mentally retarded (Folstein and Rutter, 1988; Rutter, 1988). Thus, the two groups differ in the association with obstetric and perinatal complications; in the peak age of onset of epileptic fits (adolescence in autism; infancy and early childhood in mental handicap); in neuropathology (gross cortical abnormalities being usual in severe retardation and rare in autism); in the kinds of medical conditions with which they are associated (e.g. Down's syndrome is the most frequent cause of severe mental handicap but is rarely associated with autism; similarly cerebral palsy is quite common in association with mental handicap but is rare in autism); and in patterns of cognitive deficit. It seems likely, therefore, that we must look for different aetiologies for autism than those we have found for mental retardation.

Secondly, there is a coherence to the cognitive and social deficits associated with autism in both the twin and family studies that have used comparable methods. These suggest (but certainly do not prove) that there may be one or more genetic mechanisms that connect autism with this broader-based, familial loading—mechanisms that extend across a substantial proportion of cases of autism.

Thirdly, although indeed there are real difficulties in deciding quite where and how to draw the diagnostic boundaries for autism, research findings indicate the value of making diagnostic distinctions. For example, many children with severe developmental disorders of receptive language show marked autistic features, but Rutter and Mawhood's (1991) follow-up into adult life showed that such disorders were sometimes associated with the development of florid paranoid psychoses in late adolescence, whereas this never occurred in the matched group of autistic individuals (both groups being of normal non-verbal intelligence). Similarly, many children with Rett's syndrome get misdiagnosed as autism (Witt-Engerstrom and Gillberg, 1987) but the course of Rett's syndrome (Hagberg *et al.*, 1983; Kerr and Stephenson, 1986) is quite different from that of autism. Differential diagnosis is often difficult but it is crucial to progress in science.

We may conclude, then, that the search for autism-specific genetic factors continues to be a worthwhile enterprise. However, several features create difficulties in that search. First, the history of medical genetics suggests that genetic heterogeneity is to be expected. Secondly, there are substantial uncertainties on how to define the phenotype for autism. The evidence from both twin and family studies suggests that the usually accepted criteria need to be widened somewhat to include a broader range of cognitive and social deficits that often are *un*associated with mental handicap.

Thirdly, because autistic individuals so rarely have children, vertical transmission of autism as such is not to be expected (other than very rarely). This feature will necessarily complicate the study of family patterns examining different genetic models.

Fourthly, as already noted, the tendency to stop having children after the birth of an autistic child (if there has been one normal child born previously) will also complicate family patterns and, in particular, will make the detection of recessive autosomal inheritance more difficult.

Fifthly, the empirical findings so far include several puzzling features. Thus, there is an apparent paradox in the finding of Macdonald *et al.* (1989) that the familial loading for cognitive/social deficits is least evident (if present at all) in cases of autism associated with normal intelligence, yet the affected individuals among the siblings usually show normal intelligence. This could be consistent with a multifactorial model but the small difference in familial loading between males and females with autism does not strongly support such a model. A further puzzle is presented by the apparent disparity in the findings of twin and family studies between those that are heavily weighted towards profoundly retarded autistic individuals (such as Baird and August, 1985; Steffenburg *et al.*, 1989) and those that mainly include autistic individuals with IQs above the profoundly retarded range (such as Folstein and Rutter, 1977; Le Couteur *et al.*, 1989a; Macdonald *et al.*, 1989). It is possible that autism in association with profound mental retardation may differ somewhat from the rest of autism; the possibility requires investigation.

Finally, it is necessary to consider the way ahead. It is obvious that there is a lot more mileage in pursuing the traditional genetic strategies. However, if these are to be maximally fruitful it will be essential to use discriminating, standardized methods of measurement on non-biased samples and to explore possible reasons for the puzzling aspects of the findings so far. As both Folstein and Rutter (1988) and Smalley *et al.* (1988) pointed out in their reviews, it will also be important to be on the alert for possibly meaningful subgroupings of autism. These could be marked by indices as varied as level of IQ, development of epilepsy, serotonin level, the presence of minor congenital anomalies, cognitive pattern, low-level expression of chromosomal fragile sites, cerebellar abnormalities as identified by brain imaging studies, and presence of motor clumsiness. There is also the need to exploit the use of molecular genetic techniques. Up to now, they have been little used to study polygenic factors, but that possibility is also there.

The genetic study of psychiatric disorders presents many problems but of all psychiatric conditions, autism stands out as one likely to involve a particularly strong genetic component. Although we are still a long way from having identified the genetic mechanisms involved, that should prove possible in the foreseeable future.

REFERENCES

August G. J., Stewart M. A., Tsai L. (1981). The incidence of cognitive disabilities in the siblings of autistic children. *British Journal of Psychiatry*; **138**: 416–22.

Baird T. D., August G. J. (1985). Familial heterogeneity in infantile autism. *Journal of Autism and Developmental Disorders*; **15**: 315–21.

Bartak L., Rutter M., Cox A. (1975). A comparative study of infantile autism and specific developmental receptive language disorder: I. The children. *British Journal of Psychiatry*; **126**: 127–45.

Blomquist H. K., Bohman M., Edvinsson S. O. *et al.* (1985). Frequency of the fragile X syndrome in infantile autism. *Clinical Genetics*; **27**: 113–17.

Bolton P., Rutter M., Butler L. *et al.* (1989). Fragile X and autism. Paper given at the First World Congress on Psychiatric Genetics, Churchill College, Cambridge, 3–5 August.

Brookfield J. F. Y., Pollitt R. J., Young I. D. (1988). Family size limitation: a method for demonstrating recessive inheritance. *Journal of Medical Genetics*; **25**: 181–5.

Brown W. T., Jenkins E. C., Cohen I. L. *et al.* (1986). Fragile-X and autism: a multicenter survey. *American Journal of Medical Genetics*; **23**: 341–52.

Cantwell D., Baker L., Rutter M. (1978). Family factors. In: *Autism: A Reappraisal of Concepts and Treatment* (Rutter M., Schopler E., eds.), pp. 269–96. New York: Plenum Press.

Courchesne E. (1989). Neuroanatomical systems involved in infantile autism: The implications of cerebellar abnormalities. In: *Autism: Nature, Diagnosis and Treatment* (Dawson G., ed.), pp. 119–43. New York: Guilford Press.

Cox A., Rutter M., Newman S., Bartak L. (1975). A comparative study of infantile autism and specific developmental receptive language disorder. II. Parental characteristics. *British Journal of Psychiatry*; **126**: 146–59.

Deykin E. Y., MacMahon B. (1979). The incidence of seizures among children with autistic symptoms. *American Journal of Psychiatry*; **136**: 1310–12.

Dykens E., Leckman J. F., Paul R., Watson M. (1988). Cognitive, behavioral and adaptive functioning in fragile X and non-fragile X retarded men. *Journal of Autism and Developmental Disorders*; **18**: 41–52.

Emery A. E. H. (1986). *Methodology in Medical Genetics: An Introduction to Statistical Methods* 2nd edn. Edinburgh: Churchill Livingstone.

Falconer D. S. (1965). The inheritance of liability to certain diseases, estimated from the incidence among relatives. *Annals of Human Genetics*; **29**: 51–76.

Folstein S., Rutter M. (1977). Infantile autism: a genetic study of 21 twin pairs. *Journal of Child Psychology and Psychiatry*; 18: 297–321.

Folstein S., Rutter M. (1988). Autism: familial aggregation and genetic implications. *Journal of Autism and Developmental Disorders*; 18: 3–30.

Freeman B. J., Ritvo E. R., Mason-Brothers A. *et al.* (1989). Psychometric assessment of first-degree relatives of 62 autistic probands in Utah. *American Journal of Psychiatry*; 146: 361–4.

Fryns J. P. (1986). The female and the fragile-X. A study of 144 obligate female carriers. *American Journal of Medical Genetics*; 23: 213–19.

Gillberg C., Steffenburg S. (1987). Outcome and prognostic factors in infantile autism and similar conditions: a population-based study of 46 cases followed through puberty. *Journal of Autism and Developmental Disorders*; 17: 273–87.

Gillberg C., Wahlstrom J. (1985). Chromosome abnormalities in infantile autism and other childhood psychoses: a population study of 66 cases. *Developmental Medicine and Child Neurology*; 27: 293–304.

Gurling H. (1986). Candidate genes and favoured loci: strategies for molecular genetic research into schizophrenia, manic depression, autism, alcoholism and Alzheimer's disease. *Psychiatric Developments*; 4: 289–309.

Hagberg B., Aicardi J., Dias K., Ramos O. (1983). A progressive syndrome of autism, dementia, ataxia, and loss of purposeful hand use in girls: Rett's syndrome: report of 35 cases. *Annals of Neurology*; 14: 471–9.

Hagerman R. J., Jackson A. W., Levitas A. *et al.* (1986). An analysis of autism in fifty males with the fragile X syndrome. *American Journal of Medical Genetics*; 23: 359–74.

Hanson D. R., Gottesman I. I. (1976). The genetics, if any, of infantile autism and childhood schizophrenia. *Journal of Autism and Childhood Schizophrenia*; 6: 209–33.

Hermelin B., O'Connor N. (1970). *Psychological Experiments with Autistic Children*. Oxford: Pergamon.

Hunt A., Dennis J. (1987). Psychiatric disorder among children with tuberose sclerosis. *Developmental Medicine and Child Neurology*; 29: 190–8.

Jones M. B., Szatmari P. (1988). Stoppage rules and genetic studies of autism. *Journal of Autism and Developmental Disorders*; 18: 31–40.

Kähkönen M., Alitalo T., Airaksinen R. *et al.* (1987). Prevalence of the fragile X syndrome in four birth cohorts of children of school age. *Human Genetics*; 77: 85–7.

Kanner L. (1943). Autistic disturbances of affective contact. *Nervous Children*; 2: 217–50.

Kemper M. B., Hagerman R. J., Ahmad R. S., Mariner R. (1986). Cognitive profiles and the spectrum of clinical manifestations in heterozygous fra(x) females. *American Journal of Medical Genetics*; 23: 139–56.

Kerr A. M., Stephenson J. B. P. (1986). A study of the natural history of Rett syndrome in 23 girls. *American Journal of Human Genetics*; 24: 77–83.

Kolvin I., Garside R., Kidd J. (1971). Studies in the childhood psychoses. IV. Parental personality and attitude and childhood psychoses. *British Journal of Psychiatry*; 118: 403–6.

Le Couteur A., Bailey A. J., Rutter M., Gottesman I. (1989a). An epidemiologically based twin study of autism. Paper given at the First World Congress on Psychiatric Genetics, Churchill College, Cambridge, 3–5 August.

Le Couteur A., Rutter M., Lord C. *et al.* (1989b). Autism Diagnostic Interview: a standardized investigator-based instrument. *Journal of Autism and Developmental Disorders*; 19: 363–87.

Le Couteur A., Rutter M., Summers D., Butler L. (1988). Letter: Fragile X in female autistic twins. *Journal of Autism and Developmental Disorders*; 18: 458–60.

Lennox L., Callias M., Rutter M. (1977). Cognitive characteristics of parents of autistic children. *Journal of Autism and Childhood Schizophrenia*; 7: 243–61.

Levitas A., McBogg P., Hagerman R. (1983). Behavioral dysfunction in the fragile X syndrome. In: *The Fragile X Syndrome: Diagnosis, Biochemistry and Intervention* (Hagerman R., McBogg P., eds.), pp. 153–73. Dillon, Colorado: Spectra.

Lord C., Rutter M., Goode S. *et al.* (1989). Autism Diagnostic Observation Schedule: a standardized observation of communicative and social behavior. *Journal of Autism and Developmental Disorders*; 19: 185–212.

Lotter V. (1967). Epidemiology of autistic conditions in young children. II. Some characteristics of the parents and children. *Social Psychiatry*; 1: 163–73.

Lotter V. (1974). Factors related to outcome in autistic children. *Journal of Autism and Developmental Disorders*; 4: 263–77.

Macdonald H., Rutter M., Rios P., Bolton P. (1989). Cognitive and social abnormalities in the siblings of autistic and Down's syndrome probands. Paper given at First World Congress on Psychiatric Genetics, Churchill College, Cambridge, 3–5 August.

MacGillivray I., Campbell D. M., Thompson D. (1988). *Twinning and Twins*. Chichester: Wiley.

Minton J., Campbell M., Green W. *et al.* (1982). Cognitive assessment of siblings of autistic children. *Journal of the American Academy of Child Psychiatry*; 213: 256–61.

Netley C. F., Lockyer L., Greenbaum G. (1975). Parental characteristics in relation to diagnosis and neurological status in childhood psychosis. *British Journal of Psychiatry*; 127: 440–4.

Nichols P. L. (1984). Familial mental retardation. *Behavior Genetics*; 14: 161–70.

Payton J. B., Steele M. W., Wenger S. L., Minshaw N. J. (1989). The fragile X marker in perspective. *Journal of the American Academy of Child Psychiatry*; 28: 417–21.

Pembrey M. (1991). Chromosomal abnormalities. In: *Biological Risk Factors for Psychosocial Disorders* (Rutter M., Casaer P., eds.). Cambridge: Cambridge University Press (in press).

Piven J., Gayle J., Chase G. *et al.* (1990). A family history study of neuropsychiatric disorders in the adult siblings of autistic individuals. *Journal of the American Academy of Child and Adolescent Psychiatry* 29: 177–83.

Plomin R., Rende R. D., Rutter M. (1991). Quantitative genetics and developmental psychopathology. In: *Rochester Symposium on Developmental Psychopathology*, Vol 2, Internalizing and Enternalizing Expressions of Dysfunction (Cicchetti D., ed.). Hillsdale, NJ: Lawrence Erlbaum (in press).

Reed E. W., Reed S. C. (1965). *Mental Retardation: A Family Study*. Philadelphia: Saunders.

Reiss A. L., Feinstein C., Rosenbaum K. N. (1986). Autism and genetic disorders. *Schizophrenia Bulletin*; 12: 724–8.

Reiss A. L., Hagerman R. J., Vinogradov S. *et al.* (1988a). Psychiatric disability in female carriers of the fragile-X chromosome. *Archives of General Psychiatry*; 45: 25–30.

Reiss A. L., Patel S., Kumar A. J., Freund L. (1988b). Preliminary communication: neuroanatomical variations of the posterior fossa in men with the fragile X (Martin–Bell) syndrome. *American Journal of Medical Genetics*; 31: 407–14.

Riikonen R., Amnell G. (1981). Psychiatric disorders in children with earlier infantile spasms. *Developmental Medicine and Child Neurology*; **23**: 747–60.

Ritvo E., Brothers A. M., Freeman B. J. (1988). Letter: Eleven possibly autistic parents. *Journal of Autism and Developmental Disorders*; **18**: 139–43.

Ritvo E. R., Freeman B. J., Mason-Brothers A. *et al.* (1985). Concordance for the syndrome of autism in 40 pairs of afflicted twins. *American Journal of Psychiatry*; **142**: 74–7.

Ritvo E. R., Freeman B. J., Pingree C. *et al.* (1989a). The UCLA-University of Utah epidemiologic survey of autism: prevalence. *American Journal of Psychiatry*; **146**: 194–9.

Ritvo E. R., Jorde L. B., Mason-Brothers A. *et al.* (1989b). The UCLA-University of Utah epidemiologic study of autism: recurrence risk and genetic counselling. *American Journal of Psychiatry*; **146**: 1032–6.

Rutter M. (1967). Psychotic disorders in early childhood. In: *Recent Developments in Schizophrenia* (Coppen A. J., Walk A., eds.). *British Journal of Psychiatry* Special Publication 2, pp. 133–58. Ashford, Kent: Headley Bros/RMPA.

Rutter M. (1970). Autistic children: infancy to adulthood. *Seminars in Psychiatry*; **2**: 435–50.

Rutter M. (1979). Language, cognition and autism. In: *Congenital and Acquired Cognitive Disorders* (Katzman R., ed.), pp. 247–64. New York: Raven Press.

Rutter M. (1988). Biological basis of autism: implications for intervention. In: *Preventive and Curative Intervention in Mental Retardation* (Menolascino F. J., Stark J. A., eds.), pp. 265–94. Baltimore: Paul Brookes.

Rutter M., Mawhood L. (1991). The long-term psychosocial sequelae of specific developmental disorders of speech and language. In: *Biological Risk Factors for Psychosocial Disorders* (Rutter M., Casaer P., eds.). Cambridge: Cambridge University Press (in press).

Rutter M., Bolton P., Harrington R. *et al.* (1990a). Genetic factors in child psychiatric disorders. I. A review of research strategies. *Journal of Child Psychology and Psychiatry*; **31**: 3–37.

Rutter M., Macdonald H., Le Couteur A. *et al.* (1990b). Genetic factors in child psychiatric disorders. II. Empirical findings. *Journal of Child Psychology and Psychiatry*; **31**: 30–83.

Schopler E., Loftin J. (1969). Thinking disorders in parents of young psychotic children. *Journal of Abnormal Psychology*; **74**: 281–7.

Silliman E. R., Campbell M., Mitchell R. S. (1989). Genetic influences in autism and assessment of metalinguistic performance in siblings of autistic children. In: *Autism: Nature, Diagnosis and Treatment* (Dawson G., ed.), pp. 225–9. New York: Guilford.

Smalley S. L., Asarnow R. F., Spence M. A. (1988). Autism and genetics: a decade of research. *Archives of General Psychiatry*; **45**: 953–61.

Spence M. A., Ritvo E. R., Marazota M. L. *et al.* (1985). Gene mapping studies with the syndrome of autism. *Behavior Genetics*; **15**: 1–13.

Steffenburg S., Gillberg C. (1986). Autism and autistic-like conditions in Swedish rural and urban areas: a population study. *British Journal of Psychiatry*; **138**: 416–22.

Steffenburg S., Gillberg C., Hellgren L. *et al.* (1989). A twin study of autism in Denmark, Finland, Iceland, Norway and Sweden. *Journal of Child Psychology and Psychiatry*; **30**: 405–16.

Tsai L. Y. (1987). Pre-, peri-, and neonatal factors in autism. In: *Neurobiological Issues in Autism* (Schopler E., Mesibov G. B., eds.), pp. 180–9. New York: Plenum Press.

Tsai L. Y., Beisler J. M. (1983). The development of sex differences in infantile autism. *British Journal of Psychiatry*; 142: 373–8.

Tsai L. Y., Stewart M. A., August G. (1981). Implications of sex differences in the familial transmission of infantile autism. *Journal of Autism and Developmental Disorders*; 11: 165–73.

Turner G., Robinson H., Laing S., Purvis-Smith S. (1986). Preventive screening for the fragile-X syndrome. *New England Journal of Medicine*; 315: 607–9.

Vogel F., Motulsky A. G. (1986). *Human Genetics* 2nd edn. New York: Springer-Verlag.

Wahlstrom J., Steffenburg S., Hellgren L., Gillberg C. (1989). Chromosome findings in twins with early-onset autistic disorder. *American Journal of Medical Genetics*; 32: 19–21.

Waldrop M., Halverson C. E. (1971). Minor physical anomalies and hyperactive behavior in young children. In: *The Exceptional Infant* (Hellmuth J., ed.). New York: Brunner/Mazel.

Waterhouse L., Wing L., Fein D. (1989). Re-evaluating the syndrome of autism in the light of empirical research. In: *Autism: Nature, Diagnosis and Treatment* (Dawson G., ed.), pp. 263–81. New York and London: Guilford.

Webb T. O., Bundey S., Thake A., Todd J. (1986). The frequency of the fragile X chromosome among school children in Coventry. *Journal of Medical Genetics*; 23: 396–9.

Wing L., Gould J. (1979). Severe impairments of social interaction and associated abnormalities in children: epidemiology and classification. *Journal of Autism and Developmental Disorders*; 9: 11–30.

Witt-Engerström I., Gillberg C. (1987). Letter: Rett syndrome in Sweden. *Journal of Autism and Developmental Disorders*; 17: 149–50.

Wolff S., Narayan S., Moyes B. (1988). Personality characteristics of parents of autistic children. *Journal of Child Psychology and Psychiatry*; 29: 143–54.

World Health Organization (1989). *International Classification of Diseases, ICD-10: 1989*, Draft of Chapter V, Categories F00—F99, Mental and Behavioural Disorders (including disorders of psychological development). Geneva: WHO.

16 *Learning disability and psychiatric/behavioural disorders: a genetic perspective*

A. J. HOLLAND

INTRODUCTION

Behavioural and psychiatric disorders may occur in as many as a quarter to a half of people with developmental learning disabilities (Ballinger and Reid, 1977; Corbett, 1979; Lund, 1985; Fraser *et al.*, 1986). When they do occur they can have a profound effect on the person's quality of life (Brown, 1990). The recent move to community-based facilities has highlighted the need for a greater understanding of the factors that cause and maintain behavioural and psychiatric disorders in people with learning disabilities, as well as the urgent need to develop new treatments and management strategies, and to evaluate them.

People described as having a 'learning disability' vary in their personalities and social backgrounds, as do the rest of the population, but they are also heterogeneous in the nature, severity and cause of the disability. For example, for some people their disability may be due to inheritance of a chromosomal or single-gene disorder (Evans and Hamerton, 1985), and in others it may be due to environmental factors operating during the intrauterine or perinatal period (Hagberg and Hagberg, 1984). The different causes have particular effects on brain development and function. In many cases this results in severe, developmental, intellectual impairment and marked limitations in social and living skills, and in language development. The resultant disabilities give rise to considerable disadvantage, and to the person being classified as 'mentally handicapped' (World Health Organization, 1980). At the milder end of the spectrum the learning disability may be first identified at school and may not be accompanied by any marked developmental delay or disadvantage. In the former (severe) group, sensory impairments (Ellis, 1986), epilepsy (Corbett *et al.*, 1975), and the social and language impairment characteristic of autism (Shah *et al.*, 1982) are all more common.

The potential seriousness of the problems presented by behavioural difficulties are best illustrated by one particular behaviour, that of self-injury. Oliver *et al.* (1987) reported that 12% of people resident in mental handicap hospitals within one particular health region had shown self-injurious behaviour, sufficient to cause tissue damage, in the previous month. In this region as a whole, only 2% of people with this behaviour had had any form of proper assessment or treatment programme. This type of behaviour also illustrates how diverse causes can underly apparently similar behaviours. For example, people with Lesch–Nyan syndrome are at one pole of a complex genetic/environmental continuum. In this X-linked, single-gene disorder, the self-injurious behaviour that invariably occurs is remarkable in its complexity. Those with the disorder actively seek methods of self-restraint or ask for splints as they are unable to control the impulse to injure themselves. The genetic and enzyme defect is known (Seegmiller, 1976) but as yet this has not provided an explanation of the behaviour. In those with other causes for their disability, sensory impairments and severe social and language impairments may be important risk factors in the causation of self-injurious behaviour. Inadvertent reinforcement of the behaviour by family or care staff may result in the behaviour being maintained for a long time. Understanding a particular behavioural problem, for example self-injury, requires an understanding of the biological, developmental, psychological and environmental factors that may have contributed to the cause and maintenance of the behaviour (Iwata *et al.*, 1982; Oliver and Head, 1990). The nature of the behaviour itself often gives little clue to its aetiology.

Much of the research in the field of mental handicap has focused on characterizing syndromes and identifying their causes. This work has increased the accuracy of genetic counselling and is of considerable value to parents or prospective parents. However, prenatal screening and genetic counselling can only hope to reduce the number of children born with mental handicapping disorders; they will not prevent the problem completely. Genetic and psychiatric research needs to focus on understanding the causes of disordered behaviour, and on the relationship between specific genetic syndromes or identified chromosomal abnormalities and the risk of developing particular psychiatric disorders or abnormalities of behaviour.

There are a number of examples of associations or possible associations between particular genotypes and 'behavioural' or 'psychiatric' phenotypes. Crow (1988) has argued that people with sex chromosomal abnormalities have an increased probability of developing psychiatric illness and that this observation, and the observed pattern of segregation of psychotic illness in families, suggest that a gene located in the pseudo-autosomal region of the sex chromosomes may be important as a predisposing factor for psychiatric illness. Other chromosome abnormalities have been shown to cosegregate with psychotic illness in particular families. These may also give clues to the possible genetic locus for an allele that increases the predisposition to psychotic illness (Holland and Gosden, 1990).

Although it has been shown that people with learning disabilities also have an increased risk for psychotic illness (Reid, 1972; Wright, 1982; and review by Turner, 1989) and not just psychiatric disorder in general, the reasons for this are not known. To answer the question as to whether this is related to the presence of abnormal brain development and/or the presence of the learning disability regardless of the cause requires further research.

I will now discuss two other examples that illustrate important links between genetic syndromes and psychiatric disorder or abnormalities of behaviour. First, research into the relationship between Down's syndrome and Alzheimer's disease; secondly, the relationship between severe over-eating, which occurs with people who have the Prader–Willi syndrome.

DOWN'S SYNDROME AND ALZHEIMER'S DISEASE

The search for, and localization of, the gene for familial Alzheimer's disease on chromosome 21 (St. George-Hyslop *et al.*, 1987) was directly related to the longstanding observation that people with Down's syndrome (trisomy 21) invariably develop the neuropathological changes of Alzheimer's disease as early as the third and fourth decades of life (see review by Oliver and Holland, 1986). In addition, Heston and Mastri (1977) also reported an excess number of Down's syndrome births in the families of probands with Alzheimer's disease, a finding also made by Heyman *et al.* (1983), but not by Whalley *et al.* (1982). Before the finding of linkage between a marker on chromosome 21 and early-onset Alzheimer's disease, it had been argued that the neuropathological changes observed in people with Down's syndrome were due to a number of other possible factors including the non-specific effects of having the syndrome (Epstein, 1983), abnormal immunological function (Countryman *et al.*, 1977; Epstein and Epstein, 1980), and premature ageing associated with increased activity of the enzyme superoxide dismutase, the gene for which is on chromosome 21 (Sinet, 1982).

The neuropathological findings are at odds with the clinical observations. Assessment of cognitive deterioration in people with a pre-existing intellectual impairment may be difficult, and apparent deterioration may either go unnoticed or be put down to the pre-existing mental handicap. As many as a half of people with Down's syndrome may deteriorate in ability as they become older and eventually meet the criteria for dementia, but it is equally clear that not all people develop a dementing illness (Dalton and Crapper-McLauglin, 1986). This is illustrated by comparison of computed tomography (CT) brain scans from two people with Down's syndrome, both in their early 50s: one (Fig. 16.1) had lost many of his previously acquired skills and had dementia; the other (Fig. 16.2) had no evidence of such deterioration. More recent studies of older people with Down's syndrome have demonstrated that the risk of developing Alzheimer's dementia increases with age (Lai and Williams, 1989) and is accompanied by changes in brain structure as demonstrated by CT scans (Schapiro *et al.*, 1989).

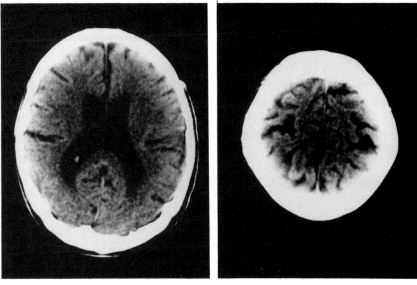

Fig. 16.1   *CT brain scan showing two cuts, one (a) at the level of the lateral ventricles and the other (b) near the top of the cerebral hemispheres of a male with Down's syndrome aged 56 years. In the clinical history and on examination there was evidence of cognitive deterioration and loss of skills. The scans show enlarged ventricles and evidence of cerebral atrophy*

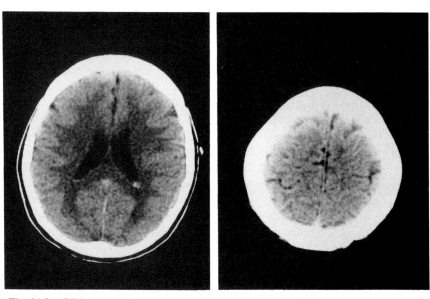

Fig. 16.2   *CT brain scan showing two cuts, one (a) at the level of the lateral ventricles and the other (b) near the top of the cerebral hemispheres of a female with Down's syndrome aged 54 years. In the clinical history and on examination there was no evidence of cognitive deterioration or loss of skills. There is no evidence of cerebral atrophy (compare with Fig. 16.1)*

Two other areas of research are of particular relevance. First, the finding of an increase in the amyloid precursor protein pre-A4 in the serum of people with Down's syndrome, as might be expected given that the gene for the A4 amyloid protein has been localized on chromosome 21 (21q11–q22). However, levels of the amyloid precursor in the serum of people with Alzheimer's disease were similar to those in controls, suggesting that if a defect in amyloid, or its precursors, is important in the aetiology of Alzheimer's disease, the mechanism is different in people with Down's syndrome and in those without (Rumble *et al.*, 1989; Selkoe, 1990). Secondly, decreases in the microviscosity of platelet membranes have been described in people with Alzheimer's disease but not in people with multi-infarct dementia (Hicks *et al.*, 1987). Lipoperoxidation levels in the erythrocytes of people with Alzheimer's disease are similar to those of controls, but there is a significant increase in the number of platelet membrane abnormalities in the platelets of those with Alzheimer's disease (Hajimohammadreza *et al.*, 1990). Post-mortem brain tissue from people who had Alzheimer's disease shows abnormalities of lipoperoxidation under a stimulated test situation but not under basal conditions (Hajimohammadreza and Brammer, 1990).

The localization of the site for the 'Alzheimer allele' on the proximal part of the long arm of chromosome 21, close to the marker D21S13, together with the localization of the amyloid gene on chromosome 21, have therefore raised a number of questions as to the cause of Alzheimer's disease in those with Down's syndrome. Both loci are outside the part of chromosome 21 that has to be inherited in triplicate to develop the Down's syndrome phenotype, and a considerable genetic distance from the locus for the gene coding for the enzyme, superoxide dismutase (SOD). The activity of this enzyme is increased by half in the brains of people with Down's syndrome, as would be anticipated from a gene dosage effect (Brooksbank and Balazs, 1983). The increased activity of SOD gives rise to an increased number of free hydroxyl radicals, which in turn are thought to be the cause of the premature ageing in people with Down's syndrome. If this is the case, the recent genetic findings and those described above suggest that the process of ageing and the aetiology of Alzheimer's disease are independent of each other, at least in Down's syndrome. This requires further investigation by, first, establishing a method for accurately and reliably diagnosing dementia in people with Down's syndrome, and secondly, correlating the presence of dementia and its age of onset with measures of ageing, such as skin and hair changes, cataract formation and measures including DNA repair, platelet microviscosity and immunological function.

THE PRADER–WILLI SYNDROME, OBESITY AND OVER-EATING

This syndrome was first described by Prader, Labhert and Willi (1956) and is characterized by neonatal hypotonia, obesity commencing in childhood, short stature, delay in normal secondary sexual development and varying degrees of learning disability. The obesity may be severe, leading to an increased morbidity and mortality. In addition, there may be disorders of sleep and behaviour (Clarke *et al.*, 1989). Characteristically, excessive intake of food starts in early childhood. The children seek out food and their parents have to respond by locking the kitchen door and food cupboards, and by taking over total control of food intake. In adult life the problems can increase, as with greater independence food is more readily available. This is illustrated in Fig. 16.3, which shows the rapid increase in weight of an 18-year-old female. At home her parents had total control over her food intake by locking all food cupboards and the refrigerator. Once in a hostel she had free access to food and she was unable to restrain herself from eating large amounts, day and night.

The clinical features and the hypogonadism in this syndrome suggest there is an abnormality of the hypothalamus; however, there have been no detailed post-mortem studies of this (Jeffcoate *et al.*, 1980). The intellec-

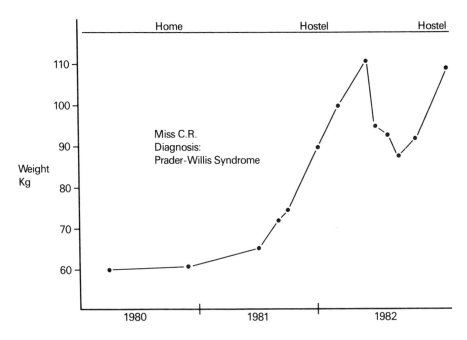

Fig. 16.3 *Graph of the weight (in kg) of a female with the Prader–Willi syndrome. At the top of the graph her place of residence is shown. After she left home and had free access to food, her weight increased rapidly, only decreasing during subsequent hospital admissions*

tual impairment also characteristic of this disorder remains unexplained. More recent studies have reported that half or more of people with this syndrome have an abnormality (usually a deletion) of the proximal long arm of chromosome 15 (15p11–13; Ledbetter *et al.*, 1981). Abnormalities of this chromosomal site are also associated with Angelman's syndrome, a disorder quite distinct from the Prader–Willi syndrome (Williams *et al.*, 1989).

The control of food intake is by a complex system involving a number of feedback mechanisms and different neuropeptides, aminoacids, prostaglandins and primary amine transmitters (Morley, 1980). Studies on animals and man have shown that cholecystokinin (Baile *et al.*, 1986), 5-hydroxytryptamine (Blundell and Hill, 1987), insulin and corticotrophin-releasing hormone (Morley and Levine, 1982) all have an inhibitory action on food intake, whereas neuropeptide Y and peptide YY (Clarke *et al.*, 1984), noradrenaline and endorphins (Morley and Levine, 1981) increase food intake above the normal physiological drive.

In humans, behavioural changes can be observed and the process of satiety and fullness after food intake measured by using linear analogue scales. Although it is well recognized that people with the Prader–Willi syndrome overeat, the behavioural and pathophysiological basis for this is not known. Studies being carried out by Dr. Janet Treasure, Janine Dallow and myself at the Institute of Psychiatry and by Dr. Ed Hillhouse at King's College Hospital have shown that people with this syndrome will continue to eat food at a steady rate and, in our experimental situation, ate on average three times more calories than a control group, stopping their intake after one hour only because the food was then removed. Figures 16.4 and 16.5 show the rates of eating of individuals in a control group, and of individuals with the Prader–Willi syndrome. During this experimental time they also fail to lose the sensation of 'hunger', as measured on a 10-cm analogue scale, to the same degree as the control group, despite eating substantially more food. From our preliminary findings we conclude that people with this syndrome continue to eat because they fail to satiate. The question remains as to what the link is between the identified abnormality on chromosome 15 and the failure to satiate. High levels of cholecystokinin were found in the serum of people with Prader–Willi syndrome during the period in which they were overeating, suggesting that the peripheral release of this hormone is normal and related to quantity eaten or to some other factor (for example, stomach distension) but that the central effect of bringing about satiety is markedly reduced. Whether a lack of sensitivity to cholecystokinin centrally, or whether abnormalities of other feedback mechanisms, as mentioned earlier, are the explanation of the observed failure to satiate requires further investigation.

The results of this type of research are important in that they may lead to new treatments, but even these preliminary findings may be of value in helping people with the syndrome and members of their family and/or care staff to understand the problem. It is all too easy to see the behaviour as

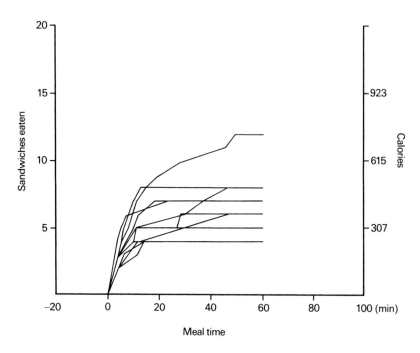

Fig. 16.4   *Graphs of the rate of eating of individuals in a control group (matched for age) who were exposed to food for one hour. The left hand axis gives the rate in sandwich quarters eaten and the right in calories*

being due to 'stubbornness' or 'wilfulness', and, as a result, any effort to help the person disappears, their weight increases and their quality of life becomes severely impaired. Appreciating that there is a very specific deficit affecting the satiation mechanism makes sense of the behaviour and allows relatives to help in a more constructive way.

FUTURE DEVELOPMENTS

Understanding the relative importance of biological and environmental factors in the aetiology and maintenance of problem behaviours or psychiatric disorder in people with a learning disability requires both knowing the cause of the learning disability and its effect on brain structure and functioning, as well as having a clear understanding of the nature of the problem behaviour. If a certain behaviour or psychiatric disorder is shown to be more common in people with a particular causation for their learning disability, this suggests that the disability itself and other factors common to people with such disabilities are unlikely to be the cause of the

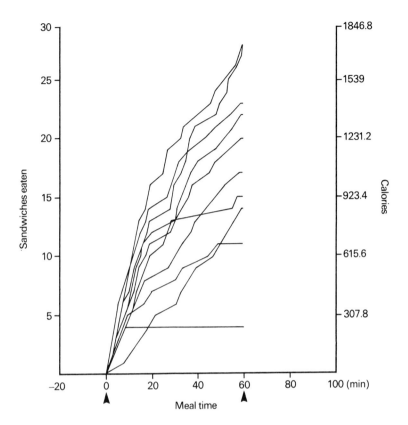

Fig. 16.5   *Graphs of the rate of eating of individuals with the Prader–Willi syndrome who were exposed to food for one hour. The left hand axis gives the rate in sandwich quarters eaten and the right in calories*

problem behaviour or psychiatric disorder. Under these circumstances it is a reasonable hypothesis that something unique to the syndrome is the cause. If the syndrome is known to be genetic, then the question remains as to how the genetic defect, the presumed abnormality of brain function and the behaviour are connected.

Animal models are being used to try and answer this question in the case of Lesch–Nyan syndrome. Models have been proposed on the basis of lesions affecting specific neuronal pathways at a particular developmental stage. Neonatal rats, whose nigrostriatal dopaminergic pathways have been destroyed by a neurotoxin, show an increased susceptibility to self-injurious behaviour, for example, self-biting (Breese *et al.*, 1984). A similar response is not elicited by dopamine antagonists in adult rats. It has therefore been suggested that abnormalities of D_1 dopamine receptors induced in animals may be a model for the self-injurious behaviour seen in people with Lesch–Nyan syndrome. Further work has examined the possible roles of other neurotransmitter systems (Sivam, 1989) and the central opiates (Herman *et al.*, 1987). Given the numerous possible causes of self-injurious behaviour in the learning-disabled population as a whole, any model relevant to the Lesch–Nyan syndrome would have to be applied in other cases with great care. A clear characterization of the behaviour would be necessary. For example, whether self-restraint was a feature, or there was a clear 'function' to the behaviour, or the presence of a mood disorder and whether the age of onset of the behaviour was in early childhood or later in life. The relevance of such models to human self-injurious behaviour could be tested by the development of ligands for specific brain receptors and the use of the new brain imaging techniques, or by the use of drugs with very specific sites of action.

The evidence that the syndrome of autism may be due to genetic factors is increasing (Bolton and Rutter, 1990). However, there remains the problem of aetiological heterogeneity. This is partly solved by looking for all known causes possibly associated with autism, for example, tuberous sclerosis (Hunt and Dennis, 1987) or possibly fragile-X syndrome (Gillberg and Wahlstrom, 1985), but also by more sophisticated ways of characterizing the deficit. Different ways of assessing the cognitive and social impairments of autism are available, which may allow a more clear definition of the phenotype (Frith, 1989; Barron-Cohen, 1990). Identifying possible susceptibility genes for autism or its spectrum disorders may be difficult because of the problems of collecting sufficiently large pedigrees, the possible sex effect on the expression of any genetic abnormality, and the lack of any clues as to the possible genetic locus. However, the use of sophisticated cytogenetic techniques, together with new molecular genetic methods of detecting submicroscopic deletions (Lamb *et al.*, 1989), may allow the detection of deletions that can give some clue to the possible localization of individual genes responsible for such neurodevelopmental disorders as autism as well as other disorders associated with mental handicap.

CONCLUSIONS

The clinical assessment of behavioural and/or psychiatric disorder in a person with a learning disability requires the same rigorous approach as should be expected in any good psychological and psychiatric practice. The relative importance of biological, developmental, psychological and environmental factors will vary between individuals and within individuals over time. Advances in genetic research allow the identification of particular genotypes and the characterization of variation at the genetic level. A number of different approaches can be used to understand the link between the established genetic defect and the propensity to abnormalities of behaviour. Such work requires sophisticated characterization of the problem behaviour or psychiatric disorder.

ACKNOWLEDGEMENTS

My thanks to Chris Oliver and Lissa Crayton for permission to show the CT scans on two subjects from an ongoing study of Down's syndrome at the Institute of Psychiatry, funded by the Wellcome Trust, and Iradj Hajimohammadreza and Michael Brammer, who are investigating the platelet and biochemical abnormalities in this group. My thanks also to Janet Treasure, Janine Dallow and Ed Hillhouse for their permission to present some of the data from a study of the Prader–Willi syndrome, partly funded by the Prader–Willi Syndrome Association, which has recently been completed. In this study, levels of cholecystokinin were kindly measured by Dr. Brazell of the Merck Sharp and Dohme research laboratories.

REFERENCES

Baile C. A., McLaughlin C. L., Della-Fera M. A. (1986). Role of cholecystokinin and opioid peptides in control of food intake. *Physiological Review*; 66: 172–234.

Ballinger B. R., Reid A. H. (1977). Psychiatric disorder in an adult training centre and a hospital for the mentally handicapped. *Psychological Medicine*; 7: 525–8.

Barron-Cohen S. (1990). Autism: a specific cognitive disorder of 'mind blindness'. *International Review of Psychiatry* 2: 81–90.

Blundell J. E., Hill J. E. (1987). Serotoninergic modulation of the pattern of eating and the profile of hunger-satiety in humans. *International Journal of Obesity*; 11: 141–55.

Bolton P., Rutter M. (1990). Genetic influences in autism. *International Review of Psychiatry* 2: 67–80.

Breese G. R., Baumeister A. A., McCown T. J. *et al.* (1984). Neonatal 6-hydroxydopamine treatment: model of susceptibility for self-mutilation in the Lesch–Nyan syndrome. *Pharmacology and Biochemical Behavior*; 21: 459–61.

Brooksbank B. W. L., Balazs R. (1983). Superoxide dismutase and lipoperoxidation in Down's syndrome fetal brain. *Lancet*; i: 881–2.

Brown R. I. (1990). Quality of life for people with learning difficulties: the challenge for behavioural and emotional disturbance. *International Review of Psychiatry* 2: 23–32.

Clarke J. J., Kalva P. S., Crowley W. L., Kalva S. P. (1984). Neuropeptide Y and human pancreatic polypeptide stimulate feeding behaviour in rats. *Endocrinology*; 115: 427–9.

Clarke D. J., Waters J., Corbett J. A. (1989). Adults with Prader–Willi syndrome: abnormalities of sleep and behaviour. *Journal of the Royal Society of Medicine*; 82: 21–4.

Corbett J. A. (1979). Psychiatric morbidity and mental retardation. In: *Psychiatric*

Illness and Mental Handicap (Snaith P., James F. E., eds.). Ashford, Kent: Headley Bros.

Corbett J. A., Harris R., Robinson R. G. (1975). Epilepsy. In: *Mental Retardation and Developmental Disabilities*, vol. VII (Wortis J., ed.). New York: Bruner Mazel.

Crow T. J. (1988). Sex chromosomes and psychosis: a pseudoautosomal locus. *British Journal of Psychiatry*; **153**: 675–83.

Countryman P. I., Heddle J. A., Crawford E. (1977). The repair of X-ray induced chromosomal damage in trisomy 21 and normal diploid lymphocytes. *Cancer Research*; **37**: 52–8.

Dalton A. J., Crapper-McLachlan D. R. (1986). Clinical expression of Alzheimer's disease in Down's syndrome. In: *Psychiatric Perspectives on Mental Retardation. Psychiatric Clinics of North America*; **9**: 659–70.

Ellis D. (1986). *Sensory Impairments in Mentally Handicapped People*. London: Croom Helm.

Epstein C. J. (1983). Down's syndrome and Alzheimer's disease; implications and approaches. In: *Biological Aspects of Alzheimer's Disease* (Katzman R., ed.), Banbury Report No. 15, pp. 169–82. New York: Cold Spring Harbor Laboratory.

Epstein L. B., Epstein C. J. (1980). T-lymphocyte function and sensitivity to interferon in trisomy 21. *Cellular Immunology*; **51**: 303–18. •

Evans J. A., Hamerton J. L. (1985). Chromosomal anomalies. In: *Mental Deficiency, the Changing Outlook* (Clarke A. M., Clarke A. D. B., Berg J. M., eds.). London: Methuen.

Fraser W. I., Leudar I., Gray J., Campbell I. (1986). Psychiatric and behaviour disturbance in mental handicap. *Journal of Mental Deficiency Research*; **30**: 49–57.

Frith U. (1989). *Autism: Explaining the Enigma*. Oxford: Blackwell.

Gillberg C., Wahlstrom J. (1985). Chromosome abnormalities in infantile autism and similar conditions: a population study of 66 cases. *Developmental Medicine and Child Neurology*; **27**: 293–304.

Hagberg B., Hagberg G. (1984). Aspects of prevention of pre-, peri and postnatal brain pathology in severe and mild mental retardation and analysis from recent Swedish epidemiological research. In: *Scientific Studies in Mental Retardation* (Dobbing J., Clarke A. D. B., Corbett J. A. *et al.*, eds.). London: Royal Society of Medicine.

Hajimohammadreza I., Brammer M. (1990). Brain membrane fluidity and lipid peroxidation in Alzheimer's disease. *Neuroscience Letters*; **112**: 333–7.

Hajimohammadreza I., Brammer M., Eagger S. *et al.* (1990). Platelet and erythrocyte membrane changes in Alzheimer's disease. *Biochimica et Biophysica Acta* (in press).

Herman B. H., Hammock M. K., Arthur-Smith A. *et al.* (1987). Naltrexone decreases self-injurious behaviour. *Annals of Neurology*; **22**: 550–2.

Heston L., Mastri A. R. (1977). The genetics of Alzheimer's disease. *Archives of General Psychiatry*; **34**: 977–81.

Heyman A., Wilkinson W. E., Hurwitz B. J. *et al.* (1983). Alzheimer's disease: genetic aspects and associated clinical disorders. *Annals of Neurology*; **14**: 507–16.

Hicks N., Brammer M. J., Hymas N., Levy R. (1987). Platelet membrane properties in Alzheimer's and multi-infarct dementias. *Journal of Alzheimer's Disease and Associated Disorders*; **1**: 90–7.

Holland A. J., Gosden C. (1990). A balanced chromosomal translocation partially segregating with psychotic illness in a family. *Psychiatry Research*; **32**: 1–8.

Hunt A., Dennis J. (1987). Psychiatric disorder among children with tuberous sclerosis. *Developmental Medicine and Child Neurology*; **29**: 190–8.

Iwata D. A., Dorsey M. F., Slifer K. J. *et al.* (1982). Towards a functional analysis of self-injury. *Analysis and Intervention in Developmental Disabilities*; **2**: 3–20.

Jeffcoate W. J., Laurance B. M., Edwards C. R. W., Besser G. M. (1980). Endocrine function in the Prader–Willi syndrome. *Clinical Endocrinology*; **12**: 81–9.

Lai F., Williams R. S. (1989). A prospective study of Alzheimer's disease in Down syndrome. *Archives of Neurology*; **46**: 849–53.

Lamb J., Wilkie A. O. M., Harris P. C. *et al.* (1989). Detection of break points in submicroscopic chromosomal translocation, illustrating an important mechanism for genetic disease. *Lancet*; **ii**: 819–24.

Ledbetter D. H., Riccardi V. M., Airhart S. D. *et al.* (1981). *Deletions of chromosome is as a cause of Prader-Willi syndrome. New England Journal of Medicine*; **304**: 325–8.

Lund J. (1985). The prevalence of psychiatric morbidity in mentally retarded adults. *Acta Psychiatrica Scandinavica*; **72**: 563–70.

Morley J. E. (1980). The neuroendocrine control of appetite: the role of the endogenous opiates, cholecystokinin, TRH, gamma aminobutyric acid and diazepam receptors. *Life Sciences*; **27**: 355–68.

Morley J. E., Levine A. S. (1981). Dynorphin (1–13) induces spontaneous feeding in rats. *Life Sciences*; **29**: 1901–3.

Morley J. E., Levine A. S. (1982). Corticotrophin releasing factor, grooming and ingestive behaviour. *Life Sciences*; **31**: 1459–64.

Oliver C., Head D. (1990). Self-injurious behaviour in people with learning difficulties: determinants and interventions. *International Review of Psychiatry* **2**: 101–115.

Oliver C., Holland A. J. (1986). Down's syndrome and Alzheimer's disease: a review. *Psychological Medicine*; **16**: 307–22.

Oliver C., Murphy G. H., Corbett J. A. (1987). Self-injurious behaviour in people with mental handicap: a total population study. *Journal of Mental Deficiency Research*; **31**: 147–62.

Prader A., Labhart A., Willi H. (1956). Ein Syndrom von Adipositas Kleinwuchs, Kryptorchismus und Oligophrenie nach myatonieartigem Zustand im Neugeborenalter. *Schweiz Medizinisch Wochenschrift*; **86**: 1260–1.

Reid A. H. (1972). Psychoses in adult mental defectives. i: manic depressive psychosis. ii: schizophrenia and paranoid psychosis. *British Journal of Psychiatry*; **120**: 205–80.

Rumble B., Retallack R., Hilbich C. *et al.* (1989). Amyloid A4 protein and its precursor in Down's syndrome and Alzheimer's disease. *New England Journal of Medicine*; **320**: 1447–52.

St. George-Hyslop P. H., Tanzi R. E., Polinsky R. J. *et al.* (1987). The genetic defect causing familial Alzheimer's disease. Maps on chromosome 21. *Science*; **235**: 885–90.

Schapiro M. B., Luxenberg J. S., Kay E. J. A. *et al.* (1989). Serial quantitative CT analysis of brain morphometrics in adult Down's syndrome at different ages. *Neurology*; **39**: 1349–53.

Seegmiller J. E. (1976). Inherited deficiency of hypoxanthine-guanine phosphoribosyltransferase in X-linked uric aciduria (the Lesch–Nyan syndrome and its variants). *Advances in Human Genetics*; **6**: 75–163.

Selko D. J. (1990). Deciphering Alzheimer's Disease: The amyloid precursor protein yields new clues. *Science*, **248**; 1058–60.

Shah A., Homes N., Wing L. (1982). Prevalence of autism and related conditions in adults in a mental handicap hospital. *Applied Research in Mental Handicap*; **3**: 303–17.

Sinet P. M. (1982). Metabolism of oxygen derivatives in Down's syndrome. *Annals of the New York Academy of Sciences*; **396**: 83–94.

Sivam S. P. (1989). D_1 dopamine receptor-mediated substance P depletion in the striatonigral neurones of rats subjected to neonatal dopaminergic denervation: implications for self-injurious behaviour. *Brain Research*; **500**: 119–30.

Turner T. H. (1989). Schizophrenia and mental handicap: a historical review with implications for further research. *Psychological Medicine*; **19**: 301–14.

Whalley L. J., Carothers A. D., Collyer S. *et al.* (1982). A study of familial factors in Alzheimer's disease. *British Journal of Psychiatry*; **140**: 249–56.

Williams C. A., Gray B. A., Hendrickson J. E. *et al.* (1989). Incidence of 15q deletions in the Angelman syndrome: a survey of twelve affected persons. *American Journal of Medical Genetics*; **32**: 339–45.

World Health Organization (1980). *International Classifications of Impairments, Disabilities and Handicaps.* Geneva: WHO.

Wright E. C. (1982). The presentation of mental illness in mentally retarded adults. *British Journal of Psychiatry*; **141**: 496–502.

17 *The genetics of the common forms of dementia*

A. F. WRIGHT

INTRODUCTION

What is it that allows some individuals to show remarkably little outward sign of cognitive impairment in old age while so many others are afflicted with varying degrees of cognitive decline? The evangelist John Wesley once stated 'I have now completed my seventy-fourth year: and by the peculiar favour of God, I find ... all my faculties of body and mind, just the same as they were at four-and-twenty' (Wesley, 1777). Twelve years later, even Wesley found 'his strength now diminished so much that he found it difficult to preach more than twice a day' (Southey, 1820). One of the major problems in this advanced age group is that both physical and mental deterioration are often compounded, producing considerable diagnostic ambiguity for the investigator. Certainly, the prevalence of dementia in the over-65 year age group is remarkably high: about 5% (1.3–6.2%) have severe dementia while 2.6 to 15.4% have a mild degree of dementia (Mortimer *et al.*, 1981; Gurland and Cross, 1982). By the ninth decade, its prevalence is at least 20% and in some surveys as high as 36% in this population (Pfeffer *et al.*, 1987). Neuropathological studies have shown that half of all cases of severe dementia are attributable to Alzheimer's disease, just under one-fifth to multi-infarct dementia, a similar proportion to mixed Alzheimer's–multi-infarct dementia, and the remainder to a variety of more specific causes (Tomlinson *et al.*, 1970; Mortimer *et al.*, 1981). The clinical signs of Alzheimer's dementia may only appear after enough senile plaques and neurofibrillary tangles have formed to constitute a threshold for clinical abnormality, so that for those fortunate enough to evade the signs of failing memory and personal decline, dementia may still lie close to the surface (Blessed *et al.*, 1968). Neuropathological surveys of the unselected elderly population show a high frequency of the same neuropathological changes as are found in Alzheimer's disease; the disease appears to differ from 'normal' ageing in degree rather than in kind (Tomlinson *et al.*, 1968; Dayan, 1971; Matsuyama and Nakumara, 1978; Ulrich, 1982).

Multi-infarct dementia is also strongly age-related in its occurrence: Akesson (1969) found that the age-specific incidence of severe multi-infarct dementia rose sharply from 3.5 to 9.6 cases per thousand between the eighth and ninth decades. Factors such as hypertension and degenerative vascular disease that predispose to this disease also increase steeply with age. The common forms of dementia therefore consist largely of these two groups, Alzheimer's disease and multi-infarct dementia, which alone or in combination probably account for over 80% of cases and both of which are strongly age-related in incidence.

The genetics of multi-infarct dementia is relatively poorly understood in comparison with that of Alzheimer's disease. Few satisfactory family studies have been carried out, although these have consistently shown an increased morbidity risk in the first-degree relatives of probands when compared with spouses or the general population (Constantinidis *et al.*, 1962; Akesson, 1969), indirectly implicating genetic factors. The problem of clinically distinguishing multi-infarct dementia from Alzheimer's disease and other types of dementia can be partially dealt with using appropriate rating scales (Hachinski *et al.*, 1975; Rosen *et al.*, 1980), although the high frequency of mixed states remains a problem. Twin studies have so far provided little evidence for or against a genetic hypothesis (Jarvik *et al.*, 1980), although predisposing factors such as hypertension are under some degree of genetic control (Mongeau, 1987). The identification of specific genes influencing multi-infarct dementia remains elusive, although rare families with an autosomal-dominant form have now been identified (Sourander and Walinder, 1977) and provide scope for the identification of such genes using 'new genetic' techniques. This approach has led to the identification of genes in other, rarer causes of dementia; a cystatin C defect in an autosomal dominant type of hereditary cerebral haemorrhage (congophilic angiopathy; Ghiso *et al.*, 1986) and prion protein gene defects in the autosomal dominant forms of spongiform encephalopathy such as Gerstmann–Straussler syndrome and Creutzfeld–Jacob disease (Collinge *et al.*, 1989).

TWIN AND FAMILY STUDIES IN ALZHEIMER'S DISEASE

Twin studies in Alzheimer's disease have not provided compelling evidence for genetic influences (Table 17.1). These studies are problematic because of the late onset, leading to small numbers of surviving twin pairs, itself introducing a bias towards pairs showing increased longevity (Jarvik *et al.*, 1972). Concordance estimates are also unreliable because of the late onset, particularly if there is wide variation in age of onset. There are always potential ascertainment problems in such studies; the presence of a significant family history of the illness may increase the likelihood both of ascertainment and of participation in such a study. Table 17.1 summarizes the twin studies: most of them are accounts of individual twin pairs but three studies of twin series have been carried out. The study by Kallman (1956) contained the largest number of twin pairs but is the least well documented. This showed a significantly higher monozygous (MZ) twin concordance (42.8%) compared with that for dizygous (DZ) twins (8%).

Table 17.1 Summary of twin studies in Alzheimer's disease. The percentage concordance in monozygous (MZ) and dizygous (DZ) twin pairs and the number (No.) of pairs are shown

Reference	Concordance (%)		No. (MZ,DZ)
	MZ	DZ	
Kallman (1956)	43	8	54
Jarvik *et al.* (1980)	50	100	7 (6,1)
Davidson and Robertson (1955)	0	—	1
Hunter *et al.* (1972)	0	—	1
Sharman *et al.* (1979)	100	—	1
Cook *et al.* (1981)	100	—	1
Embry and Lippmann (1985)	100	—	1
Nee *et al.* (1987)	41	40	22 (17,5)
Luxenberg *et al.* (1987)	0	—	1

However, a follow-up study of this series by Jarvik *et al.* (1980) failed to confirm this result, although the number of twin pairs had dwindled considerably by this time. The only other comparable study is that by Nee *et al.* (1987), who have been studying 22 twin pairs longitudinally, which showed that the MZ twin concordance was 41% while that for DZ twins was 40%—again, no compelling evidence for genetic determination of Alzheimer's disease, at least in these families.

The heritability of a character provides a measure of the proportion of the total variance in the character in a population that is directly heritable (due to additive genetic factors). It is generally applied to quantitative characteristics, but it can also be estimated in discrete characteristics, such as a disease, if one applies a threshold model (Falconer, 1965). These methods were applied to the data of Sjogren *et al.* (1952), Larsson *et al.* (1963) and Heston and Mastri (1977), with the age of onset of probands partitioned into early (less than 65 years) and late (more than 65 years) groups (Wright and Whalley, 1984; Table 17.2). The results in the families of early-onset probands showed that the heritability lies in the range 0.46 (Sjogren *et al.*) to 0.63 (Heston and Mastri), typical of a multifactorial trait. The latter, slightly higher estimate may reflect the presence of at least one family with multiple affected members, suggesting autosomal-dominant inheritance. In the families of late-onset probands, the heritability was lower at 0.32 (Larsson *et al.*, 1963), reflecting the declining difference between the incidence of Alzheimer's disease in the relatives compared with the steeply rising incidence in the general population. These results are consistent with the disease being inherited as a multifactorial or polygenic character, in which genetic differences in the population account for less of the variation in late-onset than in early-onset illness.

A number of more recent family studies are methodologically different

Table 17.2 Estimates of heritability ($\pm$ SEM) in the families of early-onset (under 65 years) and late-onset (over 65 years) probands with Alzheimer's disease (from Wright and Whalley, 1984)

Age of onset (probands)	No. of probands	No. of relatives	Heritability	Reference
Early (<65 yrs)	34	255	0.46 ± 0.09	Sjogren *et al.* (1952)
	30	167	0.63 ± 0.13	Heston and Mastri (1977)
Late (>65 yrs)	256	2421	0.32 ± 0.06	Larsson *et al.* (1963)

from the earlier ones (Heyman *et al.*, 1983; Mohs *et al.*, 1987; Breitner *et al.*, 1988; Huff *et al.*, 1988). These tend to be large, prospective studies of living rather than autopsy-confirmed probands, and which use questionnaires, standardized rating scales or structured interviews of key informants. In some cases, diagnostic criteria in secondary cases appear less than adequate (Huff *et al.*, 1988) and only in some studies was confirmatory medical evidence of a retrospective diagnosis obtained in secondary cases. Diagnoses generally relied on operational criteria for Alzheimer's disease such as those developed by the US National Institutes of Health (McKhann *et al.*, 1984), although attempts to correlate such clinical groups with neuropathological data have showed relatively poor agreement in the diagnosis, ranging from 64 to 86% (Tierney *et al.*, 1988). These recent genetic studies have corroborated the earlier ones in showing an increased, cumulative incidence rate in the relatives of Alzheimer probands compared with the general population, although they have tended to find higher, age-specific incidence rates in the oldest age groups, reaching 50% or more by the ninth decade. This has led to renewed proposals of an autosomal-dominant gene, reaching almost full penetrance by this age, as first suggested by Larsson *et al.* (1963). Larsson had pointed out that with a gene frequency of 0.06, some 55% of the population would be expected to manifest the disease given sufficient longevity. There is no easy way of directly distinguishing these two hypotheses, one claiming a declining role for genetic factors causing onset in later life, the other supporting an autosomal-dominant gene and increased penetrance with advancing age. One finding more easily explained on a complex genetic model is that the relatives of early-onset probands tend to have onset at an earlier age than the relatives of late-onset probands (Breitner *et al.*, 1988; Huff *et al.*, 1988), even although cumulative incidence by the age of 90 years may be similar in the two groups. This is consistent with the results of the early family studies which showed a higher heritability of early-onset illness in the relatives of early-onset probands (see Wright and Whalley, 1984). The early onset would appear to be the heritable factor.

A further result that is most easily explicable on a multifactorial basis is that the age of onset in relatives is substantially later than in the probands (Table 17.3). This implies bias in the ascertainment of the probands and regression towards the mean of the Alzheimer's disease population with regard to onset age in relatives. This differs markedly from the situation in familial Alzheimer's disease, which by definition is an autosomal dominant condition with early onset and in which the age of onset in relatives is very close to that in the probands (Table 17.3), implying tighter genetic control. The broad distribution of onset age in the sporadic group is consistent with a multifactorial aetiology, with increased variability due to more diverse genetic and non-genetic factors. Analysis of 44 published Alzheimer's disease families with two or more affected members shows a low positive correlation ($r = 0.167$) between the within-family mean age of onset and its standard deviation (Fig. 17.1). In older age-groups an accurate measurement of the standard deviation in onset age requires that most 'at risk' members do not die before they have a chance of manifesting the illness, therefore the correlation coefficient is probably underestimated. Standard deviations are also an inaccurate measure of variance in onset age when the number of affected members is small, as with many of the families with non-familial Alzheimer's disease.

AGEING IN ALZHEIMER'S DISEASE

An increasing body of evidence suggests that ageing can be attributed to the accumulation of errors in informational macromolecules (see Florini,

Table 17.3 Mean ($\pm$ SD) age of onset in Alzheimer's disease (AD) and familial Alzheimer's disease (FAD) probands (Op) and their affected relatives (O_R)

	Probands		*Relatives*		*Difference*	*Reference*
Disease	*Onset (Op)*	*No.*	*Onset (O_R)*	*No.*	*($O_R - Op$)*	
AD	52.3 ± 8.7	10	63.4 ± 11.9	12	11.1	Heyman *et al.* (1983)
	61.1 ± 9.3	79	74.3 ± 9.1	34	13.2	Breitner *et al.* (1988)
	66.01	25	70.8	87	4.8	Heston *et al.* (1981)
	64.6	50	72.6	23	8.0	Huff *et al.* (1988)
	65.7 ± 3.1	7	68.5 ± 5.9	10	> 2.8	Heyman *et al.* (1983)
FAD	38.3 ± 7.8	3	39.4 ± 6.4	30	1.1	Wheelan (1959), Feldman *et al.* (1963), Lowenberg and Waggoner (1934)

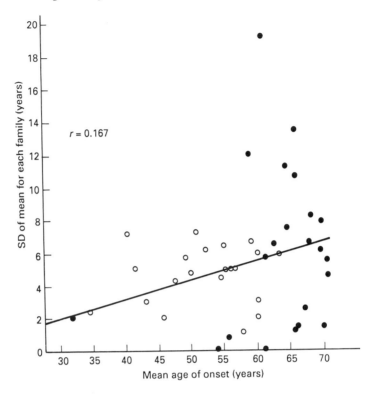

Fig. 17.1   *Mean age of onset in 22 familial Alzheimer's disease (FAD) kindreds (○) and 22 Alzheimer's disease (AD) kindreds (●) plotted against the standard deviation (SD) of the mean, for each family. The correlation coefficient (r) and regression line are shown. Data from Heyman et al. (1983), Wheelan (1959), Goate et al. (1989), St. George-Hyslop et al. (1987), Schellenberg et al. (1988), Lowenberg and Waggoner (1934)*

1981). The genetics of ageing is conveniently discussed in terms of explicit and implicit modes of inheritance (Samis, 1978). Explicit inheritance is illustrated by the effects of specific genes on the ageing process, some of which can produce diseases of premature ageing such as the progeroid syndromes (Goldstein, 1978). In Werner's syndrome, for example, some normal ageing processes are advanced by as much as 30 years (Epstein *et al.*, 1966). Similarly, in Down's syndrome an extra copy of chromosome 21 results in widespread acceleration of ageing processes including Alzheimer's disease. Martin (1977) has pointed out that this condition shows more widespread features of premature ageing even than the monogenic, premature ageing syndromes. Individually, these genetic abnormalities tend to produce not normal ageing but a caricature of it (Martin, 1977) and it is in this context that the gene for familial Alzheimer's disease might be said to represent either an acceleration of a particular type of cerebral ageing or even a 'genocopy' of this: the mechanisms might be different from those causing the age-related increase in Alzheimer's disease in the general population.

Intrinsic inheritance of ageing is more subtle but probably more important. Ageing is thought ultimately to result from the accumulation of unrepaired stochastic errors either in the DNA itself or in its products, but this must occur in the context of a specific genotype; different genotypes will age differently. Repair processes will differ, as will the gene products, in their sensitivity to error-producing processes. A major piece of evidence showing that ageing is under genetic control comes from the observed differences in longevity between mammalian species. For example, similar types of age-related change occur in rodents about 30 times faster than in man. This illustrates how heritable factors that are otherwise implicit within a species' genome can have a dramatic effect on ageing processes. The stochastic element in ageing, however, leads to the conclusion that much of ageing is due to chance, environmental or other non-genetic influences on genome structure and function. The consequences of error accumulation are not heritable except at the cellular level and then only in dividing cells. Unrepaired somatic mutation in end-differentiated cells such as neurones, or in the mitochondrial genome, which is repaired at a very low rate (Linnane *et al.*, 1989), is likely to lead to inexorable somatic decline. Because, as discussed above, Alzheimer's disease is an exaggerated or premature manifestation of cerebral ageing seen in the general population, the exponential increase in incidence with age, particularly during the eighth and ninth decades, can be seen as a likely manifestation of a complex ageing process rather than the expression of a single, dominant gene.

GENETIC LINKAGE STUDIES IN ALZHEIMER'S DISEASE

The earliest reports of families with early-onset, histologically proven Alzheimer's disease, consistent with an autosomal dominant mode of inheritance were by Schottky (1932) and Lowenberg and Waggoner (1934), since when over 50 families have been published (McKusick, 1988). Estimates of the frequency of familial Alzheimer's disease compared with the commoner, sporadic disease vary from 1% (Davies, 1986) to about 40% (Heston *et al.*, 1981). A survey of some of the large family studies shows that none of the 34 families studied by Sjogren *et al.* (1952), none out of 256 families studied by Larsson *et al.* (1963), none out of the 68 families studied by Heyman *et al.* (1983) and only one out of 125 families studied by Heston *et al.* (1981) meets the minimal criteria for autosomal dominant familial Alzheimer's disease of four or more affected members in at least two generations with mean onset age under 60 years. This suggests that as few as 0.2% of all Alzheimer's disease families have an autosomal dominant mode of inheritance.

St. George-Hyslop *et al.* (1987) studied four typical families with familial Alzheimer's disease in which, for example, 54 members were affected in eight generations in one family (FAD 1), and 48 affected in eight generations in another (FAD 4). The mean age of onset in the four families ranged from 39.9 to 52.0 years. They typed the families for 10 DNA markers on chromosome 21 and found evidence of linkage to the D21S1/S11 and D21S16 loci in chromosome region 21q21 (Table 17.4a). The closest linkage (at zero recombination) was to the most proximal marker D21S16 lying relatively close to the centromere. This result was confirmed by Goate *et al.* (1989) in six early-onset families with familial Alzheimer's disease. Schellenberg *et al.* (1988) on the other hand found significant evidence against linkage to D21S1/S11, which is located about 8 centimorgans (cM) distal to D21S16, in seven families with the familial disease of Volga German descent (Table 17.4a). Linkage was excluded for at least 15 cM on either side of the D21S1/S11 locus, even assuming a gene frequency as high as 0.06 in this inbred group. Genetic heterogeneity may therefore be present within familial Alzheimer's disease. Pericak-Vance *et al.* (1988) analysed linkage to these markers in three families with early-onset Alzheimer's disease (under 60 years of age) and in ten late-onset families (Table 17.4b). Only one family (No. 372) met the criteria for familial Alzheimer's disease described above of four or more affected members in at least two generations and mean onset before 60 years of age. This family, with five affected members and mean onset age 49 years, showed positive lod scores (Z max 0.90, 0.65) at zero recombination with both D21S1/S11 and D21S16. Autopsy confirmation of the diagnosis was only possible in five out of thirteen families. Problems of clinical diagnoses and mixed pathology are likely to be particularly significant in the older affected members of such families. The possibility that phenocopies can produce spurious recombinants may also become significant in families with an older mean age of onset. Indeed, in their late-onset, non-familial Alzheimer's disease families, the D21S1/S11 data of Pericak-Vance *et al.* (1988) were strongly negative, excluding linkage to > 20 cM on either side of this probe (Table 17.4b). Unaffected members were classified as status unknown to minimize the possibility of misclassifying individuals who may go on to develop the illness. Schellenberg *et al.* (1988) also found evidence against linkage to D21S1/S11 in six late-onset families (mean onset 69 years; Table 17.4b). The available evidence therefore provides significant evidence against linkage to proximal 21q21 markers in late-onset (more than 60 years of age), non-familial Alzheimer's disease.

CONCLUSIONS

A simple model presenting the features of Alzheimer's disease with onset in different age groups is presented in Table 17.5. Familial Alzheimer's disease is an early-onset (40–60 years of age) condition, showing autosomal dominant inheritance, which is otherwise clinically and neuropathologically similar to later-onset forms. Certain minimal operational criteria

Table 17.4 (a) Summary of linkage data in early-onset (<60 yrs) familial Alzheimer's disease kindreds. Recombination fractions and the corresponding lod scores are shown with two chromosome 21 probes (D21S1/S11 or D21S1/S72 and D21S16); (b) linkage data in late-onset (mean onset over 60 years), Alzheimer's disease families, as above

Reference	Mean onset (years)	No. of families	Recombination fraction						Locus
			0.00	0.05	0.10	0.20	0.30	0.40	
(a)									
St. George-Hyslop et al. (1987)	50	4	$-\infty$	2.26	2.35	1.81	1.05	0.37	D21S1/S11
Schellenberg et al. (1988)	51	3	2.32	2.10	1.85	1.30	0.75	0.26	D21S16
	56	7 (Volga Germans)	$-\infty$	-0.27	0.03	0.24	0.22	0.07	D21S1/S72
			$-\infty$	-5.51	-3.60	-1.61	-0.63	-0.17	D21S1/S72
			$-\infty$	-0.16	-0.11	-0.05	-0.01	0.00	D21S16
Pericak-Vance et al. (1988)	53	3	$-\infty$	0.70	0.63	0.47	0.28	0.08	D21S1/S11
			0.65	0.58	0.50	0.35	0.19	0.06	D21S16
Goate et al. (1989)	52	6	0.64	2.28	2.16	1.60	0.89	0.27	D21S1/S11
			1.79	1.61	1.42	1.01	0.60	0.21	D21S16
(b)									
Schellenberg et al. (1988)	69	6	$-\infty$	-0.81	-0.51	-0.22	-0.08	-0.02	D21S1/S72
Pericak-Vance et al. (1988)	71	10	$-\infty$	-5.71	-3.78	-2.49	-0.72	-0.18	D21S1/S11
			$-\infty$	0.14	0.11	0.05	0.01	0.01	D21S16

Table 17.5 Model summarizing the genetic features of Alzheimer's disease (AD), familial Alzheimer's disease (FAD) and the Alzheimer-type dementia of Down's syndrome (AD-DS)

Condition	Onset	Inheritance	Population prevalence (approximate)	Other features of ageing	Linkage to proximal 21q21 markers
FAD	40–60	AD	<0.1/1000	–	+/–
AD	60–70	MF	1–10/1000	+	–
AD	70+	MF/somatic	10–150/1000	+ +	–
AD-DS	>40	Chromosomal	96–98% of DS	+ + +	NA

NA, not applicable.

for the familial disease should be satisfied, such as at least four affected members in two or more generations and mean onset before the age of 60 years. Autopsy diagnosis is important in at least some affected members of a kindred, as confusion with other dominant conditions presenting with dementia is possible (e.g. Huntington's disease, Pick's disease, Gerstmann–Straussler syndrome). Familial Alzheimer's disease has a relatively low within-family variance in age of onset compared with the late-onset disease. Close linkage to proximal 21q21 markers has been identified in four families with the familial disease and confirmed in six other families, although a series of seven related Volga German families meeting the same clinico-genetic criteria were unlinked to probes from this region, suggesting genetic heterogeneity. Features of ageing outside the brain have not been reported in familial Alzheimer's disease, in contrast to Down's syndrome, in which increased expression of the amyloid β protein precursor (ABPP), located more distally on chromosome 21 and excluded as the cause of the familial disease (Tanzi *et al.*, 1987; Van Broeckhoven *et al.*, 1987), may still be a major contributor. Recent evidence of increased ABPP expression outside the brain in patients with Alzheimer's disease makes this an intriguing possibility (Joachim *et al.*, 1989). This question could be resolved by careful examination of Down's syndrome patients with partial trisomies (see Wright and Whalley, 1984), involving either the familial Alzheimer's or the ABPP region for evidence of ageing and dementia. Autopsy data in such cases will clearly be important. The percentage of all Alzheimer patients with the familial form is probably in the region 0.1 to 1% and the overall prevalence of familial Alzheimer's disease may be less than 1 per 10 000 of the general population, although this needs to be systematically investigated.

Alzheimer's disease with later onset (60–70 years) is generally a sporadic disorder, although 16 to 41% of patients have an affected first-degree relative (Sjogren *et al.*, 1952; Larsson *et al.*, 1963; Heston *et al.*, 1981; Breitner and Folstein, 1984). The consistently increased risk of recurrence observed in the relatives of Alzheimer's disease probands provides evidence for a heritable component, although this is not supported by some twin studies. Heritability estimates are in the region of 0.46 to 0.63 for early-onset, non-familial probands, consistent with a multifactorial disorder. The prevalence of Alzheimer's disease with onset in this age group is in the region of 1 to 10 per thousand of the general population.

Late-onset Alzheimer's disease (over 70 years of age) probably represents a mixture of conditions showing multifactorial inheritance and the somatic features of cerebral ageing, the latter becoming more prominent with advancing age. Mixed forms of multi-infarct and Alzheimer-type dementia become more prominent in the older age groups, reflecting the steep, age-related increases in both conditions but also the increasing role of somatic ageing. Linkage to chromosome 21q21 markers was not found in two studies of late-onset Alzheimer families (Pericak-Vance *et al.*, 1988; Schellenberg *et al.*, 1988). The problems of linkage analysis in this age group, owing to small family size, the prolonged period of onset, phenocopies, misdiagnosis in elderly individuals with multiple cerebral and extracerebral pathology, are of major concern in such studies, so that reliable replication is difficult but important.

The identification of the gene for familial Alzheimer's disease and clarification of its role in this condition and in the dementia of Down's syndrome may elucidate the neuropathological mechanisms in other, commoner forms of Alzheimer's disease and open up new therapeutic possibilities. However, the disease may be the end result of 'normal' cerebral ageing that is inevitable given sufficient longevity. Heritable differences in human populations may either hasten or postpone these changes. This may result from the action of single genes, as in the familial condition, or many genes, as in the non-familial. However, the likelihood of a rising prevalence of Alzheimer's disease in an ageing population emphasizes the point, that, like multi-infarct dementia, Alzheimer's disease is a highly complex, multifactorial disorder in which simple solutions will be hard to find.

REFERENCES

Akesson H. O. (1969). A population study of senile and arteriosclerotic psychoses. *Human Heredity*; **19**: 546–66.

Blessed G., Tomlinson B. E., Roth M. (1968). The association between quantitative measures of dementia and of senile change in the cerebral grey matter of elderly subjects. *British Journal of Psychiatry*; **114**: 797–811.

Breitner J. C. S., Folstein M. F. (1984). Familial Alzheimer dementia: a prevalent disorder with specific clinical features. *Psychological Medicine*; **14**: 63–80.

Breitner J. C. S., Silverman J. M., Mohs R. C., Davis K. L. (1988). Familial aggregation in Alzheimer's disease: comparison of risk among relatives of early- and late-onset cases, and among male and female relatives in successive generations. *Neurology*; **38**: 207–12.

Collinge J., Harding A. E., Owen F. *et al.* (1989). Diagnosis of Gerstmann–Straussler syndrome in familial dementia with prior protein gene analysis. *Lancet*; **ii**: 15–17.

Constantinidis J., Garrone G., de Ajuriaguerra J. (1962). L'heredite des demences de l'age avance. *Encephale*; **51**: 301–44.

Cook R. H., Schneck S. A., Clark D. B. (1981). Twins with Alzheimer's disease. *Archives of Neurology*; **38**: 300–1.

Davidson E. A., Robertson E. E. (1955). Alzheimer's disease with acne rosacea in one of identical twins. *Journal of Neurological Psychiatry*; **18**: 72–7.

Davies P. (1986). The genetics of Alzheimer's disease: a review and a discussion of the implications. *Neurobiology of Ageing*; **7**: 459–66.

Dayan A. D. (1971). Comparative neuropathology of ageing. Studies on the brains of 47 species of vertebrates. *Brain*; **94**: 31–42.

Embry C., Lippmann S. (1985). Presumed Alzheimer's disease beginning at different ages in two twins. *Journal of the American Geriatric Society*; **33**: 61–2.

Epstein C. J., Martin G. M., Schultz A. L., Motulsky A. G. (1966). Werner's syndrome: a review of its symptomatology, natural history, pathologic features, genetics and relationship to the natural ageing process. *Medicine (Baltimore)*; **45**: 177–221.

Falconer D. S. (1965). The inheritance of liability to certain diseases, estimated from the incidence among relatives. *Annals of Human Genetics*; **29**: 51–76.

Feldman R. G., Chandler K. A., Levy L. L., Glaser G. H. (1963). Familial Alzheimer's disease. *Neurology*; **13**: 811–24.

Florini J. R. (1981). *CRC Handbook of Biochemistry in Aging*. Florida: CRC Press.

Ghiso J., Jensson O., Frangione B. (1986). Amyloid fibrils in hereditary cerebral haemorrhage with amyloidosis of Icelandic type is a variant of γ-trace basic protein (cystatin C). *Proceedings of the National Academy of Sciences (USA)*; **83**: 2974–8.

Goate A. M., Haynes A., Owen M. J. *et al.* (1989). Predisposing locus for Alzheimer's disease on chromosome 21. *Lancet*; **i**: 352–5.

Goldstein S. (1978). Human genetic disorders that feature premature onset and accelerated progression of biological aging. In: *The Genetics of Aging* (Schneider E. L., ed.), pp. 171–224. New York: Plenum Press.

Gurland B. J., Cross P. S. (1982). Epidemiology of psychopathology in old age: some implications for clinical services. *Psychiatric Clinics of North America*; **5**: 11–26.

Hachinski V. C., Iliff L. D., Zilhka E. *et al.* (1975). Cerebral blood flow in dementia. *Archives of Neurology*; **32**: 632–7.

Heston L. L., Mastri A. R. (1977). The genetics of Alzheimer's disease. Associations with hematologic malignancy and Down's syndrome. *Archives of General Psychiatry*; **34**: 976–81.

Heston L. L., Mastri A. R., Anderson E., White J. (1981). Dementia of the Alzheimer type. *Archives of General Psychiatry*; **38**: 1085–90.

Heyman A., Wilkinson W. E., Hurwitz B. J. *et al.* (1983). Alzheimer's disease: genetic aspects and associated clinical disorders. *Annals of Neurology*; **14**: 507–15.

Huff F. J., Auerbach J., Chakravarti A., Boller F. (1988). Risk of dementia in relatives of patients with Alzheimer's disease. *Neurology*; **38**: 786–90.

Hunter R., Dayan A. D., Wilson J. (1972). Alzheimer's disease in one monozygotic twin. *Journal of Neurology, Neurosurgery and Psychiatry*; **35**: 707–10.

Jarvik L. F., Blum J. E., Varma A. O. (1972). Genetic components and intellectual functioning during senescence: a 20-year study of ageing twins. *Behavior Genetics*; **2**: 159–71.

Jarvik L. F., Ruth V., Matsuyama S. S. (1980). Organic brain syndrome and aging: a six-year follow-up of surviving twins. *Archives of General Psychiatry*; **37**: 280–6.

Joachim C. L., Mori H., Selkoe D. J. (1989). Amyloid β-protein deposition in tissues other than brain in Alzheimer's disease. *Nature*; **341**: 226–30.

Kallman F. J. (1956). Genetic aspects of mental disorders in later life. In: *Mental Disorders in Later Life* 2nd edn. (Kaplan O. J., ed.), pp. 26–46. London: Oxford University Press.

Larsson T., Sjogren T., Jacobson G. (1963). Senile dementia: a clinical, sociomedical and genetic study. *Acta Psychiatrica Scandinavica (Supplementum)* 167; **39**: 1–259.

Linnane A. W., Marzuki S., Ozawa T., Tanaka M. (1989). Mitochondrial DNA mutations as an important contributor to ageing and degenerative diseases. *Lancet*; **i**: 642–5.

Lowenberg K., Waggoner R. W. (1934). Familial organic psychosis (Alzheimer's type). *Archives of Neurology and Psychiatry (Chicago)*; 31: 737–54.

Luxenberg J. S., May C., Haxby J. V. (1987). Cerebral metabolism, anatomy, and cognition in monozygotic twins discordant for dementia of the Alzheimer type. *Journal of Neurology, Neurosurgery and Psychiatry*; 50: 333–40.

Martin G. M. (1977). Genetic syndromes in man with potential relevance to the pathology of aging. In: *Genetic Effects On Aging* (Bergsma D., Harrison D. E., eds.), pp. 5–39. New York: A. R. Liss.

Matsuyama A., Nakumara S. (1978). Senile changes in the brain in the Japanese. In: *Alzheimer's Disease: Senile Dementia And Related Disorders* (Terry R. D., Katzman R., Bick K. L., eds.). New York: Raven Press.

McKhann G., Drachmann D., Folstein M. *et al.* (1984). Clinical diagnosis of Alzheimer's disease: report of the NINCDS-ADRDA work group under the auspices of Department of Health and Human Services task force on Alzheimer's disease. *Neurology*; 34: 939–44.

McKusick V. A. (1988). *Mendelian Inheritance in Man* 8th edn. Baltimore: The Johns Hopkins University Press.

Mohs R. C., Breitner J. C. S., Silverman J. M., Davis K. L. (1987). Alzheimer's disease. Morbid risk among first-degree relatives approximates 50% by 90 years of age. *Archives of General Psychiatry*; 44: 405–8.

Mongeau J-G. (1987). Heredity and blood pressure in humans. *Pediatric Nephrology*; 1: 69–75.

Mortimer J. A., Schuman L. M., French L. R. (1981). Epidemiology of dementing illness. In: *The Epidemiology of Dementia* (Mortimer J. A., Schuman L. M., eds.), pp. 3–23. New York: Oxford University Press.

Nee L. E., Eldridge R., Sunderland T. *et al.* (1987). Dementia of the Alzheimer type: clinical and family study of 22 twin pairs. *Neurology*; 37: 359–63.

Pericak-Vance M. A., Yamaoka L. H., Haynes C. S. *et al.* (1988). Genetic linkage studies in Alzheimer's disease families. *Experimental Neurology*; 102: 271–9.

Pfeffer R. I., Afifi A. A., Chance J. M. (1987). Prevalence of Alzheimer's disease in a retirement community. *American Journal of Epidemiology*; 125: 420–36.

Rosen W. G., Terry R. D., Fuld P. A. *et al.* (1980). Pathological verification of ischemic score in differentiation of dementias. *Annals of Neurology*; 1: 486–8.

St. George-Hyslop P. H., Tanzi R. E., Polinsky R. J. *et al.* (1987). The genetic defect causing familial Alzheimer's disease maps on chromosome 21. *Science*; 235: 885–90.

Samis H. V. (1978). Molecular genetics of aging. In: *The Genetics of Aging* (Schneider E. L., ed.), pp. 7–25. New York: Plenum Press.

Schellenberg G. D., Bird T. D., Wijsman E. M. *et al.* (1988). Absence of linkage of chromosome 21q21 markers in familial Alzheimer's disease. *Science*; 241: 1507–10.

Schottky J. (1932). Uber prasenile verblodungen. *Ztschr.f.d.ges.Neurol.u.Psychiat*; 140: 333–97.

Sharman M. G., Watt D. C., Janota I., Carrasco L. (1979). Alzheimer's disease in a mother and identical twin sons. *Psychological Medicine*; 9: 771–4.

Sjogren T., Sjogren H., Lindgren A. G. H. (1952). Morbus Alzheimer and morbus Pick. A genetic, clinical and patho-anatomical study. *Acta Psychiatrica Scandinavica (Supplementum)* 82.

Sourander P., Walinder J. (1977). Hereditary multi-infarct dementia. Morphological and clinical studies of a new disease. *Acta Neuropathologica*; 39: 247–54.

Southey R. (1820). *The Life of John Wesley*, p. 340. London: Hutchinson.

Tanzi R. E., St. George-Hyslop P. H., Haines J. L. *et al.* (1987). The genetic defect in familial Alzheimer's disease is not tightly linked to the amyloid beta-protein gene. *Nature*; 329: 156–7.

Tierney M. C., Fisher R. H., Lewis A. J. *et al.* (1988). The NINCDS-ADRDA work criteria for the clinical diagnosis of probable Alzheimer's disease: a clinicopathological study of 57 cases. *Neurology*; 38: 359–64.

Tomlinson B. E., Blessed G., Roth M. (1968). Observations on the brains of non-demented old people. *Journal of Neurological Science*; 7: 331–56.

Tomlinson B. E., Blessed G., Roth M. (1970). Observations on the brains of demented old people. *Journal of Neurological Science*; 11: 205–42.

Ulrich J. (1982). Senile plaques and neurofibrillary tangles of the Alzheimer type in nondemented individuals at presenile age. *Gerontology*; 28: 86–90.

Van Broeckhoven C., Genthe A. M., Vandenberghe A. *et al.* (1987). Failure of familial Alzheimer's disease to segregate with the A4-amyloid gene in several European families. *Nature*; 329: 153–5.

Wesley J. (1777). Journals, 28th June 1777. *The Journal of the Rev. John Wesley* vol. 4, p. 105. London: Dent.

Wright A. F., Whalley L. J. (1984). Genetics, ageing and dementia. *British Journal of Psychiatry*; 145: 20–38.

18 *The molecular basis of Alzheimer's-type dementia*

JOHN HARDY

Besides age, there are two established risk factors for developing Alzheimer's-type dementia: having Down's syndrome (trisomy 21; Olsson and Shaw, 1969) or a family history of the disorder (Sjogren *et al.*, 1952). It is clear that while most cases are sporadic, familial clustering of the illness does occur: amongst these familial clusters, there are many reported pedigrees in which Alzheimer's disease appears to segregate as an autosomal-dominant disorder of presenile onset (see, for example, Nee *et al.*, 1983). These clues led St. George-Hyslop *et al.* (1987) to search for and to find evidence of genetic linkage between this form of the disorder and restriction fragment length polymorphism (RFLP) (genetic markers D21S1/S11 and D21S16) on the proximal long arm of chromosome 21. We (Goate *et al.*, 1989a) and two other groups (C. Van Broeckhoven *et al.*, unpublished and L. Heston *et al.*, unpublished) have confirmed and refined the original observation, placing the disease locus close to, or proximal to D21S16, currently the most centromeric polymorphic marker on chromosome 21 (Fig. 18.1). The locus predisposing to Alzheimer's disease is thus distinct from the beta-amyloid gene (APP; Fig. 18.1). Beta amyloid is the major proteinaceous component of the pathological feature of Alzheimer's disease, the neuritic plaque. The gene for this protein was cloned and localized to chromosome 21 at the same time as the Alzheimer's linkage was reported. Furthermore, the gene was reported to be duplicated in some cases of Alzheimer's disease. Thus, there was great excitement at the possibility that the beta-amyloid gene was the Alzheimer's gene. This is now known not to be the case and the report of beta-amyloid gene duplication has been refuted (Delabar *et al.*, 1987; Kang *et al.*, 1987; Tanzi *et al.*, 1987a,b,c; Van Broeckhoven *et al.*, 1987; Podlisny *et al.*, 1988; St. George Hyslop *et al.*, 1988). The beta-amyloid gene is now known to be some distance telomeric of this region (Van Broeckhoven *et al.*, 1987; Tanzi *et al.*, 1988; Warren *et al.*, 1989).

The four groups who have found linkage between Alzheimer's disease and markers on chromosome 21 have largely used outbred families with an early onset of illness for their analysis (St. George Hyslop *et al.*, 1987; Van Broeckhoven *et al.*, 1988, and unpublished; Goate *et al.*, 1989a; L. Heston *et al.*, unpublished). In contrast, two groups (Pericak-Vance *et al.*, 1988;

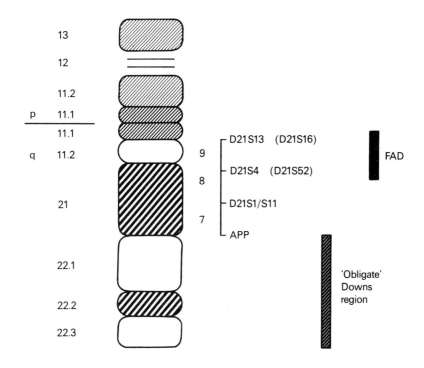

Fig. 18.1   *Diagram of human chromosome 21 showing the position of DNA markers linked to the familial Alzheimer's disease (FAD) locus, amyloid precursor protein (APP) gene and the 'obligate' Down's syndrome region*

Schellenberg *et al.*, 1988) have apparently failed to observe linkage between Alzheimer's disease and markers on chromosome 21 in families they have studied. The families they have used for their analysis have included many with a late onset of disorder (both studies) or families from a geographical isolate (the Volga Germans) with a high incidence of the familial disease and where there is a high level of inbreeding (Schellenberg *et al.*, 1988). In both studies, the data from outbred families with an early onset of disease have been consistent with the hypothesis that there is a disease locus on chromosome 21. Thus, the data from these two groups do not conflict with the view that early-onset, familial Alzheimer's disease in the general population is caused by the locus on chromosome 21: their data on the familial, late-onset disorder and on the Volga German variant of the disease do, however, need to be explained.

WHAT IS THE AETIOLOGY OF LATE-ONSET, FAMILIAL ALZHEIMER'S DISEASE?

Genetic, epidemiological investigations into the aetiology of late-onset Alzheimer's disease are extraordinarily complex for a number of reasons:

1. Diagnosis is often inaccurate and usually retrospective in many family members.
2. Complex survival curves have to be constructed to determine cumulative risks.
3. Pathological investigations suggest that most, and possibly all, clinically unaffected, very elderly individuals have some Alzheimer's disease-type changes in their brain by the time of their death. Thus the diagnosis 'unaffected' is uncertain.

For these reasons, it is not clear what proportion of late-onset disease is genetic in aetiology (see Goate *et al.*, 1989b for review). However, this information is crucial to the successful application of analyses of molecular genetic linkage to this form of the disorder. Even if late-onset disorder is predominantly non-genetic in aetiology, it will still be frequently familial among the older relations of patients, simply because of its high incidence in the general population. With this background, it is perhaps unsurprising that studies using families with a late onset of disease should fail to demonstrate linkage. We, too (unpublished) have not observed linkage to chromosome 21 markers in our population of families with a late onset of disease. Two recent analyses (Farrar *et al.*, 1989; Hardy *et al.*, 1989b) have highlighted the problems in applying linkage analysis in families with a mean age of onset of Alzheimer's disease over 60 to 65 years. Above this age, the incidence of the familial disorder would be predicted to rise steeply even if it were not genetic in aetiology (Hardy *et al.*, 1989b), simply because the disease has a greater incidence at these high ages.

WHAT IS THE AETIOLOGY OF ALZHEIMER'S DISEASE IN THE VOLGA GERMAN POPULATION?

Alzheimer's disease in the Volga German population appears to be a genetic disorder with an onset between 45 and 75 years. Linkage analysis suggests that the disease is not caused by a locus close to D21S1/S11. However, our data (Goate *et al.*, 1989a) and that of Van Broeckhoven *et al.* (1988, and unpublished), suggest that the disease locus is close to D21S16 and some distance from D21S1/S11. Schellenberg *et al.* have not yet formally excluded this chromosomal region from containing the Alzheimer's disease gene in the Volga German population (Fig. 18.2). Thus, there are two possible explanations for the result of linkage analysis in this population: either the disease locus causing all genetic cases of Alzheimer's disease is close to D21S16, or the Volga Germans represent a genetically

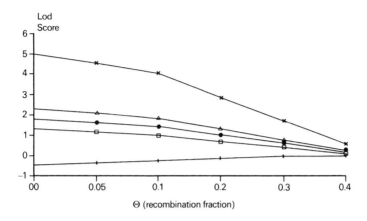

Fig. 18.2 *Evidence for Alzheimer's disease locus close to D21S16:* ●——● *Goate* et al. *(1989a);* □——□ *Pericak-Vance* et al. *(1988);* ★——★ *St. George-Hyslop* et al. *(1987);* |——| *Schellenberg* et al. *(1988);* ×——× *total material*

distinct group and disease in this group is caused at a different locus. Only more genetic analyses of these families can resolve this issue. The published data (Fig. 18.2) are at present consistent with all multiply affected families having a locus for Alzheimer's disease near D21S16.

INTERPRETATION OF RECOMBINANTS: GOING FROM LINKAGE TO GENE

The major, immediate goal of the groups working on the molecular genetics of Alzheimer's disease is to isolate and then to characterize the defective gene and its normal counterpart. Identification of linkage is thus vital but only a small step towards this goal. Once linkage has been established, the techniques of molecular and cellular genetics allow the generation of more polymorphic loci in the vicinity around the marker loci. As one gets closer to the disease locus, recombination between the new marker loci and the disease locus becomes progressively less frequent until the point is reached when a marker locus is identified that is coinherited with the disease locus in all observed meioses. At this stage, molecular techniques can be used that assist in the identification of genes in the vicinity of the marker locus: these are then candidate genes for the disease locus.

There are two serious problems with the application of this research strategy to the genetics of Alzheimer's disease.

1. One assesses whether one is getting closer to the disease locus by the occurrence of recombinants between marker loci and disease phenotype.

However, if the disease is heterogeneous (either aetiologically or genetically), or if diagnosis is uncertain, or if the disease has an age-dependent penetrance curve, then apparent recombinant events are individually uncertain. This means that the genetic resolution which can be obtained is poor: it is extremely difficult to estimate accurately how close the disease locus is to the marker locus.

2. The number of well-defined pedigrees with clearly genetic Alzheimer's disease is small, and nearly all of those which have been identified have comparatively uninformative, one-generation structures. This means that linkage phase is usually unknown (see Chapter 3) and that relatively few meioses are available in which the inheritance of the disease and marker loci can be studied.

These features, which are shared to a greater or lesser extent by other psychiatric conditions such as schizophrenia and affective disorders, mean that it is unlikely to be possible to define a small chromosomal region, for example less than 1 megabase of DNA containing the Alzheimer's disease gene (as has recently been possible for cystic fibrosis; the commonest, simple, autosomal-recessive disorder; Rommens *et al.*, 1989). Rather, genetic analysis will result in a region of DNA of the order of 10 times this size being identified as likely to contain the defective gene. Within the region defined genetically as containing the mutation causing cystic fibrosis, there appear to be only two or three genes. By analogy, therefore, the region definable as containing the Alzheimer's gene is likely to contain something of the order of 20 to 30 genes that are equally likely (on genetic grounds) to contain the mutation. It is likely that for diseases such as schizophrenia and the affective disorders, where the modes of inheritance are uncertain, the difficulties will be as great as for Alzheimer's disease, or greater. At present there are no satisfactory, elegant molecular techniques for dealing with this level of complexity of problem unless chromosomal abnormalities are discovered or those working on the pathology of the disorder generate candidate genes that map within the correct region.

IS ALZHEIMER'S DISEASE HETEROGENEOUS AT THE MOLECULAR LEVEL? A UNIFYING HYPOTHESIS

The argument as to whether Alzheimer's disease is one disorder, or should be split into many subtypes (early onset versus late onset; familial versus sporadic, with or without some particular clinical feature) has filled many pages of discussion over the last 25 years. Taken at face value, the genetic evidence I discuss above could be taken as very strongly in favour of splitting the disease into two subtypes, chromosome 21 and idiopathic. However, I wish to propose a working hypothesis concerning the aetiology of the disease which is consistent with the notion that all Alzheimer's disease has the same aetiology at the molecular level.

The example of Down's syndrome suggests that three copies (and thus, one presumes, modest over-expression) of the gene encoded at the Alzheimer's disease locus, cause the pathology of Alzheimer's disease with an onset between the ages of 30 and 55 years. Anecdotal evidence (Rowe *et al.*, 1989) suggests that some at least of the sporadic, early-onset cases may have related aetiologies such as somatic trisomy 21 mosaicism (Rowe *et al.*, 1989) or somatic mutation at the Alzheimer's disease locus (Hardy *et al.*, 1989a). I wish to suggest that the different allelic mutations (Van Duijn *et al.*, 1989) involved in the aetiology of the chromosome 21-encoded variant of the disease also involve over-expression of this locus: the greater the degree of over-expression, the earlier the onset of the disease. However, I also wish to suggest that the normal level of expression of this locus will also lead eventually to the development of the pathology of the disease over the age of 60 years. Eventually, according to this hypothesis, everyone would develop Alzheimer's disease-type changes in their brain and, at some time after the pathology had begun to accrue, they would begin to show the clinical symptoms of the disorder. This hypothesis is, therefore, a variant of the old idea that Alzheimer's disease is accelerated 'normal' ageing. This hypothesis is consistent both with the genetic data presented herein and also with pathological investigations showing that normal, very elderly individuals have similar pathology, both qualitatively and quantitatively, to demented individuals of the same age (Mann *et al.*, 1987).

REFERENCES

Delabar J. M., Goldgaber D., Lamour Y. *et al.* (1987). Beta amyloid gene duplication in Alzheimer's disease and kayotypically normal Down syndrome. *Science*; **235**: 1390–2.

Farrar L. A., Myers R. H., Cupples L. A. *et al.* (1989). Transmission and age at onset patterns in familial Alzheimer's disease; evidence for etiologic heterogeneity in late onset families. *Neurology* (in press).

Goate A. M., Haynes A. R., Owen M. J. *et al.* (1989a). Predisposing locus for Alzheimer's disease on chromosome 21. *Lancet*; i: 352–5.

Goate A. M., Owen M. J., Hardy J. A. (1989b). Genetic aetiology of Alzheimer's disease. *International Review of Psychiatry* (in press).

Hardy J. A., Goate A. M., Owen M. J. (1989a). On the aetiology of sporadic, early onset Alzheimer's disease. *Lancet* (in press).

Hardy J. A., Goate A. M., Owen M. J. *et al.* (1989b). Modelling the occurrence and pathology of Alzheimer's disease. *Neurobiological Aging* (in press).

Kang J., Lemaire H. G., Unterbec A. *et al.* (1987). The precursor of Alzheimer's disease amyloid A4 protein resembles a cell-surface receptor. *Nature*; **325**: 733–6.

Mann D. M. A., Tucker C. M., Yates P. O. (1987). The topographic distribution of senile plaques and neurofibrillary tangles in the brains of non-demented persons of different ages. *Neuropathology and Applied Neurobiology*; **13**: 123–39.

Nee L. E., Polinsky R. J., Eldridge R. *et al.* (1983). A family with histologically confirmed Alzheimer's disease. *Archives of Neurology*; **40**: 203–8.

Olsson M. I., Shaw C. M. (1969). Presenile dementia and Alzheimer's disease in mongolism. *Brain*; 92: 147–56.

Pericak-Vance M. A., Yamaoka L. H., Haynes C. S. *et al.* (1988). Genetic linkage studies in Alzheimer's disease families. *Experimental Neurology*; 102: 271–9.

Podlisny M. B., Lee G., Selkoe D. J. (1988). Gene dosage of the amyloid beta precursor protein in Alzheimer's disease. *Science*; 238: 669–71.

Rommens J. H., Iannuzzi M. C., Kerem B. S. *et al.* (1989). Identification of the cystic fibrosis gene: chromosome walking and jumping. *Science*; 245: 1059–65.

Rowe I. F., Ridler M. A. C., Gibberd F. B. (1989). Presenile dementia associated with mosaic trisomy 21 in a patient with a Down syndrome child. *Lancet*; i: 229.

St. George-Hyslop P., Tanzi R. E., Polinsky R. J. *et al.* (1987). The genetic defect causing familial Alzheimer's disease maps on chromosome 21. *Science*; 235: 885–9.

St. George-Hyslop P. H., Tanzi R. E., Polinsky R. J. *et al.* (1988). Absence of duplication of chromosome 21 genes in familial and sporadic Alzheimer's disease. *Science*; 238: 664–6.

Schellenberg G. D., Bird T. D., Wijsman E. M. *et al.* (1988). Absence of linkage of chromosome 21q21 markers to familial Alzheimer's disease. *Science*; 241: 1507–10.

Sjogren T., Sjogren J., Lindgren G. H. (1952). Morbus Alzheimer and morbus Pick. *Acta Psychiatrica Scandinavica (Supplementum)*; 82: 9–63.

Tanzi R. E., Bird E. D., Latt S. A., Neve R. L. (1987a). The amyloid beta protein gene is not duplicated in brains of patients with Alzheimer's disease. *Science*; 238: 666–9.

Tanzi R. E., Gusella J. F., Watkins P. C. *et al.* (1987b). Amyloid beta protein gene: cDNA, mRNA distribution and genetic linkage near the Alzheimer locus. *Science*; 235: 880–4.

Tanzi R. E., St. George Hyslop P. H., Haines J. *et al.* (1987c). The genetic defect in Alzheimer's disease is not tightly linked to the amyloid beta protein gene. *Nature*; 329: 156–7.

Tanzi R. E., Haines J., Watkins P. C. *et al.* (1988). Genetic linkage map of human chromosome 21. *Genomics*; 3: 129–36.

Van Broeckhoven C., Genthe A. M., Vandenberghe A. *et al.* (1987). Failure of familial Alzheimer's disease to segregate with the A4-amyloid gene in several European families. *Nature*; 329: 153–5.

Van Broeckhoven C., Van Hul W., Backhovens W. *et al.* (1988). In: *Genetics of Alzheimer's Disease* (Sinet P. M., Lamour Y., Christen Y., eds.). Berlin: Springer-Verlag.

Van Duijn C. M., Van Broeckhoven C., Hardy J. A. *et al.* (1989). Evidence for allelic heterogeneity in familial Alzheimer's disease. *Annals of Neurology* (in press).

Warren A. C., Slaugenhaupt S. A., Lewis J. G. *et al.* (1989). A genetic linkage map of 17 markers on chromosome 21. *Genomics*; 4: 579–91.

19 *Prediction and prevention in Huntington's disease*

MICHAEL J. MORRIS AND PETER S. HARPER

INTRODUCTION

Huntington's disease (HD), a progressive neuropsychiatric disorder of autosomal dominant inheritance, was delineated by George Huntington (1850–1916), a general practitioner from New England, in 1872, the year after his graduation (Huntington, 1872). Although the condition bears his name, Huntington was not the first to recognize the hereditary nature (a vital step towards prevention) of adult chorea. He was preceded by five others, all of whom were unaware of each other's work. Stevens (1972) points out that the first description of inherited adult chorea was by Elliotson in 1832, 40 years before Huntington. Waters in 1841 described, in a letter, 'markedly hereditary' chorea, while the third to describe this condition was Gorman in his doctoral thesis (now lost) in 1846. The next description was written in Norwegian by Lund and appeared in the State Medical Report of 1860, but his work did not come to wide attention until it was translated nearly a century after its first appearance (Orbeck, 1959). In 1863, Irving Lyon, a house physician at Bellevue Hospital, New York, provided the fifth account of the disease. George Huntington's contribution *On Chorea* reached a much wider audience than those of his predecessors and he was fortunate that his work was well received and translated in Europe, especially Germany. Indeed, it was a German (Huber, 1887) who proposed the eponymous term, Huntington's chorea.

PREVALENCE

Until the 1930s, the literature on HD mainly comprised individual case reports and genealogical studies, especially from North America. Interest then turned to estimating the frequency of the disorder, initially using hospital in-patient records. Panse (1942), who made an epidemiological study of the disease in the Rhineland, was one of the first to attempt to ascertain the number of choreics in the general population. Although hospital records were the prime source of his material, he also consulted government agencies concerned with eugenics, thus casting a shadow over research into HD in Germany until the present day.

The epidemiological study of HD poses major challenges but it is necessary before there can be any serious attempt at prevention. Prolonged surveillance of a well-defined population, as part of a long-term research programme, is required to accumulate an adequate series. The use of multiple sources to identify *propositi* will contribute to a more complete ascertainment but, despite persistent searches, it is almost inevitable that cases will be missed. Certain hospitals have incomplete records and doctors may fail to diagnose affected individuals. Death certification data on HD also have limitations (Hogg *et al.*, 1979). (The ninth edition of the *International Classification of Diseases* [World Health Organization, 1978] assigned a separate code, 333.4, for HD but unfortunately this is rarely used in the collection of mortality statistics.) A newly arrived, affected immigrant from another region may well be missed and families occasionally lose contact with other members. In south Wales, the majority of cases were discovered solely through the population survey method (Walker *et al.*, 1981) and this indicates that, without such a survey, there are many unrecognized sufferers in the community.

In Britain (Table 19.1), there are about 4000 sufferers and a further 20 000 at high risk of developing the disorder (Office of Health Economics, 1980). Despite various problems of diagnostic accuracy and variable levels of ascertainment, the prevalence rate of Huntington's disease in northern

Table 19.1 Prevalence rates for HD in Britain

Reference	Area	Prevalence $\times 10^{-5}$
Critchley (1934)	East Anglia/London	
Bell (1934)	Lancashire	
Spillane and Phillips (1937)	West Wales	
Bickford and Ellison (1953)	Cornwall	5.5
Pleydell (1955)	Northamptonshire	6.5
Reid (1960)	Northamptonshire	7.2
Heathfield (1967)	Essex	2.5
Oliver (1970)	Northamptonshire	6.3
Bolt (1970)	West Scotland	5.2
Heathfield and MacKenzie (1971)	Bedfordshire	7.5
Venters (1971)	South-east Scotland	6.5
Glendinning (1975)	Somerset	5.5
Stevens (1976)	Yorkshire	4.2
Harper *et al.* (1979)	South Wales	7.6
Quarrell et al. (1988)	North Wales	5.5
Quarrell et al. (1988)	South Wales	8.8
Simpson and Johnson (1989)	Grampian	10.1

Europe is about 5 to 7 per 100 000, and about half that figure in southern European countries like Italy. Very low prevalence rates exist for oriental countries like Japan and China, and no cases have been described among the indigenous Australian Aborigines, Maoris and Eskimos.

The development of a genetic register (Table 19.2) in Wales has allowed the systematic, prospective study of HD in a clearly defined population (Walker *et al.*, 1981). This population was initially in industrial south Wales but more recently the study has been extended to north Wales (Quarrell *et al.*, 1988). The aims are complete ascertainment of the disease, using extended family tracing, and the provision of medical and social support, together with non-directive genetic counselling, to individuals at high risk of developing the disorder.

Genetic counselling, even without the availability of a preclinical test, has been shown to be an important method of primary prevention. Carter *et al.* (1983) have reported a reduction in fertility of about one half among consultands at genetic clinics attending because of a family history of HD. Similarly, a study of a population at risk (Harper *et al.*, 1979) demonstrated a pronounced fall both in the number of births at risk and the predicted future incidence of HD; systematic genetic counselling and prospective follow-up may have contributed to this decline, though a comparable trend has been found in a less intensively studied area (Quarrell *et al.*, 1988).

EARLY ATTEMPTS AT PREDICTION

When the mode of inheritance of HD was recognized, it was obvious that if gene carriers ceased to reproduce, the prevalence of the condition would fall dramatically and the incidence would approach that of the mutation rate. Attention soon focused on the identification of asymptomatic heterozygotes. To Jelliffe *et al.* (1913), a method of detecting carriers before they had children would be 'of great eugenic importance'. At the beginning of the century, another motivation for the development of predictive tests (Table 19.3) was to keep immigrants from entering the United States. At that time there was considerable concern about the frequency of the disease

Table 19.2 HD in Wales: basic epidemiological data

Total individuals on register	2748
Known kindreds with HD	150
Living affected individuals	150
Living individuals at risk (risk $> 10\%$)	1307
Disease prevalence	8.5×10^{-5}
Heterozygote prevalence	30.5×10^{-5}

Table 19.3 Classification of previous attempts at predictive testing

---

Clinical studies
1. Psychiatric
   Personality inventories
   Intelligence tests
2. Neurological
   Eye movements
   Tremor
3. Dermatological
   Dermatoglyphics
   Skin fibroblasts

Biochemical/pharmacological studies
1. CSF γ-aminobutyric acid
2. Prolactin/growth hormone responses
3. L-dopa provocation test

Radiological studies
CT scan

Genetic studies
Classical markers

---

in North America and it was recognized that the disorder appeared to originate from those of European ancestry. Legislation offered a way of dealing with the problem. In the absence of a means of detecting asymptomatic heterozygotes, it was suggested (Davenport and Muncey, 1916) that the cause of death of parents and grandparents of all immigrants should be made known to the state.

Early investigators believed that premorbid personality served as a means of identifying those who would later suffer from HD. It was suggested that irritable, quick-tempered, domineering, opinionated and easily offended individuals at risk were more likely to develop the disease. Palm (1973), in a 20-year, longitudinal, follow-up study, used a wide range of tests, including Rorschach evaluations, the Minnesota Multiphasic Personality Inventory, Wechsler intelligence tests and the electroencephalogram to determine if a dichotomy of responses distinguished between 'normal' and 'abnormal' offspring of choreics. Results were conflicting and the validity of such a programme was not proven.

Detection of very early tremor was an approach that had certain merits. Methods of measuring tremor included a series of tests of steadiness, the use of a sphygmomanometer or a tremometer. Perhaps the best known of the early attempts at preclinical detection was the l-dopa provocation test (Klawans *et al.*, 1972; 1980). It was noted that chorea in patients with HD was made worse by the oral administration of l-dopa and it was suggested that the underlying defect involved an abnormal caudate response to dopamine. Administration of l-dopa to asymptomatic individuals at risk for HD produced temporary choreic movements in a proportion, but a follow-up study showed that there had been both false-positive and false-negative results; this approach has not been pursued further.

GENE MAPPING

When two genes are close to each other on the same chromosome, they will usually be inherited together during meiosis because the probability of exchange of genetic material by crossover is small. Such neighbouring genes are said to be closely linked (see also Chapters 1, 3, 4). The probability of crossover increases with increasing distance between the two genes. The same principles of genetic linkage apply between a genetic disorder and polymorphic genetic markers. A statistical assessment of the likelihood of linkage between two loci is provided by the lod (log of the odds that the two loci are linked) score. A lod score of 3 or more is conventionally considered to establish linkage in Mendelian disorders (Morton, 1956; Ott, 1974).

The classical polymorphic markers are based on variation in protein structure and activity, and include blood groups, serum proteins and red cell enzymes. Several linkage studies in HD, involving numerous classical markers (for example ABO, MNS, Rhesus), were negative (Pericak-Vance *et al.*, 1978; Hodge *et al.*, 1980; Volkers *et al.*, 1980). This picture changed dramatically with the advent of a new class of genetic markers, namely DNA polymorphisms.

In 1983, James Gusella and his colleagues at Boston discovered close genetic linkage between HD and a DNA marker (G8) which detects a locus (D4S10) on the short arm of chromosome 4. This study (Gusella *et al.*, 1983) was initially based on two large kindreds of the disease, one of which is located in and around Lake Maracaibo, Venezuela; with 7000 members, it is the largest documented kindred not just of HD but of any genetic disorder. The detection of linkage in these kindreds after investigation of only 12 polymorphisms was unexpected, both for the rapidity of its detection and for the closeness of the linkage.

It was necessary to replicate this work to exclude the existence of genetic heterogeneity (i.e. the possibility of more than one locus being involved in the aetiology of the disease). Studies in families from south Wales (Harper *et al.*, 1985), the United States (Folstein *et al.*, 1985), Sweden (Holmgren *et al.*, 1987) and Belgium (Cassiman, 1987) have confirmed that linkage is close, while an analysis of pooled data from 63 large families (57 Caucasian, 4 Black American, 2 Japanese) has shown that D4S10 and the HD locus are about 4 centimorgans (cM) apart, with no evidence of locus heterogeneity and a combined maximum lod score of 87.69 (Conneally *et al.*, 1989). The initial discovery of linkage acted as a spur to other groups and soon newer and closer markers, such as D4S95 (BS674) and D4S114 (W92), were discovered. Most of these markers were identified by systematic screening of large numbers of DNA probes to show that they derive from the region between D4S10 and the telomere (Table 19.4). Another method of identifying markers is by investigating sequences derived from libraries (see Chapter 1) constructed with DNA enriched for chromosome 4, either from chromosome sorting or by using hybrid cell lines containing specific regions of that chromosome. The clone D4S90 (D5), for example, was isolated from such a chromosome 4-specific lambda library and shown to be terminally located in the distal region of 4p16.3, the most terminal sub-band of the short arm of chromosome 4 (Youngman *et al.*, 1988; 1989).

PREDICTIVE TESTING

D4S10, the first marker locus to be discovered for HD, is highly polymorphic, with over 90% of individuals heterozygous for at least one of the restriction fragment length polymorphisms (RFLPs). D4S95 (BS674) is also highly polymorphic. Hence, these powerful new markers have allowed predictive testing to be available for the first time in this disease. The two types of predictive testing are presymptomatic testing for the individual at risk for the disease and prenatal exclusion testing, where the estimated risk to the parent is not altered (Quarrell *et al.*, 1987a,b). Predictive tests are an important advance in the prevention of HD (Quarrell and Harper, 1987). If, for example, individuals who have an adverse presymptomatic test result refrained from reproduction, the number of choreic genes born into the population would be automatically reduced. Some family members do not want risk alteration for themselves. In the exclusion test, the aim is not so much to predict the presence or absence of the gene in the person at risk but rather to give the option to such a person of having children likely to be free from a risk of the disorder. The test allows the person to have

Table 19.4 Closely linked DNA markers to the HD gene listed in probable order (proximal to telomeric)

Locus	(Probe)	Reference
D4S62	(P8)	Hayden *et al.* (1987)
D4S10	(G8)	Gusella *et al.* (1983)
D4S95	(BS674)	Wasmuth *et al.* (1988)
D4S43	(C4H)	Gilliam *et al.* (1987)
D4S114	(W92)	Whaley *et al.* (1988)
D4S98	(BS731)	Whaley *et al.* (1988)
D4S113	(102BN4.0)	Whaley *et al.* (1988)
D4S96	(BS678)	Smith *et al.* (1988)
D4S141	(2R3)	Snell *et al.* (1989b)
D4S90	(D5)	Youngman *et al.* (1988)

children in the knowledge that, if he or she subsequently developed symptoms, the risk to the offspring would remain low (Quarrell *et al.*, 1987a,b).

Figure 19.1 shows an ideal pedigree structure and distribution of genotypes required for prediction for subjects at risk of developing HD. In Fig. 19.1(a) the affected mother of the consultand (arrowed) has inherited the A genotype from her unaffected mother (i.e. the consultand's grandmother) and therefore she must have inherited the B marker from her deceased affected father in generation I. If the DNA from the consultand is typed, it will either be AA or AB. If his marker type is AA, he will probably not inherit HD but if it is AB (Fig. 19.1(b)), he would be predicted as a gene carrier, in the absence of recombination. In Fig. 19.1(c), the pedigree is uninformative and no prediction is possible. Although the individual at risk has inherited the A marker type from his affected mother, it is not known whether this came with the HD gene or from the unaffected grandparent.

There are three major technical limitations with linkage analysis using RFLPs. First, the pedigree structure must be suitable and this requirement is more easily met in the exclusion test (Harper and Sarfarazi, 1985; Harper, 1986). Second, there will be an error rate due to recombination. Although a three-generation pedigree is the ideal family structure, it is possible to do presymptomatic tests in extended, two-generation families but here the error rate will be higher because more than one crossover may have occurred. Third, an informative polymorphism must be identified.

Studies of attitudes towards presymptomatic tests among at-risk individuals have shown that 55 to 77% would wish such a test for themselves (Stern and Eldridge, 1975; Tyler and Harper, 1983; Schoenfeld *et al.*, 1984; Tyler, 1987). (There is a dearth of studies on attitudes towards the exclusion test.) In practice, the numbers entering a presymptomatic test programme are much smaller. Quaid *et al.* (1987) sent letters to 387 individuals at 50% risk announcing the availability of the test and offering presymptomatic counselling. Only 12.6% indicated they would participate in a preclinical test programme. In a similar investigation (Craufurd *et al.*, 1989), letters were sent to 110 individuals at risk inviting them to consider a presymptomatic test and the uptake was also low (15.5%).

In 1987, we began a study to evaluate presymptomatic testing in a series of individuals at risk for HD. Inclusion criteria were a 50% *a priori* risk, and age of 18 years or over and confirmed family history of HD (a potentially informative family structure). Exclusion criteria were a significant risk of suicide, a recent history of serious psychiatric disorder or a recent history of substance misuse. The protocol is summarized in Table 19.5.

There were 187 referrals for presymptomatic testing, 88 (47%) from Wales and 99 (53%) from outside Wales; 130 were accepted into the series and, to date, 38 final results have been disclosed. The main probes used were D4S10 (G8), D4S43 (C4H) and D4S95 (BS674). Age-modified risks

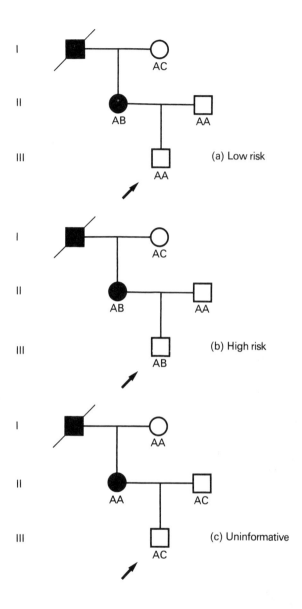

Fig. 19.1 *Pedigree structures and distribution of genotypes for predictive testing (individual requesting prediction arrowed); see text for details*

were calculated (Newcombe, 1981), and linkage analysis was done with the MLINK program (Lathrop *et al.*, 1984). In the exclusion series, there were 90 referrals; 63 were informative for the test and 24 pregnancies were tested (Quarrell *et al.*, 1987). Overall, 277 were referred for testing and 201 accepted into the series, with 62 known 'outcomes'.

Table 19.5 Wales presymptomatic testing programme for HD: summary of protocol

---

Interview one
1. Sociodemographic details
2. Confirmation of family and clinical data
3. Assessment of impact of HD
4. Assessment of knowledge of HD and presymptomatic testing
5. Reasons for requesting prediction

Interview two
1. Further explanation and counselling
2. Assessment of psychological, personality and social characteristics using standardized instruments
3. Nomination of professional supporter
4. Signature of consent form
5. Final blood sample

Interview three (held 4 weeks later)
Disclosure of results

Formal follow-up
One week
Three months
Twelve months

Several other centres (Hayden *et al.*, 1988; Meissen *et al.*, 1987; Brandt *et al.*, 1989; Brock *et al.*, 1989) have reported preliminary findings of presymptomatic testing. Our own series, while extensive, is still at an early stage regarding outcome of completed tests because the protocol involves a series of extensive counselling interviews and evaluations. Because of the great interest in identifying gene carriers since the turn of the century, some of the ethical difficulties in preclinical testing have been recognized for a long time (Gaylin, 1972). Despite careful planning and close involvement with national and international discussion on the topic, it soon became apparent that the anticipated problems were occurring in practice and several others arose that were not foreseen (Morris *et al.*, 1988a,b; Harper and Morris, 1989). As there has been little systematic documentation of clinical and laboratory problems, we have recorded those that have occurred in our extensive series of test applicants so that other centres, especially those about to embark on a predictive test programme, may be aware of these pitfalls (Morris *et al.*, 1989). It is clear that the issues surrounding predictive testing are more complex than initially expected. Some of them are now discussed in more detail and others are summarized in Table 19.6.

It is convenient to classify the problems into those occurring before, during and after laboratory testing. About 20% of referrals (38) were inappropriate, which indicates that much more professional and family education is necessary. We were particularly concerned when doctors

Table 19.6 Problems encountered during predictive testing for HD

Problems before laboratory testing	
1. Inappropriate use of the test:	
(a) referral without permission of individual	4
(b) referral of minors by parents	22
doctors	6
social workers	3
(c) request from adoption societies	7
2. Lack of clear family history of HD	15
3. Clinical status of key individuals:	
(a) applicant for testing already clinically affected	18
(b) applicant showing equivocal clinical signs	3
(c) affected relatives unknown to applicant	5
Problems during laboratory testing	
1. Refusal to donate blood sample:	
(a) affected individual	10
(b) other relative	2
2. Use of research sample for clinical application	14
3. Unintentional risk alteration possible	5
4. Anonymous testing	3
5. Problems with sample processing:	
(a) inadequate labelling	6
(b) sample wastage (tube broken in post; DNA degraded)	23
(c) inappropriate release of sample to other centre	1
(d) use of pseudonyms by applicant	1
6. Non-paternity	3
Problems after predictive testing	
1. Result requested by insurance company	1
2. Refusal to allow general medical practitioner access to result	4
3. Follow-up by testing centre refused	3

referred adult at-risk individuals without telling them. Two such patients had psychiatric symptoms and blood samples were sent to us for analysis unknown to the patient. This raises two issues: one concerns 'benevolent deception' of the patient and the second is whether predictive tests should be treated in the same way as other medical investigations. Since the Salgo ruling over 30 years ago (*Salgo* v. *Stanford University*, 1957), there is increasing recognition of patient autonomy and applicants have a legitimate right to know what use will be made of their blood samples. As for the second point, the fundamental differences between most other medical investigations and presymptomatic testing is that the applicants are generally not medically ill and samples are required not only from the applicant but also from key relatives. We have declined to test subjects without their knowledge.

The testing of children, not uncommonly requested by parents, is also an inappropriate use of the test (Harper and Clarke, 1990). There is international agreement on this point and guidelines drawn up by the World Federation of Neurology and the International Huntington Association recommend that 'the test is only available for individuals having reached the age of majority' (World Federation of Neurology/International Huntington Association, 1990). We have also declined requests to test at-risk children placed for adoption. To test a child would be to prefer the interests of a third party (the adoption society) over those of the child, who is unable to give its own consent (Morris *et al.*, 1988a,b).

PROGRESS TOWARDS IDENTIFICATION OF THE HUNTINGTON'S DISEASE GENE

The localization of the HD gene to the short arm of chromosome 4 not only provides the basis for predictive testing but also raises the possibility of isolating and characterizing the aberrant gene. This approach has become known as 'reverse genetics' (Ruddle, 1984; Rowland, 1988) because the gene product is unknown and recombinant DNA techniques are used to isolate the gene without knowledge of the primary defect. The application of reverse genetics has been successful in other genetic diseases, such as chronic granulomatous disease, the first disease for which the unknown product was revealed (Royer-Pokora *et al.*, 1986). A major application of reverse genetics led to the isolation of the Duchenne muscular dystrophy gene and its protein product, dystrophin, a substance which was previously unrecognized (Hoffman *et al.*, 1987a,b) and whose characterization has greatly enhanced our understanding of the cell biology, biochemistry and pathophysiology of the disorder. The gene and protein for cystic fibrosis have recently been identified by reverse genetics (Riordan *et al.*, 1989; Rommens *et al.*, 1989) without any chromosomal defect being available, a situation comparable to that in HD.

The reverse genetics approach is currently the only one directly applicable to HD as the underlying protein defect remains unknown despite extensive biochemical and pharmacological study (Bruyn *et al.*, 1965; Butterfield *et al.*, 1977; Caraceni *et al.*, 1977). In an effort to identify sequences flanking (i.e. one on either side of) the HD locus, many new DNA polymorphisms distal to D4S10 have been described (see Table 19.4). However, genetic mapping is less useful than physical methods for high-resolution mapping (at the level of a million base pairs and smaller) for two reasons: lack of informativeness in key family members and the need to study a large number of meiotic events. The newer physical mapping techniques, such as pulse-field gel electrophoresis (Carle and Olson, 1984; Schwartz and Cantor, 1984; see Chapter 1) complement family analyses; they allow the ordering of DNA markers and the localization of disease mutations caused by deletions or other rearrangements. Radiation mapping, another physical mapping technique, uses the fragmentation of chromosomes exposed to radiation to order genetic markers (Cox *et al.*, 1989) and the linear order of the markers constructed by using the radiation hybrid map is consistent with the available meiotic map. This technique can also define the relative order of probes that have not been ordered by meiotic mapping.

The detection of linkage disequilibrium or non-random allelic association (see Chapter 4) is another strategy for identifying the HD gene. Necessary conditions to observe this phenomenon are a marker very close to the disease locus (about 1 cM or closer), a low mutation rate for the disease and a low mutation for the polymorphic site. Although negative results for D4S10 have been reported (Youngman *et al.*, 1986), strong linkage disequilibrium has recently been detected between HD and the loci D4S95 and D4S98 (Snell *et al.*, 1989a; Theilmann *et al.*, 1989). This has three important implications. Firstly, the observed disequilibrium will help the study of the origin and spread of HD mutations in different populations. Secondly, it suggests that the HD gene is near the loci D4S95 and D4S98, which are considerably proximal to the telomere. Thirdly, linkage disequilibrium may enable a risk modification for presymptomatic test applicants from families within a population whose structure precludes genetic linkage prediction.

The discovery of linkage disequilibrium with closely linked DNA markers and the gene for cystic fibrosis (Estivill *et al.*, 1987) was an important step towards isolation of the cystic fibrosis gene. The discovery of linkage disequilibrium in HD indicates that existing markers are sufficiently close to permit cloning of the disease gene in the near future. When this occurs, it will be another major achievement of reverse genetics. Analysis of the HD mutation at the level of DNA sequence will then be possible; this will remove many of the technical limitations in presymptomatic testing and allow testing of those with an inadequate family structure, including applicants who are offspring of so-called isolated cases. Knowledge of the protein product will provide a foundation for research aimed at the true prevention of the disorder in those carrying the gene, and for therapeutic trials in those already affected. When this stage is reached, many of the currently problematic aspects of presymptomatic testing for HD will be removed.

ACKNOWLEDGEMENTS

We thank our colleagues, especially clinical geneticists, who have referred consultands for predictive testing and Audrey Tyler for helpful comments on the manuscript. Our work is supported by the Mental Health Foundation.

REFERENCES

Bell J. (1934). Huntington's chorea. In: *The Treasury of Human Inheritance* (Fisher R. A., ed.), pp. 1–77. Cambridge: Cambridge University Press.

Bickford J. A. R., Ellison R. M. (1953). High incidence of Huntington's chorea in the Duchy of Cornwall. *Journal of Mental Science*; 99: 291–4.

Bolt J. M. (1970). Huntington's chorea in the west of Scotland. *British Journal of Psychiatry*; 116: 259–70.

Brandt J., Quaid K. A., Folstein S. E. *et al.* (1989). Presymptomatic diagnosis of delayed-onset disease with linked DNA markers: the experience in Huntington's disease. *Journal of the American Medical Association*; 261: 3108–14.

Brock D. H., Mennie M., Curtis A. *et al.* (1989). Predictive testing for Huntington's disease with linked DNA markers. *Lancet*; ii: 463–6.

Bruyn G. W., Mink C. J. K., Calje J. F. (1965). Biochemical studies in Huntington's chorea. *Neurology*; 15: 455–61.

Butterfield D. A., Oeswein J. Q., Markesbery W. R. (1977). Electron spin resonance study of membrane protein alteration in Huntington's disease. *Nature*; 267: 453–5.

Caraceni T. A., Panerai A. E., Parati E. A. *et al.* (1977). Altered growth hormone and prolactin responses to dopaminergic stimulation in Huntington's chorea. *Journal of Clinical Endocrinology and Metabolism*; 44: 870–5.

Carle G. F., Olson M. V. (1984). Separation of chromosomal DNA molecules from yeast by orthogonal-field-alteration gel electrophoresis. *Nucleic Acids Research*; 12: 5647–64.

Carter C. O., Evans K. A., Baraitser M. (1983). Effect of genetic counselling on the prevalence of Huntington's chorea. *British Medical Journal*; 286: 281–3.

Cassiman J. J. (1987). DNA diagnosis of autosomal dominant and recessive diseases. In: *Genetic Risk, Risk Perception, and Decision Making* (Evers-Kiebooms G., Cassiman J.-J., Van den Berghe H., d'Ydewalle G., eds.), pp. 97–114. New York: Liss.

Conneally P. M., Haines J. L., Tanzi R. E. *et al.* (1989). Huntington's disease: no evidence for locus heterogeneity. *Genomics*; 5: 304–8.

Cox D. R., Pritchard C. A., Uglum E. *et al.* (1989). Segregation of the Huntington disease region of human chromosome 4 in a somatic cell hybrid. *Genomics*; 4: 397–407.

Craufurd D., Dodge A., Kerzin-Storrar L., Harris R. (1989). Uptake of presymptomatic predictive testing for Huntington's disease. *Lancet*; ii: 603–5.

Critchley M. (1934). Huntington's chorea and East Anglia. *Journal of State Medicine*; 42: 575–87.

Davenport C. B., Muncey E. B. (1916). Huntington's chorea in relation to heredity and eugenics. In: *Bulletin of Eugenic Records Office 7*. Washington: Carnegie Institute.

Estivill X., Scambler P. J., Wainwright B. J. *et al.* (1987). Patterns of polymorphism and linkage disequilibrium for cystic fibrosis. *Genomics*; 1: 257–63.

Folstein S. E., Phillips J. A., Meyers D. A. *et al.* (1985). Huntington's disease: two families with differing clinical features show linkage to the G8 probe. *Science*; 229: 776–9.

Gaylin W. (1972). Genetic engineering: the ethics of knowing. *New England Journal of Medicine*; 286: 1361–2.

Gilliam T. C., Bucan M., MacDonald M. E. *et al.* (1987). A DNA segment encoding two genes very tightly linked to Huntington's disease. *Science*; **238**: 950–2.

Glendinning N. (1975). A study in Huntington's chorea. Unpublished MD thesis, University of London.

Gusella J. F., Wexler N. S., Conneally P. M. *et al.* (1983). A polymorphic DNA marker genetically linked to Huntington's disease. *Nature*; **306**: 234–8.

Harper P. S. (1986). The prevention of Huntington's chorea. The Milroy lecture. *Journal of the Royal College of Physicians*; **20**: 7–14.

Harper P. S., Clarke A. (1990). Should we test children for adult genetic diseases? *Lancet*, i: 1205–6.

Harper P. S., Morris M. (1989). Predictive testing for Huntington's disease: progress and problems (Editorial). *British Medical Journal*; **298**: 404–5.

Harper P. S., Morris M. J. (1991). *Predictive and Presymptomatic Testing for Genetic Disorders: Lessons from Huntington's Disease*. London: Galton Institute (in press).

Harper P. S., Sarfarazi M. (1985). Genetic prediction and family structure in Huntington's chorea. *British Medical Journal*; **290**: 129–31.

Harper P. S., Walker D. A., Tyler A. *et al.* (1979). Huntington's chorea. The basis for long-term prevention. *Lancet*; ii: 346–9.

Harper P. S., Youngman S., Anderson M. A. *et al.* (1985). Genetic linkage between Huntington's disease and the DNA polymorphism G8 in south Wales families. *Journal of Medical Genetics*; **22**: 447–50.

Hayden M. R., Hewitt J., Maresca A., Langlois S. (1987). A polymorphic DNA probe located to human chromosome 4p16 (D4S62). *Nucleic Acids Research*; **9**: 3938.

Hayden M. R., Robbins C., Allard D. *et al.* (1988). Improved predictive testing for Huntington disease by using three linked DNA markers. *American Journal of Human Genetics*; **43**: 689–94.

Heathfield K. W. G. (1967). Huntington's chorea: investigation into the prevalence of this disease in the area covered by the North East Metropolitan Regional Hospital Board. *Brain*; **90**: 203–32.

Heathfield J. W. G., MacKenzie I. C. K. (1971). Huntington's chorea in Bedfordshire. *Guys Hospital Report*; **120**: 295–309.

Hodge S. E., Spence M. A., Crandall B. F. *et al.* (1980). Huntington disease: linkage analysis with age-of-onset corrections. *American Journal of Medical Genetics*; **5**: 247–54.

Hoffman E. P., Brown R. H., Jr., Kunkel L. M. (1987a). Dystrophin: the protein product of the Duchenne muscular dystrophy locus. *Cell*; **51**: 919–28.

Hoffman E. P., Knudson C. M., Campbell K. P., Kunkel L. M. (1987b). Subcellular fractionation of dystrophin to the triads of skeletal muscle. *Nature*; **330**: 754–8.

Hogg J. E., Massey E. W., Schoenberg B. S. (1979). Mortality from Huntington's disease in the United States. *Advances in Neurology*; **23**: 27–35.

Holmgren G., Almqvist W., Anvret M. *et al.* (1987). Linkage of G8 (D4S10) in two Swedish families with Huntington's disease. *Clinical Genetics*; **32**: 289–94.

Huber A. (1887). Chore hereditaria der Erwachsenen. *Virchows Archives of Pathology and Anatomy*; **108**: 267–85.

Huntington G. (1872). On chorea. *Medical and Surgical Reporter*; **26**: 317–21.

Jelliffe S. E., Muncey E. B., Davenport C. B. (1913). Huntington's chorea. A study in heredity. *Journal of Nervous and Mental Disease*; **40**: 796–9.

Klawans H. L., Jr., Goetz C. G., Paulson G. W., Barbeau A. (1980). Levodopa and presymptomatic detection of Huntington's disease: eight-year follow up. *New England Journal of Medicine*; **302**: 511–12.

Klawans H. L., Jr., Paulson G. W., Ringel S. P., Barbeau A. (1972). L-dopa in the detection of presymptomatic Huntington's chorea. *New England Journal of Medicine*; **286**: 1332–4.

Lathrop G. M., Lalouel J.-M., Julier C., Ott J. (1984). *Proceedings of the National Academy of Sciences (USA)*; **81**: 3443–6.

Meissen G. J., Myers R. H., Mastromauro C. A. *et al.* (1987). Predictive testing for Huntington's disease with use of a linked DNA marker. *New England Journal of Medicine*; **318**: 535–42.

Morris M., Harper P. S. (1989). Recent advances in Huntington's disease. *Royal Society of Medicine Current Medical Literature*; **5**: 67–70.

Morris M., Tyler A., Harper P. S. (1988a). Adoption and genetic prediction for Huntington's disease. *Lancet*; **ii**: 1069–70.

Morris M., Tyler A., Lazarou L. *et al.* (1989). Problems in genetic prediction for Huntington's disease. *Lancet*; **ii**: 601–3.

Morris M., Tyler A., Meredith L., Harper P. S. (1988b). Predictive testing for Huntington's disease: methods and problems. *Journal of Medical Genetics*; **25**: 640.

Morton N. E. (1956). The detection and estimation of linkage between the genes for eliptocytosis and the Rh blood group. *American Journal of Human Genetics*; **8**: 80–96.

Neel J. V. (1949). The detection of the genetic carriers of hereditary disease. *American Journal of Human Genetics*, **1**, 19–36.

Newcombe R. G. (1981). A life table for onset of Huntington's chorea. *Annals of Human Genetics*; **45**: 375–85.

Office of Health Economics (1980). *Huntington's Chorea.* OHE Report No. 67, p. 3. London: OHE.

Oliver J. E. (1970). Huntington's chorea in Northamptonshire. *British Journal of Psychiatry*; **166**: 241–53.

Orbeck A. L. (1959). An early description of Huntington's chorea. *Medical History*; **3**: 165–8.

Ott J. (1974). Estimation of the recombination fraction in human pedigrees: efficient computation of the likelihood for human linkage studies. *American Journal of Human Genetics*; **26**: 588–97.

Palm J. D. (1973). Longitudinal study of a preclinical test program for Huntington's chorea. In: *Advances in Neurology 1* (Barbeau A., Chase T. N., Paulson G. W., eds.), pp. 311–24. New York: Raven Press.

Panse F. (1942). Die Erbchorea: eine klinische-genetische Studie. *Samml. Psychiat. Neurol. Einzeldarst.*, 18.

Pericak-Vance M. A., Conneally P. M., Merritt A. D. *et al.* (1978). Genetic linkage studies in Huntington's disease. *Cytogenetics and Cell Genetics*; **22**: 640–5.

Pleydell M. J. (1955). Huntington's chorea in Northamptonshire. *British Medical Journal*; **ii**: 889.

Quaid K., Brandt J., Folstein S. E. (1987). The decision to be tested for Huntington's disease. *Journal of the American Medical Association*; **257**: 3362.

Quarrell O. W. J., Harper P. S. (1987). Is Huntington's chorea predictable and preventable? In: *More Dilemmas in the Management of the Neurological*

Patient (Warlow C., Garfield J., eds.), pp. 36–44. Edinburgh: Churchill Livingstone.

Quarrell O. W. J., Meredith A. L., Tyler A. *et al.* (1987). Exclusion testing for Huntington's disease in pregnancy with a closely linked DNA marker. *Lancet*; i: 1281–3.

Quarrell O. W. J., Tyler A., Jones M. P. *et al.* (1988). Population studies of Huntington's disease in Wales. *Clinical Genetics*; 33: 189–95.

Reid J. J. (1960). Huntington's chorea in Northamptonshire. *British Medical Journal*; ii: 650.

Riordan J. R., Rommens J. M., Kerem B.-S. *et al.* (1989). Identification of the cystic fibrosis gene: cloning and characterisation of complementary DNA. *Science*; 245: 1066–73.

Rommens J. M., Iannuzzi M. C., Kerem B.-S. *et al.* (1989). Identification of the cystic fibrosis gene: chromosome walking and jumping. *Science*; 245: 1059–65.

Rowland L. P. (1988). Dystrophin: a triumph of reverse genetics and the end of the beginning. *New England Journal of Medicine*; 318: 1392–4.

Royer-Pokora B., Kunkel L. M., Monaco A. P. (1986). Cloning the gene for an inherited human disorder—chronic granulomatous disease—on the basis of its chromosomal location. *Nature*; 322: 32–8.

Ruddle F. H. (1984). Reverse genetics and beyond. *American Journal of Human Genetics*; 36: 944–53.

Salgo v Leland Stanford Jr. University Board of Trustees (1957). Cal Dist Ct App, 317 P 2d 170.

Schoenfeld M., Myers R. H., Berkman B. *et al.* (1984). Potential impact of a predictive test on the gene frequency of Huntington disease. *American Journal of Human Genetics*; 18: 423–9.

Schwartz D. C., Cantor C. R. (1984). Separation of yeast chromosome-sized DNAs by pulsed field gradient gel electrophoresis. *Cell*; 37: 67–75.

Simpson S., Johnston A. W. (1989). The prevalence and pattern of care of Huntington's chorea in Grampian. *British Journal of Psychiatry*; 155: 799–804.

Smith B., Skarecky D., Bengtsson U. *et al.* (1988). Isolation of DNA markers in the direction of the Huntington disease gene from the G8 locus. *American Journal of Human Genetics*; 42: 335–44.

Snell R. G., Lazarou L., Youngman S. *et al.* (1989a). Linkage disequilibrium in Huntington's disease: an improved localisation for the gene. *Journal of Medical Genetics*; 26: 673–5.

Snell R. G., Youngman S., Lehrach H. *et al.* (1989b). A new probe in the region of Huntington disease. *Cytogenetics and Cell Genetics (Human Gene Mapping 10)*; 51: 1083.

Spillane J., Phillips R. (1937). Huntington's chorea in South Wales. *Quarterly Journal of Medicine*; 6: 403–23.

Stern R., Eldridge R. (1975). Attitudes of patients and their relatives to Huntington's disease. *Journal of Medical Genetics*; 12: 217–23.

Stevens D. L. (1972). The history of Huntington's chorea. *Journal of the Royal College of Physicians*; 6: 271–82.

Stevens D. L. (1976). Huntington's chorea: a demographic, genetic and clinical study. Unpublished MD thesis, University of London.

Theilmann J., Kanani S., Shiang R. *et al.* (1989). Non-random association between the alleles detected at D4S95 and D4S98 and the Huntington's disease gene. *Journal of Medical Genetics*; 26: 676–81.

Tyler A., Quarrell O. W. J., Lazaro L. P. *et al.* (1990). Exclusion testing in pregnancy for Huntington's disease. *Journal of Medical Genetics*, **27**: 488–495.

Tyler A., Harper P. S. (1983). Attitudes of subjects at-risk and their relatives towards genetic counselling in Huntington's chorea. *Journal of Medical Genetics*; **20**: 179–88.

Tyler A. (1987). Genetic counselling in Huntington's chorea. In: *Genetic Risk, Risk Perception, and Decision Making* (Evers-Kiebooms G., Cassiman J.-J., Van den Berghe H., d'Ydewalle G., eds.), pp. 85–97. New York: Liss.

Venters G. (1971). Epidemiology of Huntington's chorea. Unpublished PhD thesis, University of Edinburgh.

Volkers W. S., Went L. N., Vegter van der Vlis M. *et al.* (1980). Genetic linkage studies in Huntington's chorea. *Annals of Human Genetics*; **44**: 75–9.

Walker D. A., Harper P. S., Wells C. G. C. *et al.* (1981). Huntington's chorea in South Wales. A genetic and epidemiological study. *Clinical Genetics*; **19**: 213–21.

Wasmuth J. J., Hewitt J., Smith B. *et al.* (1988). A highly polymorphic locus very tightly linked to the Huntington's disease gene. *Nature*; **332**: 734–6.

Whaley W. L., Michiels F., MacDonald M. E. *et al.* (1988). Mapping of D4S98/S114/S113 confines the Huntington's defect to a reduced physical region at the telomere of chromosome 4. *Nucleic Acids Research*; **16**: 11769–80.

World Federation of Neurology/International Huntington's Association Working Party on Predictive Testing (1990). Ethical issues policy statement on Huntington's disease molecular genetics predictive test. *Journal of Medical Genetics*; **27**: 34–8.

World Health Organization (1978). *International Classification of Diseases* 9th edn. Geneva: WHO.

Youngman S., Sarfarazi M., Quarrell O. W. J. *et al.* (1986). Studies of a DNA marker (G8) genetically linked to Huntington disease in British families. *Human Genetics*; **73**: 333–9.

Youngman S., Shaw D. J., Gusella J. F. *et al.* (1988). A DNA probe, D5 (D4S90) mapping to human chromosome 4p16.3. *Nucleic Acids Research*; **16**: 1648.

Index